Current Concepts in Hematopathology: Applications in Clinical Practice

Guest Editor

ROBERT PAUL HASSERJIAN, MD

SURGICAL PATHOLOGY CLINICS

surgpath.theclinics.com

Consulting Editor
JOHN R. GOLDBLUM, MD

December 2010 • Volume 3 • Number 4

SAUNDERS an imprint of ELSEVIER, Inc.

W.B. SAUNDERS COMPANY
A Division of Elsevier Inc.

1600 John F. Kennedy Boulevard • Suite 1800 • Philadelphia, Pennsylvania 19103-2899

http://www.surgpath.theclinics.com

SURGICAL PATHOLOGY CLINICS Volume 3, Number 4
December 2010 ISSN 1875-9181, ISBN-13: 978-1-4377-2499-8

Editor: Joanne Husovski

Surgical Pathology Clinics (ISSN 1875-9181) is published quarterly by Elsevier Inc., 360 Park Avenue South, New York, NY 10010. Months of issue are March, June, September, and December. Business and Editorial Office: Elsevier Inc., 1600 John F. Kennedy Blvd., Ste. 1800, Philadelphia, PA 19103-2899. Accounting and Circulation Offices: Elsevier Inc., 3251 Riverport Lane, Maryland Heights, MO 63043. Periodicals postage paid at New York, NY and at additional mailing offices. Subscription prices are $170.00 per year (US individuals), $199.00 per year (US institutions), $84.00 per year (US students/residents), $213.00 per year (Canadian individuals), $225.00 per year (Canadian Institutions), $213.00 per year (foreign individuals), $225.00 per year (foreign institutions), and $104.00 per year (international & Canadian students/residents). Foreign air speed delivery is included in all *Clinics'* subscription prices. All prices are subject to change without notice. **POSTMASTER:** Send address changes to *Surgical Pathology Clinics*, Elsevier, 3251 Riverport Lane, Maryland Heights, MO 63043. Customer Service: 1-800-654-2452 (US). From outside the United States, call 1-314-453-7041. Fax: 1-314-453-5170. E-mail: JournalsCustomerServiceusa@elsevier.com (for print support) and JournalsOnlineSupport-usa@elsevier.com (for online support).

Reprints. For copies of 100 or more, of articles in this publication, please contact the Commercial Reprints Department, Elsevier Inc., 360 Park Avenue South, New York, NY 10010-1710. Tel. (212) 633-3812; Fax: (212) 462-1935; email: reprints@elsevier.com.

Printed in the United States of America.

Contributors

CONSULTING EDITOR

JOHN R. GOLDBLUM, MD
Chairman, Department of Anatomic Pathology;
Professor of Pathology, Cleveland Clinics
Lerner College of Medicine, Cleveland Clinic,
Cleveland, Ohio

GUEST EDITOR

ROBERT PAUL HASSERJIAN, MD
Associate Pathologist, Department of
Pathology, Massachusetts General Hospital;
and Associate Professor, Harvard Medical
School, Boston, Massachusetts

AUTHORS

DANIEL A. ARBER, MD
Professor and Associate Chair, Department
of Pathology, Stanford University Medical
Center, Stanford, California

JAMES R. COOK, MD, PhD
Associate Professor of Pathology; Department
of Clinical Pathology, Cleveland Clinic,
Cleveland, Ohio

LAURENCE DE LEVAL, MD, PhD
Professor of Pathology, Institute of Pathology,
Centre Hospitalier Universitaire Vaudois,
Lausanne, Switzerland

AHMET DOGAN, MD, PhD
Professor of Pathology, Division of Anatomic
Pathology, Department of Laboratory Medicine
and Pathology, Mayo Clinic, Rochester,
Minnesota

JUDITH A. FERRY, MD
Associate Professor of Pathology, Harvard
Medical School; Director of Hematopathology,
James Homer Wright Pathology Laboratories
of the Massachusetts General Hospital,
Boston, Massachusetts

TRACY I. GEORGE, MD
Assistant Professor, Department of Pathology,
Stanford University School of Medicine,
Stanford University Medical Center, Stanford,
California

ROBERT PAUL HASSERJIAN, MD
Associate Pathologist, Department of
Pathology, Massachusetts General Hospital;
and Associate Professor, Harvard Medical
School, Boston, Massachusetts

HANS-PETER HORNY, MD
Professor, Institut für Pathologie, Klinikum
Ansbach, Escherichstrasse6, Ansbach,
Germany

MATTHEW HOWARD, MD
Clinical Instructor, Division of
Hematopathology, Department of Laboratory
Medicine and Pathology, Mayo Clinic,
Rochester, Minnesota

DAN JONES, MD, PhD
Quest Diagnostics Nichols Institute, Chantilly, Virginia

ROBERT B. LORSBACH, MD, PhD
Director of Hematopathology & Associate Professor, Department of Pathology, University of Arkansas for Medical Sciences, Little Rock, Arkansas

MIHAELA ONCIU, MD
Associate Member, St Jude Faculty; Medical Director, Anatomic Pathology; Department of Pathology, St Jude Children's Research Hospital, Memphis, Tennessee

ALIYAH R. SOHANI, MD
Hematopathologist, Massachusetts General Hospital; Instructor in Pathology, Department of Pathology, Harvard Medical School, Boston, Massachusetts

SA A. WANG, MD
Department of Hematopathology and Associate Director of Clinical Flow Cytometry Laboratory, University of Texas, MD Anderson Cancer Center, Houston, Texas

OLGA K. WEINBERG, MD
Fellow, Department of Pathology, Stanford University Medical Center, Stanford, California

Contents

Follicular lymphoma is a relatively common B-cell lymphoma composed of follicle center B lymphocytes. Follicular lymphomas occurring in the pediatric population and in some extranodal sites exhibit particular clinicopathologic features and clinical behavior that are often distinct from adult nodal follicular lymphoma. A type of "in-situ" follicular lymphoma presents as intrafollicular neoplastic cells in a background of architecturally normal lymphoid tissue and may be difficult to recognize in routine sections. Accurate recognition of the morphologic variants and clinicopathologic subtypes of follicular lymphoma is important to avoid confusing them with other lymphomas and reactive processes. This article presents the overview, diagnosis, differential diagnosis, and key points of 'conventional' adult nodal follicular lymphoma and its morphologic variations, pediatric follicular lymphoma, extranodal follicular lymphomas, gastrointestinal follicular lymphoma, primary cutaneous follicle center lymphoma, testicular follicular lymphoma, and follicular lymphoma in-situ.

Chronic lymphocytic leukemia (CLL), small lymphocytic lymphoma (SLL), and monoclonal B-cell lymphocytosis (MBL) are clonal proliferations of small, mature B cells. CLL and SLL are considered neoplastic, although they are indolent and many patients with these lymphomas never require treatment. Most MBL cases share immunophenotypic and genetic features with CLL and SLL but have a small burden of clonal cells. This review focuses on the pathologic features of CLL, SLL, and MBL and their differential diagnoses. Guidelines are provided to separate the entities from one another and to avoid pitfalls in distinguishing these entities from other lymphomas and from reactive lymphoid proliferations.

The diagnosis and classification of lymphoproliferative disorders in the spleen are frequently challenging. Some lymphoproliferative disorders, such as hairy cell leukemia and splenic marginal zone lymphoma, characteristically present with primarily splenic involvement. Secondary involvement of the spleen may be seen with any lymphoma. Precise classification requires integration of the morphologic findings with clinical data, phenotypic studies, and often cytogenetic and/or molecular genetic analysis. Correlation with the findings in peripheral blood and bone marrow may also be required in some cases. This article discusses the diagnostic approach to splenic-based lymphoproliferative disorders in routine practice and describes the clinicopathologic features of lymphoid neoplasms that characteristically present in the spleen.

Lymph node–based peripheral T-cell lymphomas are rare and exhibit a morphologic spectrum that overlaps with reactive lymphoid hyperplasia, B-cell lymphomas, and Hodgkin lymphoma, presenting a diagnostic challenge. This review focuses on the major categories of lymph node–based peripheral T-cell lymphomas recognized by the 2008 World Health Organization classification of tumors of lymphoid tissues. Diagnostic strategies for approaching T-cell neoplasms using a combined clinical, morphologic, immunophenotypic, and genetic approach are presented. Practical information to aid in distinguishing peripheral T-cell lymphomas from other hematologic malignancies and benign conditions is provided.

This article reviews the spectrum of Epstein-Barr virus and Kaposi sarcoma herpesvirus (KSHV/HHV-8)-associated B-cell lymphoid proliferations, their pathologic features and clinical presentation, diagnostic criteria, and some pathogenetic aspects. Emphasis is on the differential diagnosis issues and difficulties that the pathologist may face for the correct identification and interpretation of these lesions.

Burkitt lymphoma (BL) is an aggressive B-cell neoplasm with an extremely short doubling time that mainly affects children and young adults. Despite characteristic features, none is entirely specific for BL and the differential diagnosis may include diffuse large B-cell lymphoma (DLBCL), B lymphoblastic leukemia/lymphoma, and high-grade B-cell lymphoma unclassifiable with features intermediate between DLBCL and BL. This content presents a practical approach to establish a diagnosis of BL and distinguish it from other highgrade B-cell malignancies. The authors pay particular attention to high-grade B-cell neoplasms with features intermediate between DLBCL and BL, a new diagnostic category in the 2008 World Health Organization classification system that provides a framework for categorizing challenging cases not meeting diagnostic criteria for either "classic" BL or DLBCL.

The plasma cell neoplasms are malignancies of the most terminally differentiated cells in B-cell ontogeny and are frequently associated with the production of a monoclonal immunoglobulin molecule or M protein. In this article, our discussion focuses on plasma cell myeloma. The molecular pathogenesis of plasma cell myeloma is briefly reviewed, and the general immunophenotypic properties of the plasma cell neoplasms are discussed. Particular emphasis is given to challenging variants or unusual presentations of the plasma cell neoplasms.

The evaluation of pediatric bone marrow poses specific challenges when compared with the general adult population. These challenges stem in part from the higher likelihood of congenital disorders with hematopoietic manifestations, some of which may give rise to hematologic malignancies. Familiarity with the spectrum of disorders seen in the pediatric age group allows for an appropriate and focused differential diagnosis. This review addresses the diagnostic workup of pediatric bone marrow samples, as directed by the peripheral blood and bone marrow findings in the context of the patient's clinical history. Recommendations for the appropriate use of ancillary studies in various scenarios are provided.

Diagnosis of Myelodysplastic Syndromes in Cytopenic Patients   1127

Sa A. Wang

Sustained clinical cytopenia is a frequent laboratory finding in ambulatory and hospitalized patients. For pathologists and hematopathologists who examine the bone marrow (BM), a diagnosis of cytopenia secondary to an infiltrative BM process or acute leukemia can be established based on morphologic evaluation and flow cytometry immunophenotyping. It can be more challenging to establish a diagnosis of myelodysplastic syndromes (MDS). In this article, the practical approaches for establishing or excluding a diagnosis of MDS (especially low-grade MDS) in patients with clinical cytopenia are discussed along with the current diagnostic recommendations provided by the World Health Organization and the International Working Group for MDS.

Acute Myeloid Leukemia with Myelodysplasia-Related Changes: A New Definition   1153

Olga K. Weinberg and Daniel A. Arber

Acute myeloid leukemia (AML) with multilineage dysplasia was introduced in the 2001 World Health Organization (WHO) classification to encompass cases of AML characterized by myelodysplastic syndrome-like features. The 2008 WHO classification revised this group into a new category, AML with myelodysplasia-related changes (AML-MRC). The category now includes patients with at least 20% blasts in peripheral blood or bone marrow and any of the following: (1) AML arising from a previous MDS or mixed MDS/myeloproliferative neoplasm, (2) AML with a specific MDS-associated cytogenetic abnormality and/or (3) AML with multilineage dysplasia. Up to 48% of all patients with AML are encompassed within the AML-MRC subgroup. AML-MRC patients have worse prognosis compared with patients with AML, not otherwise specified. This article presents microscopic features, diagnosis, diagnostic algorithm, differentials, and clinical features of AML-MRC.

Histiocytic and Dendritic Cell Neoplasms   1165

Dan Jones

This article covers myelomonocytic lineage tumors and dendritic cells (DCs) of myeloid-derived, plasmacytoid, and follicle-associated types. The morphologic and immunophenotypic features in this group of neoplasms is featured, including mature/fully differentiated neoplasms such as Langerhans cell histiocytosis, its malignant counterpart Langerhans cell sarcoma, and S100-negative histiocytic proliferations. More immature/precursor malignancies in this group include myeloid and monocytic leukemias presenting in extramedullary tissues, and the newly codified blastic plasmacytoid dendritic cell neoplasm. Although likely not related histogenetically to myeloid-related DC, mesenchymal-type lymph node tumors including follicular dendritic cell and fibroblastic reticulum sarcomas are discussed. All of these neoplasms can exhibit a range of immunophenotypic and morphologic features likely reflecting the plasticity of the nonneoplastic precursors from which they are derived.

An unusual disease, mastocytosis challenges the pathologist with a variety of morphologic appearances and heterogeneous clinical presentations ranging from skin manifestations (pruritis, urticaria, dermatographism) to signs and symptoms indicative of mast cell mediator release, including flushing, hypotension, headache, and anaphylaxis among others. In this article, the focus is on recognizing the cytology, histopathology, clinical features, and prognostic implications of systemic mastocytosis, a clonal and neoplastic mast cell proliferation infiltrating extracutaneous organ(s) with or without skin involvement. Diagnostic pitfalls are reviewed with ancillary studies to help unmask the mast cell and exclude morphologic mimics.

Surgical Pathology Clinics

RELATED INTEREST

Myelodysplastic Syndromes
Benjamin L. Ebert, MD, *Guest Editor*
Hematology/Oncology Clinics of North America, April 2010

THE CLINICS ARE NOW AVAILABLE ONLINE!

Access your subscription at:
www.theclinics.com

Preface
Diagnostic Hematopathology: Aiming at a Moving Target

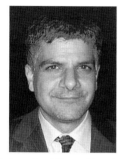

Robert Paul Hasserjian, MD
Guest Editor

The field of hematopathology is an ever-changing discipline: as our clinical colleagues develop and implement increasingly sophisticated therapies, we pathologists are constantly refining our ability to effectively diagnose the diseases they are treating. Many current therapies aim to target oncogenic pathways deregulated in particular neoplasms, requiring us to interrogate diseases with tools that tease out these specific pathways. While these ancillary tools often inform us about the tumor biologies, they add to the large amounts of (sometimes contradictory) data that we must digest and synthesize in each case. The goal of this issue is to present the current state-of-the-art diagnostic approaches in several particular areas of hematopathology. I have chosen areas that my colleagues and I feel are particularly challenging, have undergone changes and refinements, and/or have been influenced by evolving concepts in our field. This issue thus both provides guidelines to apply in practice as well as reviews current changes to the field of hematopathology.

Splenic B-cell lymphomas/leukemias, nodal peripheral T-cell lymphomas, histiocytic and dendritic neoplasms, systemic mastocytosis, and diseases affecting the bone marrow of pediatric patients are not frequently encountered by most pathologists. Such unfamiliar diagnostic arenas can be particularly challenging; for example, nodal T-cell lymphomas and pediatric bone marrow neoplasms are notorious for their difficult differential diagnosis with reactive processes. This issue provides practical diagnostic approaches to these diseases that integrate salient morphologic and clinical features with the appropriate use of ancillary testing. Such approaches are designed to help the pathologist correctly diagnose and classify these relatively uncommon neoplasms and avoid potential pitfalls. Conversely, plasma cell neoplasms and bone marrow interpretation in cytopenic patients represent areas in diagnostic hematopathology that are relatively commonly encountered by the practicing pathologist: anemia is the most common indication for bone marrow sampling in most practices and plasma cell myeloma is one of the most common hematologic malignancies. Again, the authors in this issue provide guidance on how pathologists should handle these scenarios and indicate what diagnostic information is currently necessary to provide our clinical colleagues so that they can develop an appropriate treatment plan for each patient.

As the field of hematopathology continues to advance, the diagnostic criteria of certain diseases have changed. In particular, definitions of acute myeloid leukemia with myelodysplasia-related changes, chronic lymphocytic leukemia/small lymphocytic leukemia, and Burkitt lymphoma have undergone modifications in the 2008 WHO Classification of Tumours of Hematopoietic and Lymphoid Tissues. These changes reflect evolving concepts in hematopathology, where disease categorization is increasingly driven by our understanding of tumor biology and, in some cases, clinical behavior and/or response to therapy. The authors in this issue review the rationale behind the refinements to these diagnostic categories

Surgical Pathology 3 (2010) xi–xii
doi:10.1016/j.path.2010.09.011

surgpath.theclinics.com

and suggest the appropriate use of ancillary studies to correctly classify the disease entities. The topic of B-cell proliferations related to herpesviruses (EBV and HHV8) reviews several recent changes in the classification of virus-associated lymphomas and lymphoproliferative disorders and also compares and contrasts the various diseases caused by herpesviruses. Finally, the current state-of-the-art diagnostic approach to "conventional" follicular lymphoma is described and new disease variants are reviewed: these variants reflect our increasing realization that the category of follicular lymphoma is likely more complex and heterogeneous than previously thought.

Each topic has been organized in order to maximize its practical utility: there are summary lists of key features as well as challenging pitfalls for each disease or disease category. Most of the topics are organized so as to present the clinical, morphologic, phenotypic, and genetic features of each disease, with sections on differential diagnosis and prognosis. Differential diagnoses are put forth either as lists for each entity (with key distinguishing features) or as tables summarizing a disease category. Approaches to pediatric bone marrow interpretation and the diagnosis of myelodysplasia in cytopenic patients are organized differently: the differential diagnoses and diagnostic algorithms are presented for particular scenarios based on the basic bone marrow appearance and clinical findings. All articles are extensively illustrated with images that underscore the salient features of the diseases discussed in the text and provide up-to-date references.

I am deeply indebted to the all authors who have contributed to this issue. Their collective wealth of experience in these challenging areas of diagnostic pathology is truly an invaluable resource. I hope that this issue will serve as both an update on the current state of diagnostic hematopathology and also a useful resource to pathologists in their daily practice.

Robert Paul Hasserjian, MD
Department of Pathology
Massachusetts General Hospital
and Harvard Medical School
55 Fruit Street
Boston, MA 02114, USA

E-mail address:
rhasserjian@partners.org

RECENT ADVANCES IN FOLLICULAR LYMPHOMA: PEDIATRIC, EXTRANODAL, AND FOLLICULAR LYMPHOMA IN SITU

Judith A. Ferry, MD[a,b,*]

KEYWORDS

- Follicular lymphoma • Follicular lymphoma in situ • Pediatric • Extranodal • Differential diagnosis

ABSTRACT

Follicular lymphoma is a relatively common B-cell lymphoma composed of follicle center B lymphocytes. Follicular lymphomas occurring in the pediatric population and in some extranodal sites exhibit particular clinicopathologic features and clinical behavior that are often distinct from adult nodal follicular lymphoma. A type of "in-situ" follicular lymphoma presents as intrafollicular neoplastic cells in a background of architecturally normal lymphoid tissue and may be difficult to recognize in routine sections. Accurate recognition of the morphologic variants and clinicopathologic subtypes of follicular lymphoma is important to avoid confusing them with other lymphomas and reactive processes; in addition, some of these subtypes of follicular lymphoma display unusually indolent clinical behavior that warrant their separation from "conventional" follicular lymphoma.

OVERVIEW OF FOLLICULAR LYMPHOMA

Follicular lymphoma is a neoplasm composed of follicle center B lymphocytes. Among B-cell lymphomas, it is the second most common type, following diffuse large B-cell lymphoma. Follicular lymphoma occurs most often in middle-aged and older adults who present with lymphadenopathy;

Key Features
FOLLICULAR LYMPHOMA

- Neoplasm of follicle center B cells
- Mainly affects middle-aged and older adults, females more often than males
- Lymphoma is usually widespread at diagnosis
- Lymph nodes replaced by crowded, ill-defined follicles with or without diffuse areas
- Typical immunophenotype: CD20+, CD5−, CD10+, CD43−, bcl6+, bcl2+, Ki67 low
- Genetic/cytogenetic features: clonal *IGH*, t(14;18) involving *IGH* and *BCL2*

disease is widespread in most cases. In most cases, the lymphoma is low grade. The neoplastic cells express pan-B-cell antigens, markers of germinal centers and, usually, bcl2. The underlying genetic abnormality is typically a translocation involving the immunoglobulin heavy chain gene and *BCL2*. The course is usually indolent and patients may have long survival. Occasionally the clinical or pathologic features of follicular lymphoma deviate from the classic pattern. Although follicular lymphoma rarely occurs in children, when it does, its features differ from those found in adults: disease is often localized,

[a] Harvard Medical School, 25 Shattuck Street, Boston, MA 02115, USA
[*,b] James Homer Wright Pathology Laboratories of the Massachusetts General Hospital, 55 Fruit Street, Boston, MA 02114, USA
E-mail address: jferry@partners.org

Surgical Pathology 3 (2010) 877–906
doi:10.1016/j.path.2010.08.002

large cells may be numerous within neoplastic follicles, bcl2 protein is usually not expressed, and rearrangement of *BCL2* is usually absent. The uncommon follicular lymphomas arising in extranodal sites are heterogeneous. In some instances they share many features with low-grade lymph nodal follicular lymphomas, whereas in others their clinical and pathologic features are quite different. In cases of so-called follicular lymphoma in situ, neoplastic follicles are present without distortion of the underlying tissue architecture.

In this article, the clinical and pathologic features and the differential diagnosis of follicular lymphoma are discussed. The characteristics of pediatric follicular lymphoma, extranodal follicular lymphomas, and follicular lymphoma in situ are contrasted with the more common low-grade, lymph node–based follicular lymphomas occurring in adults.

'CONVENTIONAL' ADULT NODAL FOLLICULAR LYMPHOMA AND ITS MORPHOLOGIC VARIATIONS

CLINICAL FEATURES

Follicular lymphoma is a common type of lymphoma, representing 20% of all lymphomas worldwide; it is more prevalent in the United States and Western Europe than elsewhere. Nearly all patients are adults, with a median age in the sixth decade. Women are slightly more often affected than men. The most common presentation is with lymphadenopathy, which is often widespread. Staging commonly reveals involvement of the bone marrow. Rare patients present with prominent peripheral blood involvement (leukemic presentation of follicular lymphoma).

DIAGNOSIS: GROSS AND MICROSCOPIC FEATURES

Lymph nodes involved by follicular lymphoma are usually enlarged, being partially or entirely replaced by a proliferation of lymphoid follicles that are usually poorly delineated and crowded. Follicles often invade the nodal capsule; this may be associated with fibrous thickening, splitting, and reduplication of the capsule. Neoplastic follicles sometimes invade perinodal fat and vascular invasion can be seen (**Fig. 1**). The cellular composition varies from case to case, but the neoplastic follicles are typically occupied by a monotonous population of centrocytes (small cleaved cells) with a variable admixture of centroblasts (large noncleaved cells). In a small minority of cases, centroblasts predominate. Traditionally, follicular lymphomas have been graded as 1, 2, or 3 of 3, with grade 1 cases having

an average of 0 to 5 centroblasts per high-power field (hpf), in a count of 10 hpfs. Grade 2 follicular lymphomas have 6 to 15 centroblasts per hpf, and grade 3 follicular lymphomas have more than 15 centroblasts per hpf. In the 2008 World Health Organization (WHO) Classification,[1] a change to the grading scheme of follicular lymphoma was introduced. Because of a lack of a clear biologic difference between grade 1 and grade 2 follicular lymphoma, reporting the grade as "grade 1–2" for any follicular lymphoma with 0 to 15 centroblasts per average hpf is acceptable (see **Fig. 1**).[1] In addition, grade 3 follicular lymphomas are subdivided: those cases with more than 15 centroblasts per hpf but with an admixture of centrocytes are designated grade 3A, whereas those with solid aggregates of centroblasts are designated grade 3B (**Fig. 2**). Some investigators suggest that follicular lymphoma, grade 3A, is immunophenotypically and genetically more like follicular lymphoma, grade 1–2, whereas follicular lymphoma, grade 3B is distinct, and may be more closely related to diffuse large B-cell lymphoma.[2] In addition to reporting the grade of the follicular lymphoma, the pattern should be reported: the pattern is "follicular" if the architecture of the lymphoma is greater than 75% follicular; "follicular and diffuse" if its architecture is greater than 25% but less than 75% follicular; "focally follicular" if less than 25% follicular; and "diffuse" if entirely diffuse. For example, a low-grade follicular lymphoma (fewer than 15 centroblasts/hpf) that is entirely follicular would be reported as, "follicular lymphoma, follicular pattern, grade 1–2 of 3." A diffuse component in a grade 3A or 3B follicular lymphoma is considered to represent diffuse large B-cell lymphoma.[1]

DIAGNOSIS: ANCILLARY STUDIES

The usual immunophenotype of follicular lymphoma is monotypic surface immunoglobulin (sIg)+, CD20+, CD10+, bcl6+, CD5–, CD43– (**Fig. 3**). Neoplastic follicles are associated with CD21+ and CD23+ dendritic meshworks. Bcl2 protein is expressed in 85% to 90% of low-grade follicular lymphomas (see **Fig. 3D**), but in only 50% of grade 3 follicular lymphomas. The proliferation index is typically low (see **Fig. 3E**). The immunoglobulin heavy chain gene (*IGH*) is clonally rearranged. The immunoglobulin genes of follicular lymphoma are sometimes so altered by somatic hypermutation that primers used for PCR may not recognize the lymphoma's DNA sequences, leading to a false negative result. The t(14;18) (q32;q21), involving the genes *IGH* and *BCL2,* is found in up to 90% of cases, although it is less often found in grade 3 follicular lymphomas,

Fig. 1. Follicular lymphoma, follicular pattern, grade 1–2 of 3. (*A*) The lymph node is replaced by ill-defined, darkly stained follicles. (*B*) Neoplastic follicles invade the nodal capsule, with thickening and reduplication of the capsule. (*C*) Neoplastic follicles invade perinodal fat.

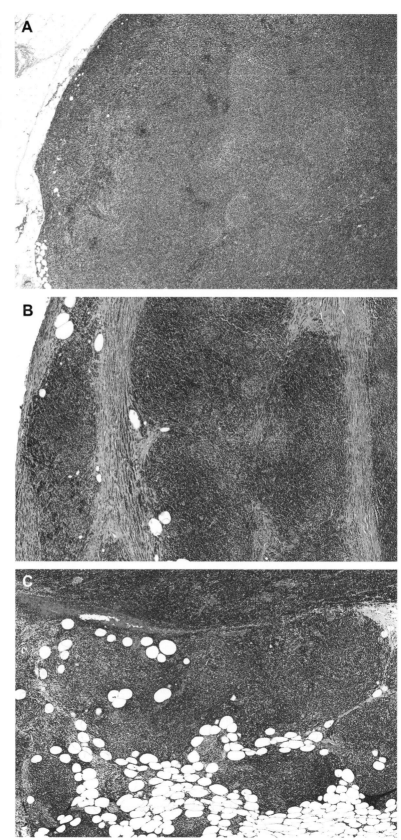

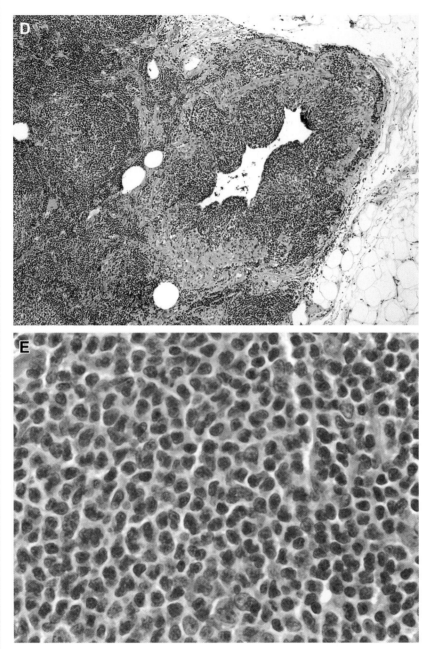

Fig. 1. Follicular lymphoma, follicular pattern, grade 1–2 of 3. (*D*) Neoplastic follicles show vascular invasion. (*E*) High power shows a nearly pure population of centrocytes with irregular nuclei and scant cytoplasm, indicating histologic grade 1–2 of 3.

among which it is identified in about half of cases.[3] The translocation is identified much more frequently in grade 3A than in grade 3B follicular lymphoma.[2] As with other low-grade B-cell lymphomas, such as marginal zone lymphoma, small lymphocytic lymphoma/chronic lymphocytic leukemia, and lymphoplasmacytic lymphoma, high-grade transformation to diffuse large B-cell lymphoma may occur.[1]

In recent years, investigators have focused on better characterizing those follicular lymphomas that lack bcl2 protein expression and/or the t(14;18).

Apparent failure of a follicular lymphoma to express bcl2 may be attributable to lack of an underlying t(14;18), but in some instances, it may be attributable to mutations in the *BCL2* gene, so that the protein expressed is abnormal and not recognized by the antibody used to detect bcl2.[4] Some follicular lymphomas that lack the t(14;18) do express bcl2 protein; however, this is often associated with increased copies of chromosome 18, so that increased copy number of the *BCL2* gene may result in

Fig. 2. Follicular lymphoma, follicular pattern, grade 3B. Large lymphoid cells with vesicular nuclei occupy almost the entire follicle (*upper right portion of image*). Their nuclei are at least twice the nuclear diameter of the small extrafollicular lymphocytes at the bottom of the image.

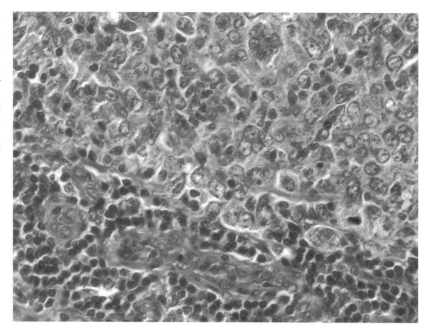

overexpression of bcl2.[5] In a study of localized (stage I) follicular lymphomas, those lacking t(14;18) were less likely to express bcl2 or CD10, more likely to present at extranodal sites, and had superior overall and disease-specific survival compared with localized follicular lymphomas with t(14;18).[6] Follicular lymphomas without the t(14;18) are genetically diverse, but among the most common abnormalities encountered are those involving the *BCL6* gene; both translocation and amplification of *BCL6* may be encountered.[5,7]

MORPHOLOGIC VARIATIONS

Some otherwise typical follicular lymphomas have unusual morphologic or immunophenotypic features. Signet ring cell lymphoma is a rare morphologic variant of non-Hodgkin's lymphoma in which some neoplastic cells contain clear cytoplasmic vacuoles or homogeneous eosinophilic globules filling much of the cytoplasm and compressing the nucleus to the periphery of the cell. This entity was first described in 1978, when Kim and colleagues[8] published a series of 7 cases of B-cell lymphoma with signet ring cells. Four cases had clear vacuoles and expressed IgG, whereas 3 cases contained periodic acid-Schiff (PAS)-positive, IgM+ inclusions resembling Russell bodies. Since that first report, a number of other cases of signet ring cell lymphoma have been described, usually in lymph nodes, but occasionally in extranodal sites.[9] Two main types of B-cell lymphomas

may have signet ring cells: low-grade B-cell lymphomas with plasmacytic differentiation, such as lymphoplasmacytic lymphoma, and follicular lymphomas (**Fig. 4**). In the former group, the cytoplasmic material is usually thought to be immunoglobulin, resulting in eosinophilic cytoplasm that is often PAS+. Among follicular lymphomas, signet ring cell cytoplasm is usually clear and ultrastructural studies typically reveal the presence of empty vacuoles. The diagnosis of follicular lymphoma with signet ring cells may not be difficult when a large biopsy specimen is available for evaluation and when the abnormal follicular architecture is readily appreciable. On a small biopsy, however, the diagnosis could be difficult, and metastatic signet ring cell carcinoma, fatty tumors, and even histiocytic proliferations could be considered in the differential diagnosis.

b) Follicular lymphoma infrequently shows marginal zone or monocytoid B-cell differentiation. Neoplastic follicles in follicular lymphomas with marginal zone differentiation have a perifollicular rim of small to medium-sized cells with moderate to abundant clear cytoplasm.[1,10] An interfollicular pattern of involvement by marginal zone cells is also described.[10] The presence of marginal zone differentiation in follicular lymphomas with t(14;18) appears to be associated with additional cytogenetic abnormalities of the type that may be seen in extranodal marginal zone lymphoma, especially trisomy 3.[10] c) A small proportion of follicular lymphomas have variably extensive plasmacytic

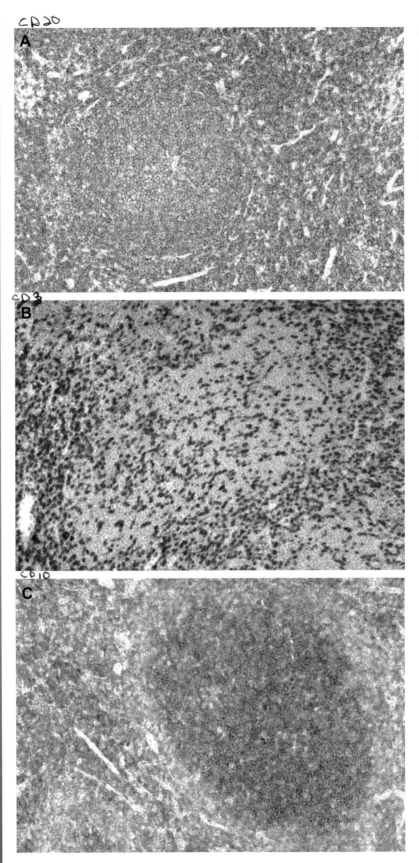

CD20

CD3

CD10

Fig. 3. Follicular lymphoma with usual immunopheno-type. (*A*) This ill-defined follicle and many neoplastic cells outside the follicle are CD20+ B cells. (*B*) CD3+ T cells are scattered in the in-terfollicular area and also within the follicle. (*C*) CD10 is brightly expressed in the follicle and dimly expressed in B cells outside the follicle.

Fig. 3. Follicular lymphoma with usual immunopheno-type. (*D*) The neoplastic B cells both within and outside the follicle coexpress bcl2. (*E*) The proliferation marker Ki67 stains less than 10% of lymphoid cells. (*A–E*, immunoperoxidase technique on paraffin sections.)

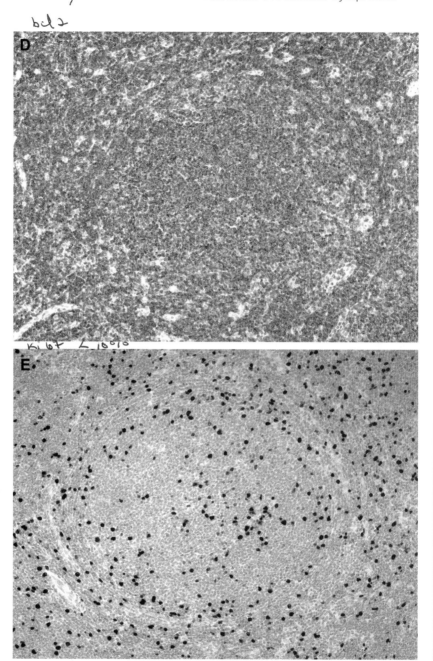

differentiation, estimated to be 3.5% in one large series. In a few cases, marginal zone and plasmacytic differentiation are both present.[12] Follicular lymphoma of any grade may have plasmacytic differentiation, although it appears to be present more often in higher grade follicular lymphomas.[2,11,12] The plasma cells may be found predominantly in the interfollicular area, in an intra- or perifollicular distribution, or in a combination of these patterns. The appearance of the plasma cells ranges from small and mature to somewhat atypical.[11,12] Some plasma cells contain Dutcher bodies, intranuclear pseudoinclusions of cytoplasm containing immunoglobulin (**Fig. 5**A). The immuno-phenotype is similar to that of cases without plasmacytic differentiation, except that plasma cells express monotypic immunoglobulin (see **Fig. 5**B, C). *BCL2* rearrangement is commonly detected; *BCL6* rearrangement is found in fewer cases. In one study, those lymphomas with a *BCL2* rearrangement by fluorescent in situ hybridization (FISH) were more likely to have preferential

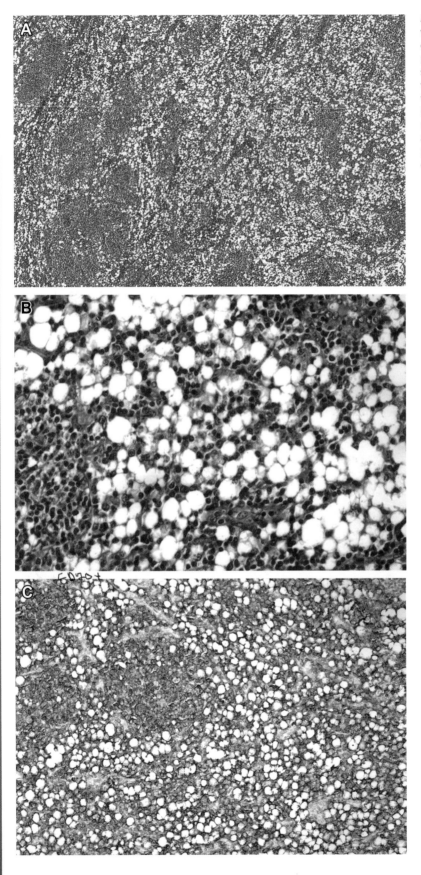

Fig. 4. Follicular lymphoma with numerous signet ring cells. (*A*) Low power shows poorly delineated, darkly stained follicles alternating with loose collections of vacuolated signet ring cells. (*B*) High power shows that many follicle center cells are distorted by large cytoplasmic vacuoles. (*C*) Most cells are CD20+ B cells.

Fig. 4. Follicular lymphoma with numerous signet ring cells. (*D*) CD3 highlights T cells in an interfollicular pattern, facilitating recognition of the follicular pattern of the lymphoma. (*E*) The immunophenotype of this lymphoma is similar to that of other follicular lymphomas, including bcl2 expression shown here. (*C–E*, immunoperoxidase technique on paraffin sections.)

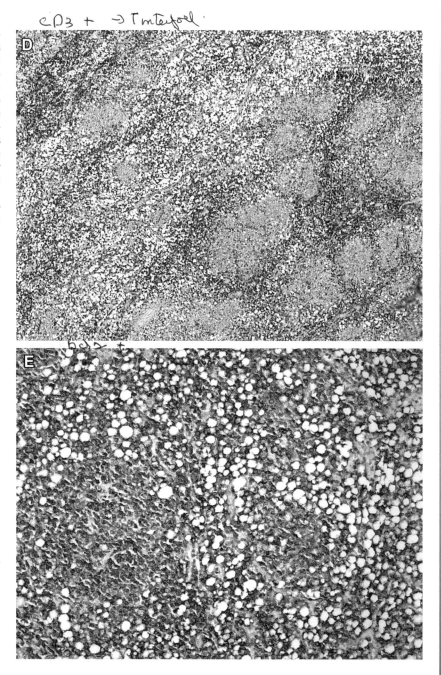

CD3 + → T interfoll.

bcl2 +

localization of the plasma cells in the interfollicular area, whereas those lacking *BCL2* rearrangement were more likely to have plasma cells in an intra- or perifollicular pattern.[12] The latter was also found in one case with concurrent *BCL2* and *BCL6* rearrangement. The main entity in the differential diagnosis of follicular lymphoma with marginal zone and/or plasmacytic differentiation is marginal zone lymphoma with infiltration and replacement of reactive follicles (follicular colonization), as marginal zone lymphomas (whether nodal, splenic, or extranodal) by definition contain marginal zone cells and often show plasmacytic differentiation. The presence of a monotonous population of follicle center cells with scant cytoplasm coexpressing bcl2 favors follicular lymphoma. If evaluated by flow cytometry, monotypic immunoglobulin expression by CD10+ B cells favors follicular lymphoma. Identifying a t(14;18) and/or *IGH-BCL2* fusion also favors follicular lymphoma.

The floral variant of follicular lymphoma is characterized by neoplastic follicles infiltrated and broken up by small lymphocytes; the follicular fragments are reminiscent of the petals of a flower.

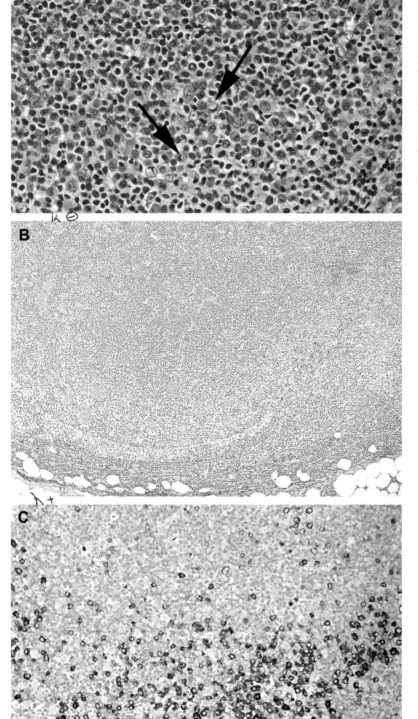

Fig. 5. Follicular lymphoma with plasmacytic differentiation (a low-power image of this lymphoma is illustrated in **Fig. 1A**). (*A*) Rare follicles contain many plasma cells, sometimes with Dutcher bodies (*arrows*), at the periphery of the follicle. (*B*) The plasma cells are negative for κ light chain. (*C*). Plasma cells show monotypic staining for λ light chain; the same monotypic λ light chain was demonstrated on the B cells by flow cytometry. (*B* and *C*, immunoperoxidase technique on paraffin sections).

Fig. 6. Follicular lymphoma, floral variant. (*A*) The lymphoma is composed of expansile, irregularly shaped follicles. (*B*) Individual follicles are composed of multiple small, "petal-like" aggregates of neoplastic follicle center cells. (*C*) The aggregates contain mostly centrocytes with rare centroblasts, in a background of small lymphocytes.

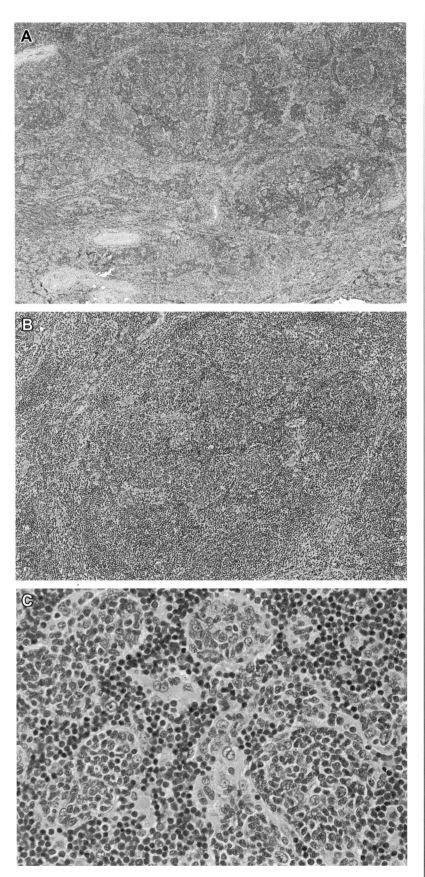

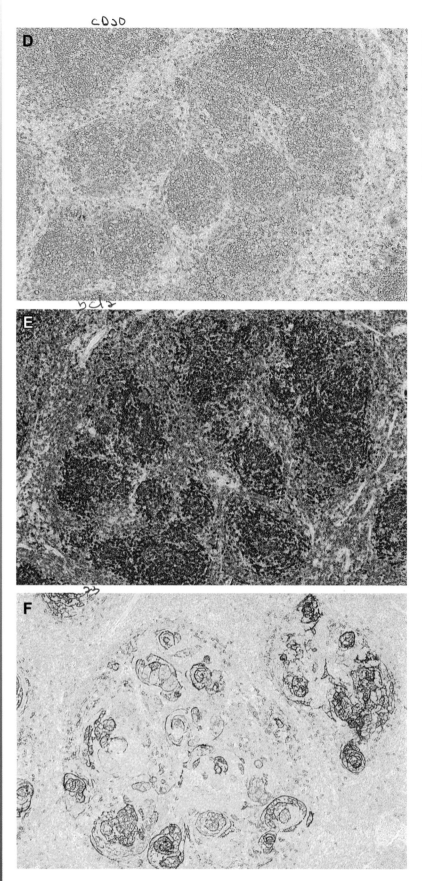

Fig. 6. Follicular lymphoma, floral variant. (*D*) The "petals" are composed of CD20+ B cells. (*E*) The neoplastic B cells coexpress and bcl2. (*F*) An immunostain for CD23 highlights the fragmented dendritic meshwork associated with this neoplastic follicle. (*D–F,* immunoperoxidase technique on paraffin sections.)

⚠️⚠️ *Differential Diagnosis*
FOLLICULAR LYMPHOMA

Diagnosis	Follicular Lymphoma	Reactive Hyperplasia	CLL/SLL	Mantle Cell Lymphoma
Patients	Older, M<F	Any age, often young	Older, M>F	Older, M≫F
Lymphadenopathy	Widespread	Localized, sometimes widespread	Widespread	Widespread
Leukemic involvement	Rare	No	Almost always	Occasional
Histology	Follicular ± diffuse areas. Centrocytes and centroblasts	Preserved architecture. Well-defined follicles with polarization	Small cells. Scattered proliferation centers with larger cells	Vaguely nodular and/or diffuse or mantle pattern. Monotonous, small irregular cells
Usual immunophenotype	CD20+, CD5−, CD10+, CD23±, bcl6+, bcl2+, Ki67 low	Follicle centers: CD20+, CD10+, bcl6+, bcl2−, Ki67 high	CD20dim+, CD5+, CD10−, bcl2+, CD23+	CD20+, CD5+, CD10−, CD23-, bcl2+, cyclin D1+, λ>κ light chain
Progression	May progress to DLBCL	Usually resolves spontaneously	May progress to DLBCL	May progress to blastoid variant of mantle cell lymphoma, not to DLBCL
Prognosis	Usually long survival	Excellent	Usually long survival	Median survival <5 years

Abbreviations: CLL/SLL, chronic lymphocytic leukemia/small lymphocytic lymphoma; DLBCL, diffuse large B-cell lymphoma; PLL, prolymphocytic leukemia.

The composition of the "petals" is similar to that of usual follicular lymphoma (**Fig. 6A−C**). The immunophenotype is also similar to other follicular lymphomas (see **Fig. 6**D, F), although in one study, 4 of 11 cases expressed CD5,[13] a finding that is quite uncommon in follicular lymphomas. There is usually an *IGH-BCL2* rearrangement.[13–15] The differential diagnosis includes reactive hyperplasia with follicle lysis, because the fragmented follicles of follicle lysis have a similar pattern. However, follicle lysis typically occurs in the background of florid follicular hyperplasia; moreover, the lysed follicles have a polymorphous composition, with many mitoses and tingible body macrophages, and do not express bcl2 protein.

DIFFERENTIAL DIAGNOSIS

The differential diagnosis of follicular lymphomas using clinical and microscopic features as well as information from ancillary studies is detailed in the Table for the Differential Diagnosis of Follicular Lymphomas.

FOLLICULAR LYMPHOMA VERSUS FOLLICULAR HYPERPLASIA

Differentiating reactive lymphoid hyperplasia with follicular hyperplasia from follicular lymphoma can be challenging. On low-power examination, a bean-shaped lymph node with an intact hilus favors reactive hyperplasia, whereas a spherical or irregularly enlarged lymph node is more suspicious for malignancy. In reactive hyperplasia, the components of the lymph node (the follicles, paracortex, medullary cords, sinuses, and hilus) should be identifiable, assuming the lymph node has been sectioned properly, and should be present in reasonable proportion to one another. Obliteration of the architecture or marked expansion of one component over the others is suspicious for

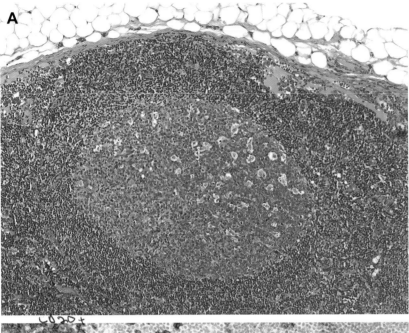

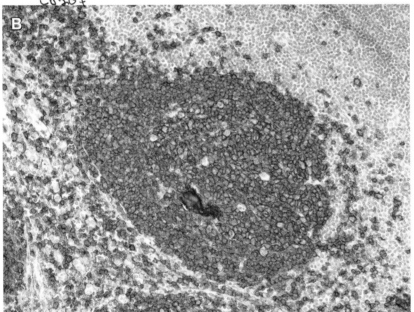

Fig. 7. Follicular hyperplasia. (*A*) This reactive follicle shows polarization with a dark zone (*top part of follicle*) and a light zone. The dark zone contains highly proliferative follicle center cells and many scattered tingible-body macrophages. The mantle is well preserved and the interface between follicle center and mantle is sharp. (*B*) The follicle is composed of CD20+ B cells; few B cells are present outside follicles.

a significant abnormality. Lymphoid follicles are normally in the cortex, arranged around the periphery of the lymph node beneath the capsule. They may be primary, quiescent follicles, composed of small aggregates of small lymphocytes, or they may be secondary, reactive follicles, with a germinal center. To assess follicles, one should note their size and shape, their location (confined to the cortex or present throughout the lymph node), presence or absence of crowding, their composition, and their mantles. A follicle center with a polymorphous composition, polarization into a dark zone and a light zone, frequent mitoses, and scattered tingible-body macrophages, is likely reactive (**Fig. 7A**). In contrast, follicles with a monotonous population of follicle center cells would suggest follicular lymphoma. A well-defined, intact mantle zone is typical of reactive follicles. Attenuation or loss of mantles may be seen in some florid reactive processes, (such as HIV-associated lymphoid hyperplasia), but can also be a clue to the diagnosis

Fig. 7. Follicular hyperplasia. (*C*) CD3+ T cells predominate outside follicles. A thin layer of T cells is also present around the periphery of the follicle center. (*D*) The follicle center is negative for bcl2, whereas the mantle zone B cells and the interfollicular T cells are bcl2+. (*B–D*, immunoperoxidase technique on paraffin sections.)

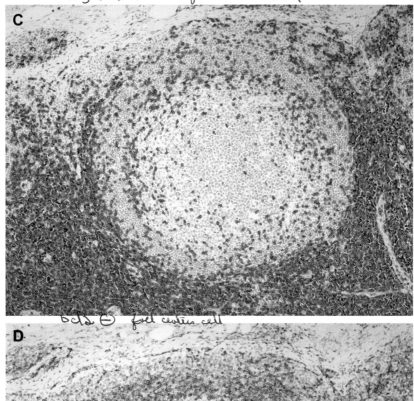

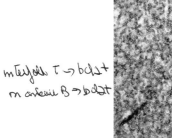

of follicular lymphoma. A thin, fibrous capsule normally surrounds the lymph node. It can be thickened in both reactive conditions, such as chronic lymphadenitis, and in some neoplastic processes, including follicular lymphoma. Invasion of the nodal capsule and invasion of follicles into perinodal fat are unusual in reactive hyperplasia and are a clue to follicular lymphoma.

B cells in lymph nodes are normally present in follicles and in a thin layer along sinuses. B cells are also scattered in small numbers in the paracortex and can be more numerous in certain reactive conditions, such as infectious mononucleosis. Numerous B cells outside follicles should raise the question of B-cell lymphoma, particularly if they express CD10 or bcl6 (see **Fig. 3**). T cells normally predominate in the paracortex and also comprise a minority of cells in the follicle center. The medullary cords contain a mixture of B and T cells. Reactive follicles have follicle centers that are CD20+, CD10+, bcl6+, and bcl2−, with a high proliferation fraction (close to 100%) that often shows some

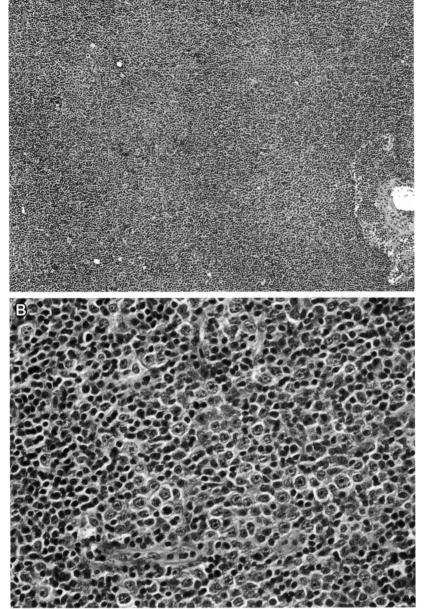

Fig. 8. Small lymphocytic lymphoma/chronic lymphocytic leukemia. (*A*) The lymph node is replaced by a diffuse proliferation of small lymphocytes with scattered ill-defined, slightly paler proliferation centers: this appearance has been likened to a "cloudy sky." (*B*) High power of a proliferation center shows that it comprises a loose collection of medium-sized and large lymphoid cells with round to oval nuclei (prolymphocytes and paraimmunoblasts) present in a background of small lymphocytes.

degree of polarization (see **Fig. 7**B–D). B cells are not usually numerous outside follicles. CD10+, bcl6+ B cells should be rare to absent outside follicles; if present in substantial numbers, the possibility of follicular lymphoma should be considered. Primary follicles (follicular structures that lack germinal centers) are CD20+, CD10−, bcl6−, and bcl2+, with a relatively low Ki67 proliferation index. Bcl2 expression in primary follicles is normal and should not suggest follicular lymphoma.

FOLLICULAR LYMPHOMA VERSUS OTHER SMALL B-CELL LYMPHOMAS

The differential diagnosis of follicular lymphoma also includes other B-cell lymphomas, in particular small lymphocytic lymphoma/chronic lymphocytic leukemia and mantle cell lymphoma. Small lymphocytic lymphoma/chronic lymphocytic leukemia sometimes has prominent proliferation centers with prolymphocytes and paraimmunoblasts that may potentially mimic follicles; however, those

Fig. 9. Mantle cell lymphoma, a small B-cell lymphoma that may histologically mimic a follicular lymphoma. (*A*) This lymph node is replaced by a nodular proliferation of small lymphoid cells, reminiscent of the pattern seen in follicular lymphoma. (*B*) Higher power shows a proliferation of small to medium-sized, irregular, darkly stained, monotonous lymphoid cells with scant cytoplasm. There is a remnant of a reactive follicle center composed of slightly larger cells with interspersed apoptotic debris (*arrows*). (*C*) The atypical cells are CD20+ B cells.

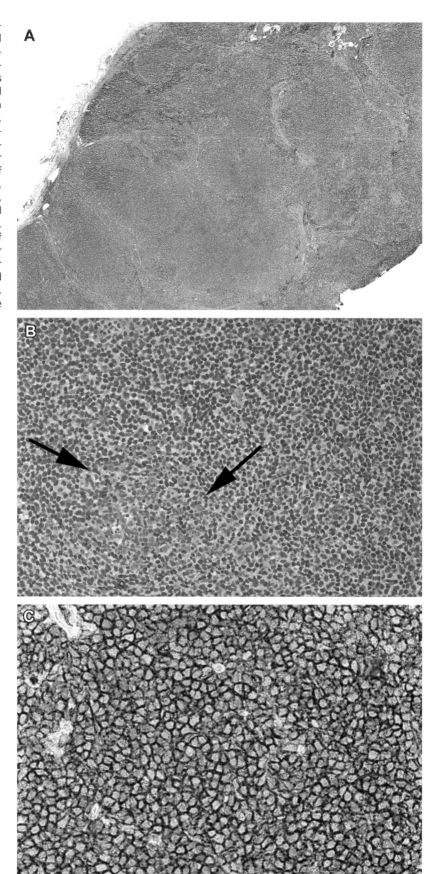

CD5 + bright → T cell (N)
CD5 + pale → manteau

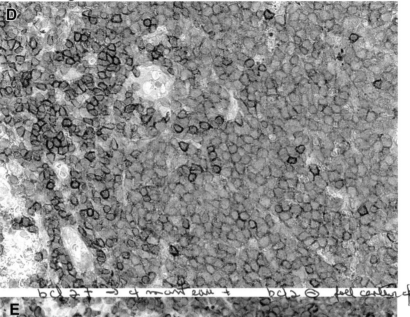

Fig. 9. Mantle cell lymphoma, a small B-cell lymphoma that may histologically mimic a follicular lymphoma. (*D*) The neoplastic mantle cells dimly coexpress CD5; the bright CD5+ cells are nonneoplastic T cells. (*E*) The neoplastic mantle cells are bcl2+, whereas the residual reactive follicle center cells (*upper left corner of image*) are negative for bcl2. (*F*) The neoplastic cells are cyclinD1+; residual reactive follicle center cells (*right side of image*) are negative. (*C–F*, immunoperoxidase technique on paraffin sections.)

bcl 2 + → ct manteau +   bcl 2 ⊖ foll center cell

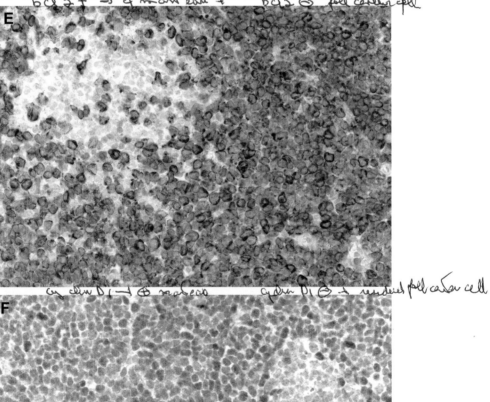

cy clin D1 → ⊕ manteau   cyclin D1 ⊖ → residual foll center cell

proliferation centers are typically more ill defined than the neoplastic follicles of follicular lymphoma and the neoplastic small lymphocytes, prolympho-cytes, and paraimmunoblasts typically have less irregular nuclei than centrocytes (**Fig. 8**). In early stages of nodal involvement, mantle cell lymphoma may have a mantle zone pattern, with neoplastic cells surrounding reactive germinal centers, or a nodular pattern, with neoplastic mantle cells re-placing follicles (**Fig. 9**). Mantle zone lymphoma with a nodular pattern may mimic follicular lymphoma, grade 1 of 3. However, mantle cell lymphoma has a more monotonous cellular compo-sition than is usual for follicular lymphoma, which usually contains at least a few centroblasts. Immu-nophenotyping is very helpful in distinguishing among these lymphomas. The differential of follic-ular lymphoma with marginal zone lymphoma was discussed previously in the section on follicular lymphoma with marginal zone/plasmacytic differentiation.

PROGNOSIS

Most follicular lymphomas are low-grade lymphomas that behave in an indolent manner. Grade 3 follicular lymphomas may behave in a more aggressive manner. Low-grade follicular lymphoma may undergo progression to an aggres-sive lymphoma with histologic features of diffuse large B-cell lymphoma or a high-grade lymphoma resembling Burkitt lymphoma; these transformed lymphomas have a poor prognosis.[16] Occasionally, low-grade follicular lymphomas have a proliferation index that is higher than would be anticipated in a low-grade lymphoma. Neoplastic follicles with greater than 30% of cells being Ki67+ have been suggested as indicating a high proliferation index,[17] but additional studies addressing this issue would be helpful in validating this threshold. These low-grade/high proliferation index follicular lymphomas may behave in a more aggressive manner than those with a low proliferation index.[17] Some lymph nodes involved by follicular lymphoma may have one or more residual reactive follicles; the presence of such reactive follicles appears to correlate with lower stage[18] and may be of prognostic importance.

PEDIATRIC FOLLICULAR LYMPHOMA

CLINICAL FEATURES

When follicular lymphoma occurs in children and adolescents (pediatric follicular lymphoma) it has distinctive clinical and pathologic features. Pedi-atric follicular lymphoma is designated as a variant of follicular lymphoma in the WHO Classification.[1]

Studies of this entity have used an upper age limit of 21 years,[19,20] but children as young as 2 years old have been affected, with a median age of 10 to 11 years. Pediatric follicular lymphoma preferen-tially affects boys (male:female ratio of approxi-mately 3:1),[19] who typically present with localized peripheral lymphadenopathy, most often in the cervical region or with tonsillar involvement.[20] Other sites, including appendix[19] and testes may be involved; testicular follicular lymphoma is dis-cussed separately later in this article.

DIAGNOSIS: MICROSCOPIC FEATURES AND ANCILLARY STUDIES

Microscopic examination shows very large, ex-pansile follicles that in many cases contain enough centroblasts to qualify for grade 3. The follicles are CD10+, bcl6+, and CD43−/+, but in contrast with most follicular lymphomas in adults, they are bcl2−. The proliferation index is often high (**Fig. 10**). *IGH* is clonally rearranged, but *BCL2* is usually not rearranged.

DIFFERENTIAL DIAGNOSIS

The differential diagnosis includes florid follicular hyperplasia and nodal marginal zone lymphoma with follicular colonization. There are rare cases of florid follicular hyperplasia, mainly in boys or young adults, in which a population of CD10+ clonal B cells can be found by flow cytometry[21]; follow-up in these patients has been uneventful. A diagnosis of pediatric follicular lymphoma should not be made unless the histologic features are atypical enough to warrant such a diagnosis.[1,22]

PROGNOSIS

The prognosis appears to be excellent[19]: patients typically do not experience relapses and are without persistent disease on follow-up. In a few instances, however, bcl2+ follicular lymphomas occur in children. These bcl2+ pediatric follicular lymphomas do not appear to have such a favorable prognosis, and may behave more like adult follic-ular lymphomas.[20]

EXTRANODAL FOLLICULAR LYMPHOMAS

A minority of follicular lymphomas arise in extrano-dal sites rather than lymph nodes. Among the more common sites are the skin[23] and the gastro-intestinal tract[24]; other sites include Waldeyer's ring,[25] testis,[26] ocular adnexa,[27] salivary glands,[28] thyroid,[29] gallbladder[30,31] and extrahepatic biliary tract,[32,33] female genital tract,[25] and others. Follic-ular lymphoma arising in the skin (primary

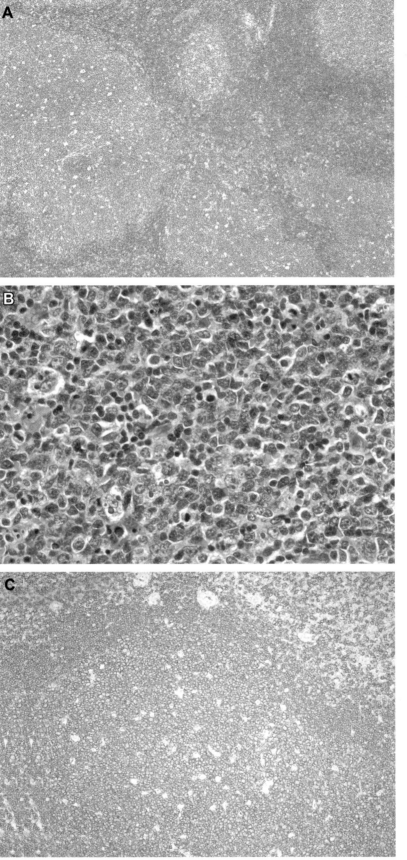

Fig. 10. Pediatric follicular lymphoma. (*A*) Very large irregular follicles distort the nodal architecture; many pale tingible body macrophages are scattered among the atypical lymphoid cells. (*B*) High power shows medium-sized and large atypical lymphoid cells with frequent mitoses and tingible body macrophages containing apoptotic debris, sharing some histologic features with a reactive follicle. (*C*) This markedly enlarged follicle is composed of CD20 + B cells.

Fig. 10. Pediatric follicular lymphoma. (*D*) The atypical B cells are positive for CD10. (*E*) Unlike most follicular lymphomas occurring in adults, the neoplastic B cells are negative for bcl2. (*F*) The proliferation index, as assessed with Ki67, is high (compare with Fig. 3E, a grade 1–2 follicular lymphoma occurring in an adult). (*C–F*, immunoperoxidase technique on paraffin sections.)

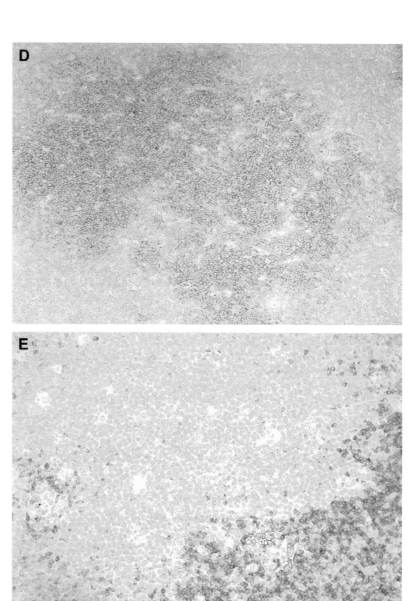

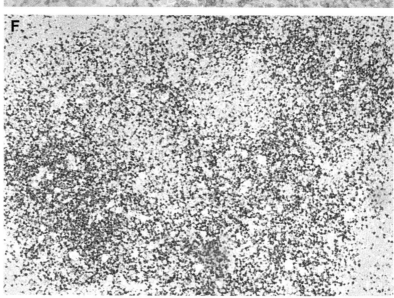

cutaneous follicle center lymphoma) is the most common primary cutaneous B-cell lymphoma.[23] With this exception, follicular lymphoma accounts for only a minority of lymphomas arising in extranodal sites. Other types of lymphoma, most often diffuse large B-cell lymphoma or extranodal marginal zone (MALT) lymphoma, are more common than follicular lymphoma in most extranodal sites. In certain extranodal sites, such as the central nervous system, follicular lymphoma is vanishingly rare, if it occurs at all. Taken together, extranodal follicular lymphomas tend to present with localized disease, less often express bcl2, less often have a translocation involving *BCL2* [t(14;18)], and may have better survival than lymph nodal follicular lymphoma.[25] However, the characteristics of follicular lymphomas appear to vary somewhat from one site to another. Follicular lymphomas that occur at several extranodal sites display particular clinicopathologic features and appear to represent distinct entities, which are discussed in the following sections.

GASTROINTESTINAL FOLLICULAR LYMPHOMA

CLINICAL FEATURES

Follicular lymphoma of the gastrointestinal tract is uncommon: fewer than 4% of all primary gastrointestinal lymphomas are follicular lymphomas.[24] However, gastrointestinal follicular lymphoma appears to be a distinct clinicopathologic entity and accordingly, primary intestinal follicular lymphoma is recognized as a variant of follicular lymphoma in the 2008 WHO Classification.[1,34] In one study of 222 gastrointestinal lymphomas, 13 duodenal lymphomas and 8 follicular lymphomas were identified; 5 of the 8 follicular lymphomas arose in the duodenum, all in its second portion, in the vicinity of the ampulla of Vater. The 5 patients were all women, aged 37 to 66 years (median, 52), with follicular lymphoma, grade 1 of 3, producing small polypoid masses and protrusions, or mucosal irregularities. Two patients had partial involvement of regional lymph nodes by follicular lymphoma. All patients were alive and well 2 to 50 months after diagnosis.[24] Several subsequent studies have also found that patients with gastrointestinal follicular lymphoma are mostly middle-aged adults,[35–38] and a female preponderance in most series.[35,36,39] The small intestine is most often involved, with duodenum most commonly involved,[35,37–39] although stomach and colorectum may be affected. On endoscopy, nodularity of the mucosa is usually seen; cases with the appearance of multiple lymphomatous polyposis are also described.[35,38,40] Taken together, the results of these studies suggest that a high proportion of duodenal lymphomas are follicular lymphoma and that a high proportion of gastrointestinal follicular lymphomas arise in the duodenum.

DIAGNOSIS: MICROSCOPIC FEATURES AND ANCILLARY STUDIES

On microscopic examination, the vast majority are grade 1 of 3, with a few grade 2 and rare grade 3 follicular lymphomas (**Fig. 11**). The follicular lymphomas typically have an immunophenotype similar to that found in nodal follicular lymphomas occurring in adults (CD20+, CD10+, bcl2+, bcl6+).[34–37,39] Immunoglobulin heavy and light chain genes are clonally rearranged and *BCL2* rearrangement is identified in most cases.[36,41,42] In-depth evaluation of these lymphomas does reveal some pathologic features that diverge from those of lymph nodal follicular lymphoma, however. Gastrointestinal follicular lymphoma frequently expresses α4β7, the mucosal homing receptor, suggesting an origin from antigen-responsive B cells residing in intestinal mucosa.[43] One study described that, in contrast with lymph nodal follicular lymphomas, intestinal follicular lymphomas are associated with "hollowed out," rather than intact, follicular dendritic cell meshworks.[42] Intestinal follicular lymphomas are reported to lack expression of activation-induced cytidine deaminase (AID).[42] Biased usage of immunoglobulin heavy chain variable region genes (*IGVH*) has been described, with disproportionate use of VH4, in particular VH4-34.[38,42] These observations suggest subtle differences in the pathologic features of intestinal and lymph nodal follicular lymphoma; they also suggest an antigen-driven component in the pathogenesis of intestinal follicular lymphoma.[38,42]

DIFFERENTIAL DIAGNOSIS

The differential diagnosis is mainly with reactive lymphoid aggregates and with other types of small B-cell lymphomas, similar to the differential of lymph nodal follicular lymphoma. In the gastrointestinal tract, the differential diagnosis also includes extranodal marginal zone lymphoma of mucosa-associated lymphoid tissue (MALT lymphoma). Compared with follicular lymphoma, marginal zone lymphoma typically has a more diffuse pattern, is composed of cells with more abundant pale cytoplasm, lacks expression of CD10 and bcl6, and may show evidence of plasmacytic differentiation in the form of a plasma

Fig. 11. Small intestinal follicular lymphoma. Multiple crowded, poorly delineated follicles lacking mantles distort the normal architecture of the small bowel.

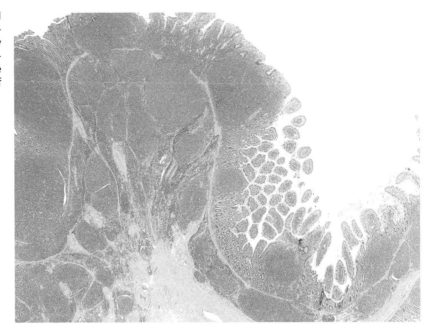

cell component expressing monotypic cytoplasmic immunoglobulin.

PROGNOSIS

The prognosis of primary gastrointestinal follicular lymphoma appears favorable. At last follow-up, most patients are free of disease and a minority are alive with disease. Death attributable to gastrointestinal follicular lymphoma appears to be very uncommon.[35,40,44]

PRIMARY CUTANEOUS FOLLICLE CENTER LYMPHOMA

CLINICAL FEATURES

Primary cutaneous follicle center lymphoma is defined as a primary cutaneous tumor composed of neoplastic follicle center cells.[23] It primarily affects adults older than 30, with a median age in the sixth or seventh decade.[23,45–47] Men are affected slightly more often than women. The lymphoma takes the form of red or violaceous plaques, nodules, or tumors, which in some instances are longstanding, having been present for years.[23,47] Lesions are found most often on the head and neck, whereas the trunk is affected less often; involvement of extremities is uncommon.

DIAGNOSIS: MICROSCOPIC FEATURES AND ANCILLARY STUDIES

The lymphoma is composed of a nodular and/or diffuse proliferation of small and large centrocytes

with a varying admixture of centroblasts in a pattern that may be follicular, follicular and diffuse, or diffuse. When a follicular pattern is present, the follicles are often ill defined and may become confluent. The follicle may be partly delineated by mantle zones composed of small B cells and are sometimes centered on adnexal structures. The lymphoma may infiltrate the surrounding dermis in an interstitial pattern and can be associated with sclerosis. In some instances, the neoplastic cells may have a spindled or lobated appearance. The lymphoma involves the dermis and often extends to involve the subcutaneous tissue, but typically spares the epidermis (**Fig. 12**). Because grading is not considered to have clinical significance, it is not necessary to grade primary cutaneous follicular lymphoma. In addition, it is not necessary to note the pattern (follicular vs diffuse) in the diagnosis, in contrast to follicular lymphoma in other anatomic sites. The neoplastic B cells are CD20+, bcl6+. The proportion of cases that are CD10+ varies among series, but overall approximately 80% of cases are CD10+; CD10 is more likely to be expressed in cases with a follicular pattern. The proportion of cases with bcl2+ neoplastic cells is even more variable among different studies. Some authorities describe absent or weak bcl2 staining in most cases,[23] whereas others report most cases to be bcl2+.[45–47] Admixed T cells may be abundant. CD21+ or CD23+ dendritic meshworks are often identified. Clonal rearrangement of *IGH* can often be detected. When *BCL2* has been evaluated using polymerase chain reaction (PCR) or FISH,

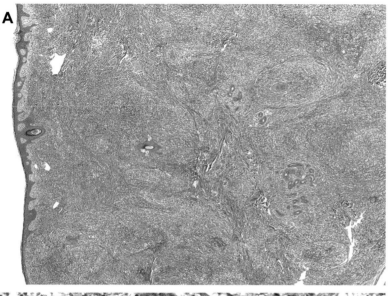

Fig. 12. Primary cutaneous follicle center lymphoma. (*A*) Low-power image shows multiple large, irregular, sometimes confluent aggregates of atypical lymphoid cells filling the dermis. (*B*) A large, poorly delineated follicle with an attenuated mantle zone fills the lower left portion of the image. Atypical cells surround eccrine glands in the right portion of the image. (*C*) The neoplastic cells have irregular, twisted, elongated nuclei, inconspicuous nucleoli, and scant cytoplasm. The epidermis is spared.

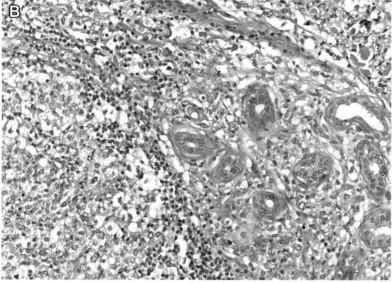

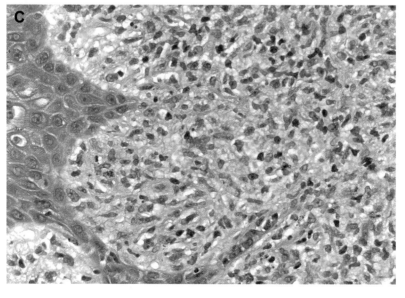

rearrangement is usually detected in only a minority of cases.[45-47]

DIFFERENTIAL DIAGNOSIS

The differential diagnosis includes a reactive lymphoid infiltrate and a primary extracutaneous follicular lymphoma with secondary cutaneous involvement. Careful morphologic and immunophenotypic study, augmented by molecular evaluation in difficult cases, can help distinguish reactive and neoplastic lymphoid follicles. Staging studies can exclude an extracutaneous primary. Bcl2 expression and *BCL2* rearrangement are more common in lymph nodal follicular lymphoma than in primary cutaneous follicle center lymphoma, and these findings would suggest the possibility of an extracutaneous primary follicular lymphoma.[23,47] The differential diagnosis also includes cutaneous marginal zone lymphoma. Cutaneous follicle center lymphoma is typically composed of cells with more irregular nuclei and less abundant cytoplasm than marginal zone lymphoma. Marginal zone lymphomas lack CD10 and bcl6 expression and often show plasmacytic differentiation.

PROGNOSIS

The prognosis of primary cutaneous follicle center lymphoma is excellent.[23] In most series, nearly all patients are alive at last follow-up and most are free of disease, whereas a minority are alive with persistent disease. Patients may develop cutaneous relapses, but spread beyond the skin to lymph nodes is very uncommon.[45-47]

TESTICULAR FOLLICULAR LYMPHOMA

CLINICAL FEATURES

Testicular lymphoma is predominantly a disease of older adults, and in adults the lymphomas are nearly always diffuse large B-cell lymphomas and only rarely follicular lymphomas.[48,49] Conversely, primary testicular lymphoma in boys is rare, but when it occurs it is most often follicular lymphoma.[26,48] Based on the small number of cases reported, patients are mostly young adults[26] or boys, mostly younger than 10 years, who present with unilateral testicular enlargement.

DIAGNOSIS: GROSS AND MICROSCOPIC FEATURES AND ANCILLARY STUDIES

The lymphomas are firm to fleshy lesions that replace all or part of the testis.[50-55] Microscopically, the lymphoma consists of crowded, poorly delineated follicles composed of atypical lymphoid cells, sometimes with diffuse areas. Large cells are often sufficiently numerous for a diagnosis of follicular lymphoma, grade 3. There may be associated sclerosis. The neoplastic cells are positive for CD20 and often express CD10 and bcl6,[26,50-55] but are negative for bcl2 and for p53 protein.[26,50,51,54,55] Proliferation index as assessed by Ki67 is high.[51,55] *BCL2* rearrangement has been reported to be absent, although clonal rearrangement of the *IGH* gene can usually be demonstrated. Individual cases with rearrangement of the *BCL6* gene[51] and mutations of the *BCL6* gene have been described.[55]

DIFFERENTIAL DIAGNOSIS

The main entity in the differential diagnosis is orchitis, particularly in cases with prominent sclerosis. Careful attention to cytologic features will facilitate performing appropriate confirmatory immunostains and establishing a diagnosis of lymphoma.

PROGNOSIS

Patients almost always have localized disease: lymphoma may be confined to the testis or may spread to involve the epididymis. Patients have been treated with surgery and chemotherapy[26,51-53] or with orchiectomy alone.[50] Disease-free survival and prognosis appear excellent, although relatively few cases have been reported and follow-up has been relatively short.[26,52,53] In contrast with lymph nodal follicular lymphoma occurring in adults, testicular follicular lymphoma preferentially affects younger patients, presents with localized disease, is typically grade 3, lacks bcl2 expression, lacks *BCL2* rearrangement, and may be curable with currently available therapy. Thus, it shares many features with pediatric follicular lymphoma presenting with lymph node involvement, as discussed previously.

FOLLICULAR LYMPHOMA IN SITU

CLINICAL FEATURES

Follicular lymphoma "in situ" is an unusual condition in which follicles containing abnormal, clonal, bcl2 brightly positive cells are present in a background of architecturally normal lymphoid tissue.[56] Relatively few cases have been reported, but patients have been mostly middle-aged to older adults with women affected more often than men.[56,57]

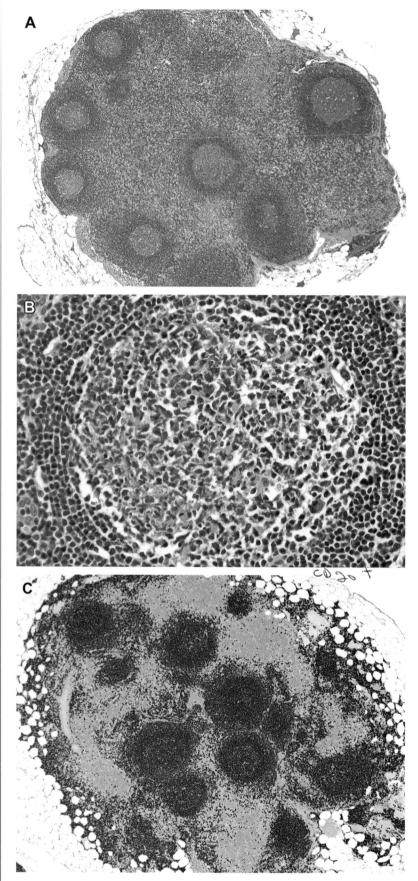

Fig. 13. Follicular lymphoma in situ involving mesenteric lymph nodes, associated with concurrent, clonally related diffuse large B-cell lymphoma of the ileum (not shown). (*A*) The mesenteric lymph node has normal architecture: follicles are normally distributed and have intact mantle zones. (*B*) This follicle has a monotonous-appearing follicle center surrounded by a well-preserved mantle zone. (*C*) CD20+ B cells are present mainly in follicles.

bcl2 + ds g?o foell partition are totalent +

T < pue sa 1/2

Fig. 13. Follicular lymphoma in situ involving mesenteric lymph nodes, associated with concurrent, clonally related diffuse large B-cell lymphoma of the ileum (not shown). (*D*) A number of follicle centers are partly or mostly occupied by cells expressing very bright bcl2. (*E*) This follicle center is almost entirely replaced by bcl2+ B cells; the bcl2 expression is much brighter than in the surrounding cells. (*C–E*, immunoperoxidase technique on paraffin sections).

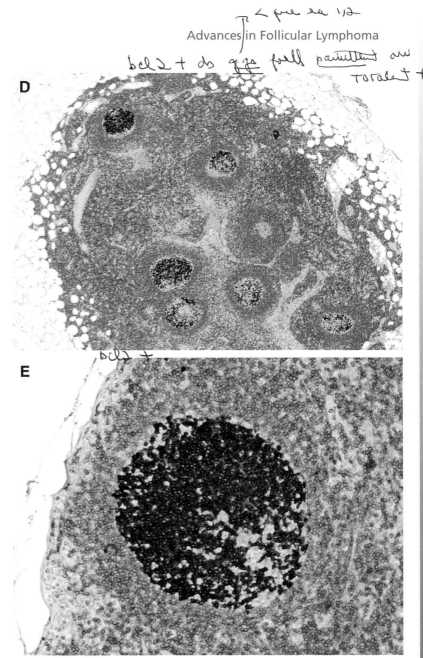

bcl2 +

DIAGNOSIS: MICROSCOPIC FEATURES AND ANCILLARY STUDIES

On microscopic examination, affected lymph nodes closely resemble reactive lymph nodes, except that some follicles may have monotonous-appearing follicle centers with intact mantles (**Fig. 13**). These monotonous follicles have an immunophenotype like that of other follicular lymphomas, except that bcl2 is consistently very bright (usually considerably brighter than the aberrant bcl2 expression found in typical follicular lymphomas). Occasionally the abnormal follicles closely resemble reactive follicles histologically, and are recognizable as abnormal only because of the strong bcl2 expression.[57] The number of abnormal follicles varies from case to case, but in most cases fewer than half of all follicles in the involved lymph nodes are abnormal. In addition, some follicles are only partially replaced by abnormal follicle center cells. Clonal *IGH* rearrangement and *BCL2* rearrangement are present in most cases, although detection using microdissected tissue or combined immunohistochemistry and FISH appears to be more sensitive than using whole sections of tissue, as the abnormal cells are present in relatively small numbers.[56,57]

DIFFERENTIAL DIAGNOSIS

The main problem in differential diagnosis is that the relatively subtle histologic changes of follicular lymphoma in situ may not be recognized on routinely stained sections. Obtaining an immunostain for bcl2 in lymph nodes with monotonous-appearing follicles (see **Fig. 13**D, E) will help to avoid overlooking the diagnosis.

PROGNOSIS

In several reported cases, follicular lymphoma in situ has been present in lymph nodes involved concurrently by another B-cell lymphoma ("composite lymphoma").[56,57] The clinical significance of this finding is variable, as some patients have follicular lymphoma in other sites at diagnosis,[56,57] others develop follicular lymphoma on follow-up, and others have no other evidence of lymphoma on follow-up. There is a tendency for lymph nodes with larger numbers of follicles showing follicular lymphoma in situ to be more likely to have overt follicular lymphoma in other

sites.[56] It is possible that follicular lymphoma in situ represents a preneoplastic change, or a very early stage in the development of follicular lymphoma that may or may not progress to clinically evident lymphoma; more recently, the terminology "In-situ involvement by follicular lymphoma-like B cells" has been suggested for this entity, given that many of these patients never develop overt lymphoma on follow-up. For those who do have evident lymphoma, the picture of follicular lymphoma in situ could possibly be produced by "seeding" of reactive follicles by neoplastic cells originating from the lymphoma.[56] We have seen a case of small intestinal diffuse large B-cell lymphoma in which mesenteric lymph nodes were free of large cell lymphoma, but did show follicular lymphoma in situ (see **Fig. 13**). When lymphoma in the two sites was analyzed by PCR, clonal peaks were found at the same location, consistent with a common clonal origin for the follicular lymphoma in situ and the diffuse large B-cell lymphoma. The latter may thus represent large cell transformation of the former in this particular case.

REFERENCES

1. Harris N, Nathwani B, Swerdlow SH, et al. Follicular lymphoma. In: Swerdlow S, Campo E, Harris N, et al, editors. WHO classification tumours of haematopoietic and lymphoid tissues. 4th edition. Lyon (France): IARC; 2008. p. 220–6.
2. Ott G, Katzenberger T, Lohr A, et al. Cytomorphologic, immunohistochemical, and cytogenetic profiles of follicular lymphoma: 2 types of follicular lymphoma grade 3. Blood 2002;99:3806–12.
3. Nguyen PL, Zukerberg LR, Benedict WF, et al. Immunohistochemical detection of p53, bcl-2, and retinoblastoma proteins in follicular lymphoma. Am J Clin Pathol 1996;105:538–43.
4. Schraders M, de Jong D, Kluin P, et al. Lack of Bcl-2 expression in follicular lymphoma may be caused by mutations in the BCL2 gene or by absence of the t (14;18) translocation. J Pathol 2005;205:329–35.
5. Horsman DE, Okamoto I, Ludkovski O, et al. Follicular lymphoma lacking the t(14;18)(q32;q21): identification of two disease subtypes. Br J Haematol 2003;120:424–33.
6. Goodlad JR, Batstone PJ, Hamilton DA, et al. BCL2 gene abnormalities define distinct clinical subsets of follicular lymphoma. Histopathology 2006;49: 229–41.
7. Karube K, Guo Y, Suzumiya J, et al. CD10-MUM1+ follicular lymphoma lacks BCL2 gene translocation and shows characteristic biologic and clinical features. Blood 2007;109:3076–9.

Pitfalls
FOLLICULAR LYMPHOMA

! Bcl2 protein expression is not specific for follicular lymphoma. It is normally found in primary follicles, normal follicle mantles, other types of low-grade B-cell lymphomas, and T cells. Only when bcl2 is coexpressed by follicle center cells does it support a diagnosis of follicular lymphoma.

! Some follicular lymphomas are negative for bcl2, in particular some grade 3 follicular lymphomas, pediatric follicular lymphoma, and some extranodal follicular lymphomas, leading to difficulty recognizing their follicles as neoplastic.

! Follicular lymphoma in situ is difficult to recognize on routine sections; an immunostain for bcl2 is required to make the diagnosis.

! The floral variant of follicular lymphoma has unusually shaped follicles that may mimic reactive follicles.

! Follicular lymphoma with many signet ring cells may be mistaken for a nonlymphoid proliferation, particularly on a small biopsy.

8. Kim H, Jacobs C, Warnke R, et al. Malignant lymphoma with a high content of epithelioid histiocytes: a distinct clinicopathologic entity and a form of so-called "Lennert's lymphoma". Cancer 1978;41:620–35.

9. Allevato P, Kini S, Rebuck J, et al. Signet ring cell lymphoma of the thyroid: a case report. Hum Pathol 1985;16:1066–8.

10. Torlakovic EE, Aamot HV, Heim S. A marginal zone phenotype in follicular lymphoma with t(14;18) is associated with secondary cytogenetic aberrations typical of marginal zone lymphoma. J Pathol 2006; 209:258–64.

11. Keith TA, Cousar JB, Glick AD, et al. Plasmacytic differentiation in follicular center cell (FCC) lymphomas. Am J Clin Pathol 1985;84:283–90.

12. Gradowski JF, Jaffe ES, Warnke RA, et al. Follicular lymphomas with plasmacytic differentiation include two subtypes. Mod Pathol 2010;23:71–9.

13. Tiesinga JJ, Wu CD, Inghirami G. CD5+ follicle center lymphoma. Immunophenotyping detects a unique subset of "floral" follicular lymphoma. Am J Clin Pathol 2000;114:912–21.

14. Kojima M, Yamanaka S, Yoshida T, et al. Histological variety of floral variant of follicular lymphoma. APMIS 2006;114:626–32.

15. Goates JJ, Kamel OW, LeBrun DP, et al. Floral variant of follicular lymphoma. Immunological and molecular studies support a neoplastic process. Am J Surg Pathol 1994;18:37–47.

16. Snuderl M, Kolman OK, Chen YB, et al. B-cell lymphomas with concurrent IGH-BCL2 and MYC rearrangements are aggressive neoplasms with clinical and pathologic features distinct from Burkitt lymphoma and diffuse large B-cell lymphoma. Am J Surg Pathol 2010;34:327–40.

17. Wang S, Wang L, Hochberg E, et al. Low histologic grade follicular lymphoma with high proliferation index: morphologic and clinical features. Am J Surg Pathol 2005;29:1490–6.

18. Adam P, Katzenberger T, Eifert M, et al. Presence of preserved reactive germinal centers in follicular lymphoma is a strong histopathologic indicator of limited disease stage. Am J Surg Pathol 2005;29: 1661–4.

19. Pinto A, Hutchison R, Grant L, et al. Follicular lymphomas in pediatric patients. Mod Pathol 1990; 3:308–13.

20. Lorsbach R, Shay-Seymore D, Moore J, et al. Clinicopathologic analysis of follicular lymphoma occurring in children. Blood 2002;99:1959–64.

21. Kussick SJ, Kalnoski M, Braziel RM, et al. Prominent clonal B-cell populations identified by flow cytometry in histologically reactive lymphoid proliferations. Am J Clin Pathol 2004;121:464–72.

22. Swerdlow S. Pediatric follicular lymphomas, marginal zone lymphomas and marginal zone hyperplasia. Am J Clin Pathol 2004;122(Suppl 1):S98–109.

23. Willemze R, Swerdlow SH, Harris N, et al. Primary cutaneous follicle centre lymphoma. In: Swerdlow S, Campo E, Harris N, et al, editors. WHO classification tumours of haematopoietic and lymphoid tissues. 4th edition. Lyon (France): IARC; 2008. p. 227–8.

24. Yoshino T, Miyake K, Ichimura K, et al. Increased incidence of follicular lymphoma in the duodenum. Am J Surg Pathol 2000;24:688–93.

25. Goodlad JR, MacPherson S, Jackson R, et al. Extranodal follicular lymphoma: a clinicopathological and genetic analysis of 15 cases arising at non-cutaneous extranodal sites. Histopathology 2004;44:268–76.

26. Bacon C, Ye H, Diss T, et al. Primary follicular lymphoma of the testis and epididymis in adults. Am J Surg Pathol 2007;31:1050–8.

27. Ferry J, Fung C, Zukerberg L, et al. Lymphoma of the ocular adnexa: a study of 353 cases. Am J Surg Pathol 2007;31:170–84.

28. Kojima M, Nakamura S, Ichimura K, et al. Follicular lymphoma of the salivary gland: a clinicopathological and molecular study of six cases. Int J Surg Pathol 2001;9:287–93.

29. Bacon CM, Diss TC, Ye H, et al. Follicular lymphoma of the thyroid gland. Am J Surg Pathol 2009;33:22–34.

30. Willingham DL, Menke DM, Satyanarayana R. Gallbladder lymphoma in primary sclerosing cholangitis. Clin Gastroenterol Hepatol 2009;7:A26.

31. Ono A, Tanoue S, Yamada Y, et al. Primary malignant lymphoma of the gallbladder: a case report and literature review. Br J Radiol 2009;82:e15–9.

32. Christophides T, Samstein B, Emond J, et al. Primary follicular lymphoma of the extrahepatic bile duct mimicking a hilar cholangiocarcinoma: case report and review of the literature. Hum Pathol 2009;40:1808–12.

33. Sugawara G, Nagino M, Oda K, et al. Follicular lymphoma of the extrahepatic bile duct mimicking cholangiocarcinoma. J Hepatobiliary Pancreat Surg 2008;15:196–9.

34. Misdraji J, del Castillo C, Ferry J. Follicle center lymphoma of the ampulla of Vater presenting with jaundice. Am J Surg Pathol 1997;21:484–8.

35. Misdraji J, Harris N, Ferry J. Follicular lymphoma of the gastrointestinal tract. Ann Oncol 2007;18(s):109A.

36. Damaj G, Verkarre V, Delmer A, et al. Primary follicular lymphoma of the gastrointestinal tract: a study of 25 cases and a literature review. Ann Oncol 2003;14:623–9.

37. Shia J, Teruya-Feldstein J, Pan D, et al. Primary follicular lymphoma of the gastrointestinal tract. Am J Surg Pathol 2002;26:216–24.

38. Sato Y, Ichimura K, Tanaka T, et al. Duodenal follicular lymphomas share common characteristics with mucosa-associated lymphoid tissue lymphomas. J Clin Pathol 2008;61:377–81.

39. Poggi MM, Cong PJ, Coleman CN, et al. Low-grade follicular lymphoma of the small intestine. J Clin Gastroenterol 2002;34:155–9.

40. Kodama T, Ohshima K, Nomura K, et al. Lymphomatous polyposis of the gastrointestinal tract, including mantle cell lymphoma, follicular lymphoma and mucosa-associated lymphoid tissue lymphoma. Histopathology 2005;47:467–78.

41. Rosty C, Briere J, Cellier C, et al. Association of a duodenal follicular lymphoma and hereditary nonpolyposis colorectal cancer. Mod Pathol 2000;13:586–90.

42. Takata K, Sato Y, Nakamura N, et al. Duodenal and nodal follicular lymphomas are distinct: the former lacks activation-induced cytidine deaminase and follicular dendritic cells despite ongoing somatic hypermutations. Mod Pathol 2009;22:940–9.

43. Bende R, Smit L, Bossenbroek J, et al. Primary follicular lymphoma of the small intestine: alpha4beta7 expression and immunoglobulin configuration suggest an origin from local antigen-experienced B cells. Am J Pathol 2003;162:105–13.

44. Huang WT, Hsu YH, Yang SF, et al. Primary gastrointestinal follicular lymphoma: a clinicopathologic study of 13 cases from Taiwan. J Clin Gastroenterol 2008;42:997–1002.

45. Aguilera NS, Tomaszewski MM, Moad JC, et al. Cutaneous follicle center lymphoma: a clinicopathologic study of 19 cases. Mod Pathol 2001;14:828–35.

46. de Leval L, Harris NL, Longtine J, et al. Cutaneous B-cell lymphomas of follicular and marginal zone types: use of Bcl-6, CD10, Bcl-2, and CD21 in differential diagnosis and classification. Am J Surg Pathol 2001;25:732–41.

47. Kim BK, Surti U, Pandya A, et al. Clinicopathologic, immunophenotypic, and molecular cytogenetic fluorescence in situ hybridization analysis of primary and secondary cutaneous follicular lymphomas. Am J Surg Pathol 2005;29:69–82.

48. Darby S, Hancock BW. Localised non-Hodgkin lymphoma of the testis: the Sheffield lymphoma group experience. Int J Oncol 2005;26:1093–9.

49. Ferry JA, Harris NL, Young RH, et al. Malignant lymphoma of the testis, epididymis, and spermatic cord. A clinicopathologic study of 69 cases with immunophenotypic analysis. Am J Surg Pathol 1994;18:376–90.

50. Heller KN, Teruya-Feldstein J, La Quaglia MP, et al. Primary follicular lymphoma of the testis: excellent outcome following surgical resection without adjuvant chemotherapy. J Pediatr Hematol Oncol 2004;26:104–7.

51. Finn L, Viswanatha D, Belasco J, et al. Primary follicular lymphoma of the testis in childhood. Cancer 1999;85:1626–35.

52. Pakzad K, MacLennan GT, Elder JS, et al. Follicular large cell lymphoma localized to the testis in children. J Urol 2002;168:225–8.

53. Moertel CL, Watterson J, McCormick SR, et al. Follicular large cell lymphoma of the testis in a child. Cancer 1995;75:1182–6.

54. Lu D, Medeiros L, Eskenazi A, et al. Primary follicular large cell lymphoma of the testis in a child. Arch Pathol Lab Med 2001;125:551–4.

55. Pileri S, Sabattini E, Rosito P, et al. Primary follicular lymphoma of the testis in childhood: an entity with peculiar clinical and molecular characteristics. J Clin Pathol 2002;55:684–8.

56. Cong P, Raffeld M, Teruya-Feldstein J, et al. In situ localization of follicular lymphoma: description and analysis by laser capture microdissection. Blood 2002;99:3376–82.

57. Roullet MR, Martinez D, Ma L, et al. Coexisting follicular and mantle cell lymphoma with each having an in situ component: a novel, curious, and complex consultation case of coincidental, composite, colonizing lymphoma. Am J Clin Pathol 2010;133:584–91.

CHRONIC LYMPHOCYTIC LEUKEMIA, SMALL LYMPHOCYTIC LYMPHOMA, AND MONOCLONAL B-CELL LYMPHOCYTOSIS

Robert Paul Hasserjian, MD

[handwritten margin note: peut se transformer → diffuse large B cell lymph[oma] ou → classique Hodg. l.]

KEYWORDS

- Chronic lymphocytic leukemia • Small lymphocytic lymphoma • Lymphocytosis
- Lymphoproliferative

ABSTRACT

Chronic lymphocytic leukemia (CLL), small lymphocytic lymphoma (SLL), and monoclonal B-cell lymphocytosis (MBL) are clonal proliferations of small, mature B cells. CLL and SLL are considered neoplastic, although they are indolent and many patients with these lymphomas never require treatment. Most MBL cases share immunophenotypic and genetic features with CLL and SLL but have a small burden of clonal cells. This review focuses on the pathologic features of CLL, SLL, and MBL and their differential diagnoses. Guidelines are provided to separate the entities from one another and to avoid pitfalls in distinguishing these entities from other lymphomas and from reactive lymphoid proliferations.

OVERVIEW

Chronic lymphocytic leukemia (CLL)/small lymphocytic lymphoma (SLL) represents a relatively common indolent B-cell lymphoma that may present as a leukemia (CLL) or as lymphadenopathy without significant lymphocytosis (SLL). CLL and SLL are otherwise biologically similar and thus distinguished entirely by their clinical presentation. Although these are indolent diseases with median survivals in excess of 10 years, transformation to high-grade lymphoma (typically diffuse large B-cell lymphoma or, less commonly, classical Hodgkin lymphoma) may occur as an adverse event. The 2008 World Health Organization (WHO) Classification of Tumours of Haematopoietic and Lymphoid Tissues recently revised the diagnostic criteria of CLL to require a minimal neoplastic peripheral blood lymphocyte count of 5×10^9/L, thus creating a new disease of a clonal CLL-like lymphoid proliferation, termed monoclonal B-cell lymphocytosis (MBL). Although MBL seems to represent a precursor lesion of CLL, the majority of patients with MBL never develop CLL, SLL, or any hematologic malignancy.[1,2] MBL is not considered equivalent to a diagnosis of lymphoma, but patients should be followed clinically for development of sufficient peripheral lymphocyte numbers and/or lymphadenopathy that is diagnostic of CLL/SLL. The relationship of MBL to CLL/SLL is, therefore, analogous to the relationship of monoclonal gammopathy of undetermined significance (MGUS) to plasma cell myeloma.

CHRONIC LYMPHOCYTIC LEUKEMIA

CLINICAL FEATURES

CLL has a median age of diagnosis of approximately 70 years and a male predominance. Patients are often asymptomatic and are diagnosed when lymphocytosis is found on routine blood testing. Symptomatic patients usually

Department of Pathology, Massachusetts General Hospital and Harvard Medical School, 55 Fruit Street, Boston, MA 02114, USA
E-mail address: rhasserjian@partners.org

Surgical Pathology 3 (2010) 907–931
doi:10.1016/j.path.2010.09.009

Key Features
OF CHRONIC LYMPHOCYTIC LEUKEMIA

1. Indolent lymphoid neoplasm of small, mature lymphocytes that presents with involvement of blood and bone marrow and often with enlargement of lymph nodes and spleen.

2. Diagnosis requires the presence of at least 5 × 10⁹/L clonal B cells with the characteristic immunophenotype in the peripheral blood or the presence of symptoms related to bone marrow infiltration.

3. Characteristic immunophenotype is CD20 dim+, monotypic surface immunoglobuin dim+, CD5+, CD23+, CD10−, and cyclin D1−.

4. Most cases have cytogenetic abnormalities detectable by fluorescence in situ hybridization (FISH), with the common abnormalities being 13q deletion, trisomy 12, 11q deletion, and 17p deletion; these genetic abnormalities have prognostic significance.

present with fatigue, symptoms related to splenomegaly, and/or lymphadenopathy.[3] Autoimmune thrombocytopenia, hemolytic anemia, or both (Evans syndrome) may be present at diagnosis or develop later in the course of disease. By definition, there is absolute lymphocytosis and by flow cytometry, the absolute level of clonal CLL cells must be at least 5 × 10⁹/L in the peripheral blood. The range of lymphocyte counts at diagnosis is highly variable and may exceed 100 × 10⁹/L in some patients. A diagnosis of CLL may be made with <5 × 10⁹/L peripheral blood CLL-phenotype B cells provided the patient has cytopenias or other symptoms attributable to the neoplastic B-cell proliferation[4]; in such cases, a bone marrow examination should be performed and other B-cell lymphomas should be excluded.

DIAGNOSIS: MICROSCOPIC FEATURES

The diagnosis of CLL can usually be established on the basis of a clonal B-cell population in the peripheral blood (absolute count greater than 5 × 10⁹/L) with characteristic morphology and flow cytometry immunophenotype; thus, a bone marrow sample is not required for a primary diagnosis of CLL. However, it is recommended that a bone marrow biopsy be performed before initiating therapy to establish the baseline level of disease and evaluate the success of subsequent therapeutic interventions. Bone marrow examination

may also be performed in CLL patients with thrombocytopenia to distinguish between extensive bone marrow infiltration and a paraneoplastic immune thrombocytopenic purpura. (http://www.nccn.org/professionals/physician_gls/PDF/nhl.pdf [accessed April 12, 2010]).

On peripheral blood smears, CLL cells resemble small lymphocytes, with regularly condensed chromatin; absent or small nucleoli; and scant, pale cytoplasm (**Fig.** 1A, B). Although the regular "soccer ball−like" pattern of chromatin condensation in CLL cells is subtly different from the more irregularly condensed chromatin of normal circulating lymphocytes, this may be difficult to appreciate on most smear preparations. Smudge cells (ruptured cell nuclei devoid of cytoplasm, see **Fig.** 1A) are frequently seen in peripheral blood smears from CLL patients and may comprise most of the white cells in the smear; preparation of the smear by hand rather than by an automated method or the addition to albumin to the blood abrogate the tendency of the CLL cells to smudge, enabling a more accurate peripheral blood white cell differential count. Smudge cells are by no means specific to CLL and can frequently be seen with other circulating lymphoma cells, blasts, or even reactive atypical lymphocytes. Prolymphocytes represent the proliferating compartment in CLL and are usually present at low levels in the peripheral blood (see **Fig.** 1C). Prolymphocytes are at least twice the diameter of small lymphocytes and have a round nucleus, somewhat dispersed nuclear chromatin (less condensed than that of small lymphocytes but also less finely dispersed than that of blasts), and a prominent central nucleolus; the cytoplasm is moderately abundant and is usually lightly basophilic. Prolymphocytes are rare in the blood of most CLL cases but but and should be enumerated: if prolymphocytes comprise greater than 55% of the circulating lymphocytes at presentation, a diagnosis of prolymphocytic leukemia is made. Cells intermediate between small lymphocytes and prolymphocytes, with variably prominent nucleoli and somewhat increased size may be frequent in CLL cases and such cells not be counted among the prolymphocytes (see **Fig.** 1D). Although the CLL lymphocytes usually exhibit round nuclear contours, a subset of cases may show cells with irregular or even clefted nuclei and/or distinct nucleoli. These cases are termed "atypical CLL" lightly and may have a more aggressive course.[5] Other cases may have unusually abundant pale cytoplasm or show plasmacytic differentiation. In spite of the wide cytomorphologic spectrum manifested by CLL, atypical morphologic features do not seem to have independent prognostic impact and the

Fig. 1. CLL in the peripheral blood. (*A*) There are many mature-appearing lymphocytes with scant cytoplasm, as well as expanded, pale smudge cells. (*B*) The lymphocytes of CLL are similar in size to normal lymphocytes and have scant pale cytoplasm; the nucleus contains many deeply stained areas of condensed chromatin.

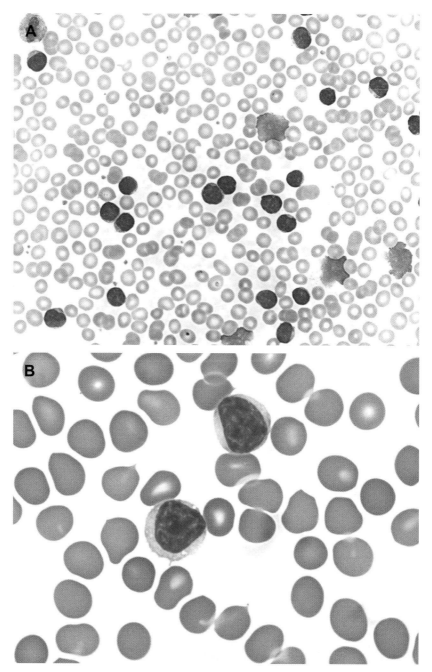

2008 WHO classification does not recognize any morphologic subtypes of CLL. The previous category of CLL/PL (CLL with 10% to 55% prolymphocytes) has been eliminated in the current classification.[4]

The lymphocytes in the bone marrow aspirate from CLL patients resemble those in the peripheral blood smear (**Fig. 2**A). Estimation of disease burden is usually based on the bone marrow biopsy and expressed as the percentage of CLL cells occupying the total intertrabecular marrow space. In the bone marrow biopsy, CLL may manifest any infiltration pattern (nodular nonparatrabecular, interstitial, diffuse, or occasionally intrasinusoidal) except for paratrabecular.[6] The most common patterns are nodular and interstitial.

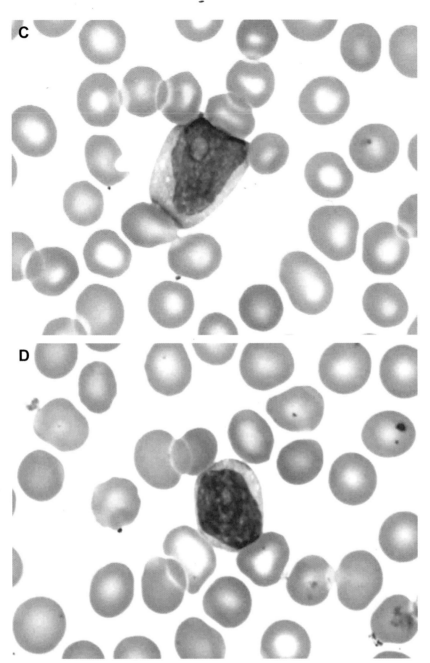

Fig. 1. CLL in the peripheral blood. (*C*) Prolymphocytes, which are rare in the blood of most cases of CLL, are much larger than small lymphocytes, with more abundant cytoplasm, more dispersed chromatin, and a prominent central nucleolus. (*D*) Slightly enlarged small lymphocytes with distinct nucleoli should not be included among prolymphocytes.

Nonparatrabecular nodules are spherical, confluent aggregates of lymphocytes (see **Fig. 2**B). Although these may occur adjacent to bone trabeculae and may even be closely opposed to the bone surface, unlike true paratrabecular aggregates that characterize follicular lymphoma, they have a spherical rather than a linear configuration and do not extend along the trabecular surface. Nodular nonparatrabecular aggregates are not specific to CLL, because they can occur in nearly all lymphoma subtypes as well as in reactive bone marrow lymphoid infiltrates. The bone marrow nodules in CLL consist of monotonous small lymphocytes with occasional admixed

Fig. 2. CLL involving the bone marrow. (*A*) Bone marrow aspirate extensively involved by CLL, with only rare erythroid and myeloid elements. (*B*) Bone marrow biopsy containing a nonparatrabecular nodule, with a round shape that pushes away adjacent adipocytes.

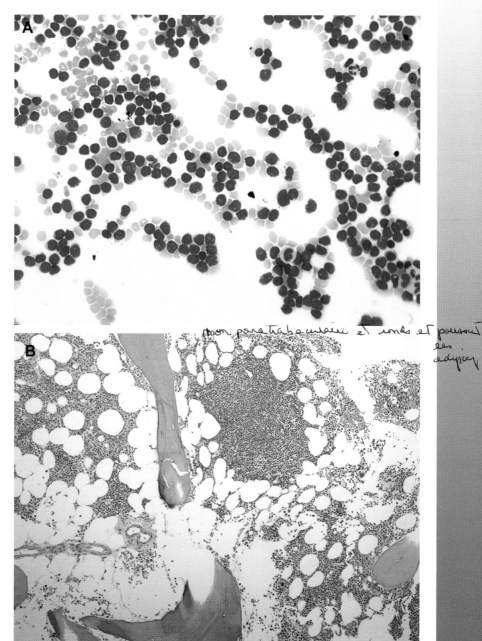

larger, nucleolated cells. Unlike bone marrow nodules in other types of lymphoma, reticulin staining is usually not significantly increased in CLL nodules.[7] Interstitial lymphoid infiltrates, in which the lymphocytes occur as single cells or small cell clusters not forming visible aggregates, are also common in CLL (see **Fig. 2**C). This pattern may difficult to appreciate on routine histology, because normal bone marrow resident lymphocytes occupy the marrow in an interstitial pattern and typically comprise 10% to 20% of the marrow cells. In contrast to the B-cell lineage of the interstitial CLL infiltrates, however, normal marrow lymphocytes are predominantly T cells (typically with a 2:1 to 3:1 ratio of T cells to B cells).[8,9] In diffuse bone marrow infiltrates, the lymphocytes form confluent

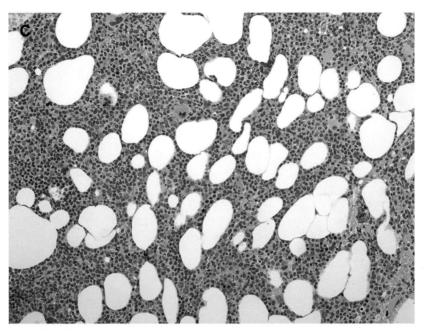

Fig. 2. CLL involving the bone marrow. (*C*) Interstitial pattern of CLL, in which the neoplastic small, irregular lymphocytes percolate among the hematopoietic elements but do not form discrete nodules and do not disturb the randomly distributed adipocytes; this pattern can be difficult to appreciate on routine histology. (*D*) Diffuse marrow involvement by CLL, in which the neoplastic lymphocytes form sheets that obliterate both adipocytes and areas of hematopoiesis.

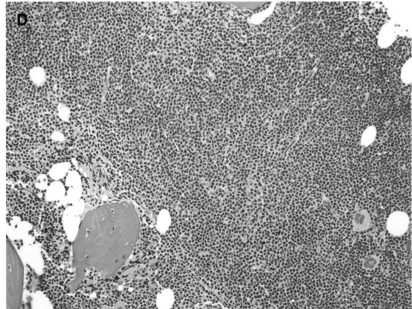

sheets of cells that displace the fat and hematopoietic cells and completely occupy at least one intertrabecular marrow space (see **Fig. 2**D). Intervening hematopoietic cells may be present, but they make up the minority of the cells; adipocytes are rare or absent in the involved areas. A diffuse pattern of involvement is present in approximately 20% of biopsied CLL patients and has been associated with adverse prognosis,[6,10] but this does not seem to be independent of other risk factors, such as genetic features (discussed later).[11] Proliferation centers, commonly seen in extramedullary tissues involved by CLL or SLL, may also be seen in the diffuse pattern of marrow involvement and rarely within nodular marrow aggregates of CLL.[12]

DIAGNOSIS: ANCILLARY STUDIES

Immunophenotypic analysis of blood and/or bone marrow is a cornerstone of CLL diagnosis. CLL has a characteristic immunophenotype, typically with expression of CD19; dim expression of CD20 and CD22; monotypic surface immunoglobulin light chain; and coexpression of CD5 (usually at a somewhat dimmer level than that of T cells), CD43, and CD23 (**Fig. 3**). Rare CLL cases (0.5% to 3%) may coexpress the T-cell marker CD8.[13] FMC7, which recognizes an epitope of CD20 and is associated with bright expression of this protein, is usually dim or negative in CLL, as is CD79b.[14,15] CD20 and surface immunoglobulin expression may be so low that they are undetectable by flow cytometry; investigation of permeabilized cells by flow cytometry usually discloses monotypic expression of cytoplasmic immunoglobulin in such cases. The hairy cell markers CD103 and CD25 are negative, although CD11c may be expressed in a subset of cases. Because it is a common disease, it is not surprising that there is some immunophenotypic variability: atypical immunophenotypes include lack of CD5, lack of CD23, and strong CD20 and/or surface immunoglobulin expression. Scoring systems have been developed to reconcile such deviations from the classic CLL phenotype.[15] In ambiguous cases, assessment for characteristic CLL aberrations by FISH (discussed later) may prove useful. Immunohistochemistry is usually not required if full flow cytometric immunophenotyping has been performed. However, it is prudent to perform cyclin-D1 immunostaining if mantle cell lymphoma has not been excluded by cytogenetics and/or FISH for a t(11;14) translocation; some cases of mantle cell lymphoma may express CD23 or demonstrate other immunophenotypic features mimicking CLL.[16]

DIFFERENTIAL DIAGNOSIS

The differential diagnosis of CLL includes other small B-cell lymphomas as well as some nonmalignant conditions. Among the lymphomas, mantle cell lymphoma can bear a close morphologic resemblance to CLL and can present as a leukemia. Immunophenotypic analysis is critical in showing the bright expression of CD20 and surface immunoglobulin and the lack of CD23 characteristic of mantle cell lymphoma. The gold standard of mantle cell diagnosis is demonstration of cyclin-D1 expression by immunohistochemistry and/or a t(11;14) by cytogenetics, FISH, or polymerase chain reaction (PCR) on a bone marrow or blood sample. Some cyclin-D1 expression may be detected within the proliferation centers of CLL, but this is not strong and

△△ Differential Diagnosis of CLL

CLL Versus	Helpful Distinguishing Features
Prolymphocytic leukemia	• Circulating lymphocytes are large with prominent nucleoli • CD20 and surface immunoglobulin are usually bright • CD5 and/or CD23 are often negative
Mantle cell lymphoma	• Circulating lymphocytes more irregular than CLL cells and/or have prominent nucleoli • CD23−, bright CD20 and surface immunoglobulin • Cyclin D1+ and CCND1 rearrangement
Follicular lymphoma	• Circulating lymphocytes usually clefted • CD5− and usually CD10+ • BCL2 rearrangement • Bone marrow aggregates are paratrabecular
Splenic marginal zone lymphoma	• Circulating lymphocytes have more abundant cytoplasm with surface projections • Usually CD5−with bright surface immunoglobulin and CD20 expression
Lymphoplasmacytic lymphoma	• Most cases lack lymphocytosis • CD5− with bright surface immunoglobulin and CD20 expression • Spectrum of small lymphocytes and plasmacytoid forms in bone marrow

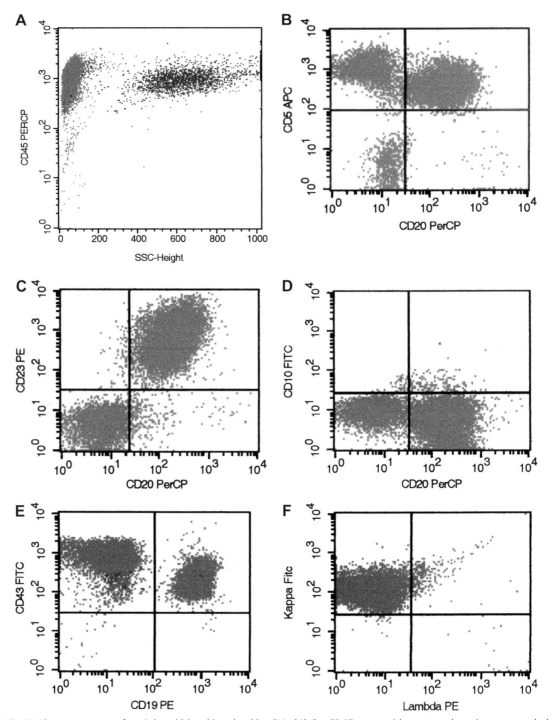

Fig. 3. Flow cytometry of peripheral blood involved by CLL. (*A*) On CD45 versus side scatter, there is an expanded population of lymphocytes (*red*). The B cells express dim CD20 with co-expression of CD5 (*B*) and CD23 (*C*) but are negative for CD10 (*D*). The CD19+ B cells also coexpress CD43 (*E*). Gating on the CD19+ B cells shows that they express monotypic surface immunoglobulin κ light chain (*F*).

uniform like the cyclin-D1 expression in mantle cell lymphoma.[17] Marginal zone lymphomas rarely demonstrate CD5 expression mimicking CLL,[18] and conversely some CLL cases have abundant cytoplasm mimicking the villous lymphocytes of splenic marginal zone lymphoma; splenomegaly is also common in CLL. The lymphocyte count in CLL is usually higher than in splenic marginal zone lymphoma and on well-prepared smears, the characteristic regularly condensed chromatin of CLL is a clue to the diagnosis. In difficult cases, FISH analysis can be helpful, because splenic marginal zone lymphomas do not exhibit the common cytogenetic abnormalities of CLL and may show other distinct abnormalities, such as a del(7q). Cases of CLL with abundant cytoplasm on smear preparations may raise the differential of hairy cell leukemia. However, CLL cells in bone marrow sections do not show the abundant pale cytoplasm that characterize almost all hairy cell leukemia cases and also lack expression of CD103 and CD25. Although CD5 may be expressed in some cases of lymphoplasmacytic lymphoma, it is usually dimmer and less uniform than in CLL. Lymphoplasmacytic lymphoma also shows brighter CD20 and surface immunoglobulin expression than CLL.[19] A small subset of extranodal marginal zone lymphomas express CD5 and these CD5+ cases may have a higher propensity for bone marrow involvement.[20] CLL cases with increased prolymphocytes may raise the differential diagnosis of B-cell prolymphocytic leukemia (B-PLL). The prol0ymphocytes in CLL more often show CD5 expression than B-PLL, although CD23 may be lost in CLL cases with increased prolymphocytes. When many circulating prolymphocytes are present, eliciting a prior history of CLL is critical in excluding a diagnosis of de novo B-PLL.

The main nonmalignant disorder that may be confused with CLL is monoclonal B-lymphocytosis (MBL); this differential is discussed later. If confirmatory peripheral blood or bone marrow flow cytometry is not available, the nonparatrabecular aggregates in CLL may overlap with reactive lymphoid aggregates. Reactive lymphoid aggregates are more common in elderly patients and can also be seen in bone marrow from patients with autoimmune diseases, infections (including HIV), aplastic anemia, and some myeloid neoplasms.[7,21] Features that favor neoplastic aggregates include the presence of many aggregates, large size, and poor circumscription with infiltration of lymphocytes into the adjacent interstitium.[7,22] Location of aggregates within subcortical fatty marrow (nonhematopoietic marrow immediately underlying the superficial iliac cortex) also favors a neoplastic cause.[7] Reactive lymphoid aggregates have a mixture of T cells and B cells. Although small T cells may be admixed with the neoplastic B cells in CLL aggregates, close inspection of the CD5 stain relative to the stains for B-cell and other T-cell markers, such as CD3, can be helpful at disclosing the malignant B-cell population in CLL: the latter usually shows dimmer staining for CD5 than the admixed normal T cells.[23,24]

PROGNOSIS

CLL is an indolent disease, with patients often dying of unrelated causes and median survivals of 10 to 15 years. Rare cases have even been reported to regress spontaneously.[25] Approximately one-third of patients have stable disease and do not require treatment, whereas approximately two-thirds of patients require treatment either at diagnosis or after disease progression.[26] The traditional Rai[27] and Binet[3] clinical staging systems have been used for decades to risk-stratify CLL patients. These clinical staging systems are based on the presence or absence of lymphadenopathy (as well as the number of sites affected), organomegaly, and cytopenias; the Rai and Binet stages correlate with patient survival. One recent study found that a low percentage ($\leq$20%) of smudge cells on the peripheral smears of CLL patients represented an adverse prognostic marker.[28]

Cytogenetic and molecular genetic factors are important prognostic factors at diagnosis. Routine cytogenetic analysis of CLL is often uninformative due to poor growth of CLL cells in culture. Interphase FISH study on the neoplastic lymphocytes from the blood, bone marrow, or involved extramedullary tissues can be used to identify several recurring abnormalities associated with CLL that have important prognostic implications and 80% of CLL cases exhibit at least one such abnormality.[29] The most common abnormality is del(13q), associated with a favorable prognosis provided it is the only detected abnormality, whereas the less frequent abnormalities del(11q), del(17p), and del(6q) are associated with an inferior prognosis and trisomy 12 is associated with an intermediate prognosis.[29] In particular, del(17q) that results in loss of the TP53 tumor suppressor gene predicts a relatively aggressive clinical course. Rare cases of CLL (<1%) harbor a t(2;14) translocation involving a BCL11A gene; such cases often have atypical, plasmacytoid morphology, but their prognosis is uncertain.[30] Adverse cytogenetic markers not present at diagnosis may develop in patients as the disease progresses.[31] An important molecular genetic prognostic marker is the mutational status of the IGH gene variable region: cases showing

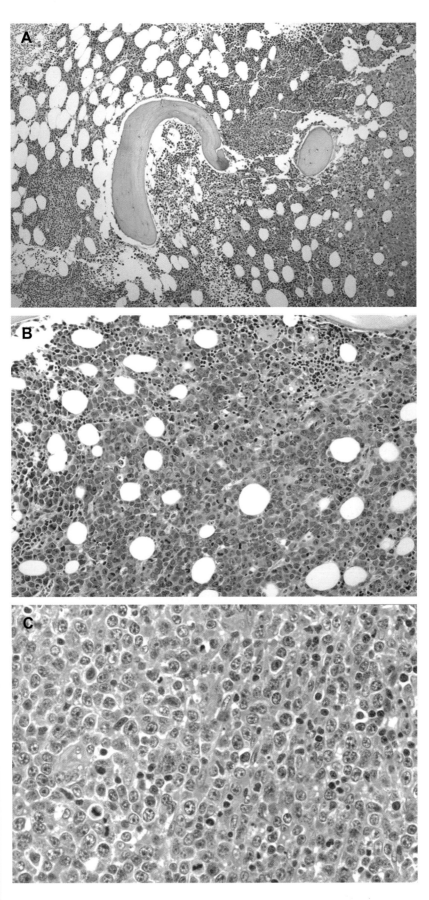

Fig. 4. Richter's syndrome. (*A*) This bone marrow biopsy contains nodular aggregates of small lymphocytes representing involvement by CLL; in the right part of the image is a sheet of large cells. (*B*) On high power, the large cells have vesicular nuclei, prominent nucleoli, and abundant cytoplasm, features of diffuse large B-cell lymphoma. (*C*) Richter's syndrome presenting as a rapidly increasing breast mass, with sheets of large cells vastly outnumbering the residual small lymphocytes. (*Image courtesy of* Dr Judith Ferry, Massachusetts General Hospital, Boston, MA.)

high levels of somatic hypermutation (<98% homology with the germline variable region, implying origin from a lymphocyte that is germinal center or postgerminal center) comprise approximately half of CLL and exhibit a significantly better prognosis than cases that lack somatic hypermutation (implying origin from a naïve, pregerminal center lymphocyte).[32] Usage of the *IGH* variable V (H)3-21 family is also a marker of a poorer prognosis irrespective of the mutational status.[33] Assessment of mutational status is a specialized test that requires sequencing and is not available in most laboratories. Immunophenotypic surrogates that correlate with unmutated (poor prognosis) CLL are expression of ZAP-70 on greater than 20% of the tumor cells by flow cytometry[34,35] or immunohistochemistry[36] and CD38 expression on greater than 30% of the tumor cells by flow cytometry.[37] Although these markers do not correlate perfectly with the mutational status, they do provide significant prognostic information. More recently, microRNA expression patterns have been shown to be associated with prognosis in CLL.[38]

Adverse events in CLL include development of a predominant population of prolymphocytes (>55% of all lymphocytes) in the blood and Richter's syndrome. Richter's syndrome represents progression of CLL to a diffuse large B-cell lymphoma, usually accompanied by abruptly worsening clinical symptoms and lymphadenopathy, and is associated with an aggressive clinical course and poor prognosis (**Fig. 4**).[39] Rare cases of CLL may transform to a picture resembling classical Hodgkin lymphoma, with Reed-Sternberg cells that are often positive for EBV. Because Reed-Sternberg—like cells can be seen in the proliferation centers of nontransformed CLL, a diagnosis of Hodgkin lymphoma requires the presence of the polymorphous background cell population typical of classical Hodgkin lymphoma. In Richter's or Hodgkin lymphoma transformations of CLL, the transformed neoplasm is frequently clonally unrelated to the background CLL.[40] The presence of enlarged lymph nodes (≥3 cm) and lack of the favorable genetic marker del(13q) in CLL are associated with an increased likelihood of developing Richter's syndrome.[41]

SMALL LYMPHOCYTIC LYMPHOMA

CLINICAL FEATURES

A diagnosis of SLL is made in patients who have peripheral lymphadenopathy or splenomegaly due to a neoplastic infiltrate of cells identical to those of CLL but with less than 5×10^9/L CLL cells in the peripheral blood. Patients with SLL usually

Key Features
OF SMALL LYMPHOCYTIC LYMPHOMA

1. Indolent lymphoid neoplasm of small, mature lymphocytes that is morphologically, immunophenotypically, and genetically similar to CLL and presents with enlargement of lymph nodes and/or spleen without significant lymphocytosis (<5 × 10⁹/L).

2. Morphology in lymph nodes is typically a diffuse proliferation of small lymphocytes with round nuclei and condensed chromatin and many pale proliferation centers.

3. Proliferation centers comprise the proliferating cells of small lymphocytic lymphoma, which are mostly medium-sized prolymphocytes as well as scattered large, nucleolated paraimmunoblasts.

present with generalized lymphadenopathy and more than 80% of patients are Ann Arbor stage III or IV. The median age at presentation is approximately 60 years and there is a male predominance, similar to CLL patients.[42,43] Almost all patients with SLL show low-level peripheral blood involvement by neoplastic cells with a CLL phenotype[44] and bone marrow involvement is identified in 70% of patients.[43]

DIAGNOSIS: MICROSCOPIC FEATURES

Lymph nodes involved by SLL most commonly show total architectural effacement by sheets of small lymphocytes with condensed chromatin and scant cytoplasm, similar to those seen in the bone marrow of CLL (**Fig. 5A—C**). When preserved germinal centers and/or sinuses are present, they are usually small, attenuated, and focal.[42] A characteristic feature is the presence of pseudofollicular proliferation centers, which are collections of enlarged CLL cells (medium-sized prolymphocytes and large paraimmunoblasts with vesicular nuclei) that appear pale on low power examination among the small, dark blue CLL lymphocytes (see **Fig. 5D, E**). The relative proportions of small lymphocytes, prolymphocytes, and paraimmunoblasts as well as the size and number of the proliferation centers are variable among SLL cases; however, cases with diffuse sheets of large cells should be diagnosed as diffuse large B-cell lymphoma. Lymph nodes involved by CLL (ie, accompanied by >5 × 10⁹/L monotypic CLL cells in the peripheral blood) are histologically

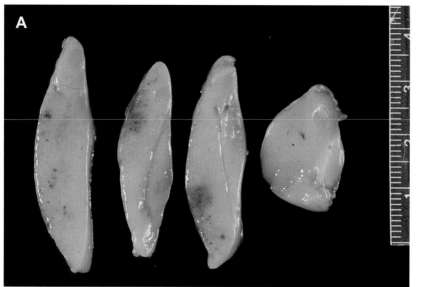

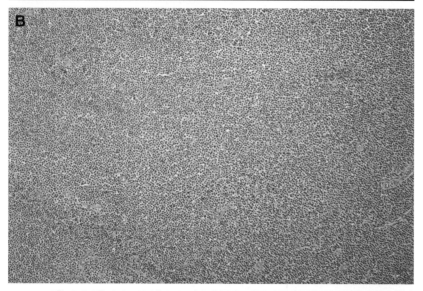

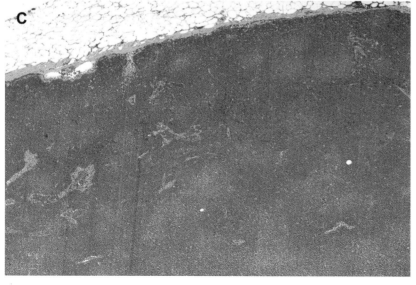

Fig. 5. Small lymphocytic lymphoma. (*A*) Gross image of lymph node involved by SLL, showing a diffuse "fish-flesh" appearance and marked nodal enlargement. (*B*) The normal nodal architecture is totally effaced by diffuse sheets of lymphocytes; proliferation centers are not evident in this case. (*C*) This case of SLL shows many pale proliferation centers, with a few patent sinuses (*left*).

Fig. 5. Small lymphocytic lymphoma (*D*) Proliferation centers are best appreciated at low power and appear as vague pale nodules within the dense mass of dark blue small lymphocytes. (*E*) On high power, proliferation centers comprise prolymphocytes that are slightly larger than the surrounding small lymphocytes (*left lower corner*) and occasional large paraimmunoblasts with vesicular nuclei and prominent nucleoli. (*F*) SLL and CLL involve the splenic white pulp, giving rise to innumerable small, irregular white nodules in this gross section of a splenectomy specimen.

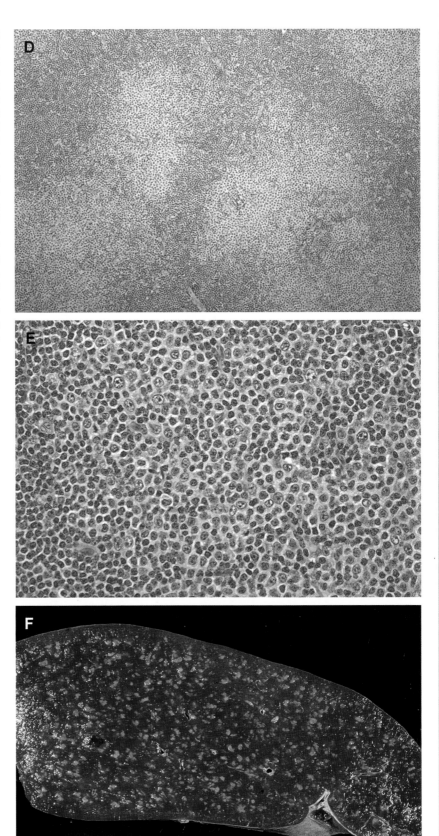

indistinguishable from those involved by SLL. In the spleen, SLL involves the white pulp as innumerable small nodules (see **Fig. 5F**). In more advanced splenic involvement, the red pulp may be diffusely involved, but the proliferation centers remain associated with areas of white pulp.[45]

DIAGNOSIS: ANCILLARY STUDIES

Although the pattern of a diffusely effaced lymph node with proliferation centers is highly suggestive of SLL, confirmatory immunohistochemical stains (and/or flow cytometry of fresh lymph node tissue) are recommended to confirm the diagnosis. The phenotype of SLL cells is identical to CLL and the classical immunoprofile (CD20+, CD5+, CD23+, CD43+, CD10−) can be readily demonstrated in paraffin sections (**Fig. 6**).[46] Most cases of CLL also express BCL2 but are BCL6 negative. Due to the characteristically dim CD20 expression, CD20 may appear weak or negative in paraffin section immunohistochemistry, requiring the use of other

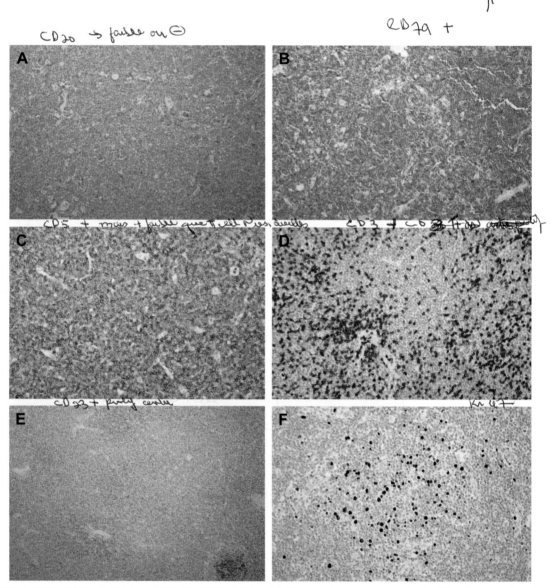

Fig. 6. Immunohistochemistry of SLL. (*A*) CD20 staining is often weak or even negative in SLL, whereas other B-cell markers, such as CD79a (*B*) or PAX5 (not shown), are more uniformly positive. (*C*) The CD5 expression level on SLL and CLL cells is weaker than that of the more darkly staining residual normal T cells, as revealed by comparison with the T-cell marker CD3 (*D*). The proliferation centers in SLL often stain more intensely for CD23 than the surrounding small lymphocytes (*E*) and also show accentuated staining for the proliferation marker Ki67 (*F, center*), which is low in the surrounding nonproliferating areas of SLL.

B-cell markers, such as CD19, CD79a, or PAX5 (see **Fig. 6**A, B). The expression of CD5 is SLL typically appears dimmer than that of the non-neoplastic T cells (see **Fig. 6**C, D), whereas CD23 expression is often limited to the proliferation centers (see **Fig. 6**E).[45] The Ki67 proliferation index in SLL is usually low (<10%), with a slightly higher index within the proliferation centers (see **Fig. 6**F).

DIFFERENTIAL DIAGNOSIS

Some SLL cases may display an interfollicular growth pattern, with preserved or even prominent germinal centers and intact sinuses (**Fig. 7**A, B).[46,47] These cases have a similar clinical behavior to SLL cases with total nodal effacement, but may be misdiagnosed as reactive hyperplasia.

Fig. 7. SLL with interfollicular involvement. (*A*) There are many residual germinal centers, with pale interfollicular and perifollicular proliferation centers in the intervening region. This pattern may be confused with reactive paracortical hyperplasia. (*B*) The monotonous interfollicular infiltrate in this case completely surrounds a residual germinal center, leading to possible confusion with a mantle or marginal zone lymphoma.

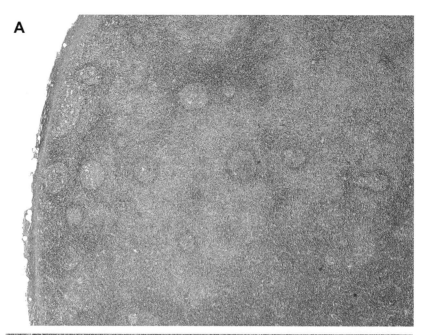

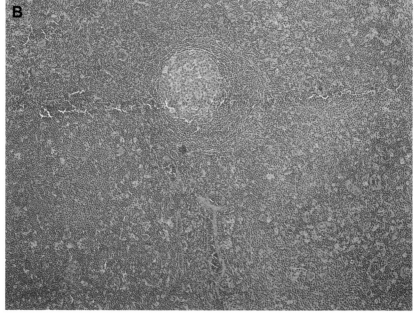

PAX5 +

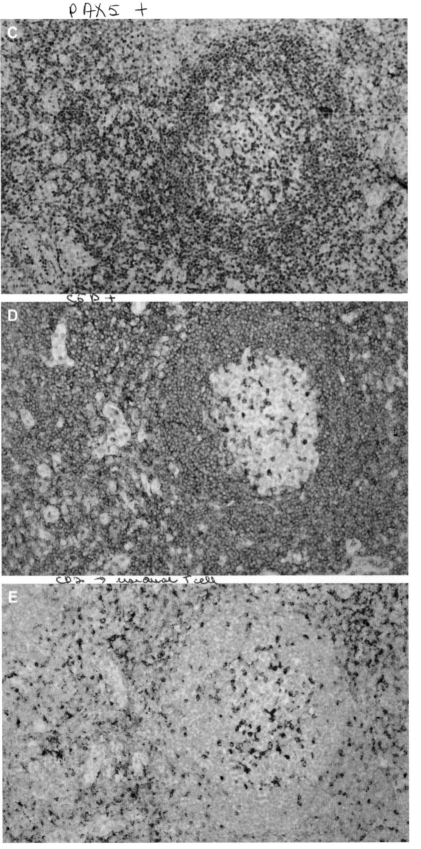

CD5 +

CD2 → residual T cell

aussi
CD23 ⊕
cyclin D1 ⊖

Fig. 7. SLL with inter-follicular involvement. Immunostains help confirm the diagnosis of SLL, because the neoplastic perifollicular and interfollicular cells are positive for PAX5 (*C*) and coexpress CD5 (*D*) compared with the scant residual T cells staining for CD2 (*E*). The neoplastic B cells in this case also expressed CD23 and were negative for cyclin D1 (not shown).

△△ Differential Diagnosis of SLL

SLL Versus	Helpful Distinguishing Features
Reactive paracortical hyperplasia	• Lack of discrete proliferation centers containing prolymphocytes and paraimmunoblasts • Small T cells rather than B cells predominate in the paracortex
Marginal zone lymphoma	• Pale areas surrounding germinal centers are composed of marginal zone cells rather than prolymphocytes and paraimmunoblasts • Neoplastic B cells are usually CD5−
Follicular lymphoma	• Neoplastic follicles are usually better-defined than the pseudo-follicles (proliferation centers) of CLL • Follicles contain CD21+ follicular dendritic cell meshworks • Follicle cells are BCL6+, CD10+, and CD5−

Recognition of proliferation centers and the abnormal prevalence of CD5+ B cell in the interfollicular region help confirm a diagnosis of SLL. In some cases of SLL, the proliferation centers may surround the reactive germinal centers in a so-called perifollicular pattern and may even show infiltration of germinal centers in a pattern reminiscent of the germinal center colonization seen in marginal zone lymphomas.[46] In such cases of SLL, the perifollicular regions are composed of prolymphocytes and paraimmunoblasts typical of proliferation centers, rather than the small monocytoid cells with abundant pale cytoplasm that characterize marginal zone lymphomas. The immunophenotype is also distinct, because marginal zone lymphomas are seldom CD5 positive (see Fig. 7C–E).

PROGNOSIS

Small lymphocytic lymphoma is an indolent lymphoma, with overall survival similar to or longer than CLL.[42] Like many other B-cell lymphomas, the clinical International Prognostic Index (IPI) score predicts overall survival in SLL patients; among patients with low IPI scores, a low hemoglobin level and B symptoms are associated with adverse outcome.[43] Neither the size of the proliferation centers, degree of architectural effacement, nor the presence of atypical histologic features, such as nuclear irregularities, are correlated with patient outcome.[42,48,49] Cytogenetic abnormalities are similar to those found in CLL. Like CLL, the presence of unmutated immunoglobulin heavy chain variable region and expression of ZAP-70 by immunohistochemistry in SLL are adverse prognostic factors.[48,50]

MONOCLONAL B-CELL LYMPHOCYTOSIS

CLINICAL FEATURES

Monoclonal B-cell lymphocytosis (MBL) is a clonal or oligoclonal proliferation of B cells that usually have a similar immunophenotype as CLL but are present in insufficient numbers ($<5 \times 10^9$/L in the blood, without extramedullary tissue involvement) to warrant a diagnosis of CLL. MBL is in many ways analogous to MGUS in that it is common in older adults and can progress to CLL over time. Although most patients with MBL do not develop CLL, a recent retrospective study has shown that almost all cases of CLL are preceded by MBL, with monotypic B cells detected in archived blood samples up to 6.4 years before the diagnosis of

Key Features
OF MONOCLONAL B-CELL LYMPHOCYTOSIS

1. Clonal proliferation of B lymphocytes in the blood at a level lower than required to diagnose CLL ($<5 \times 10^9$/L) and lacking lymphadenopathy or splenomegaly that would qualify for a diagnosis of SLL.

2. Most cases are immunophenotypically and genetically similar to CLL and only differ with respect to the peripheral blood clonal cell burden.

3. Almost all cases of CLL seem to be preceded by MBL; however, conversely, most patients with MBL have stable disease and never progress to CLL.

CLL.[1] In large general population-based studies, MBL is detected in approximately 3% of adults. Like MGUS, the incidence of MBL increases with age: MBL is present in only 0.3% of adults age 18 to 40 years but in more than 5% of individuals over age 60 years.[51] Its prevalence is increased to between 13.5% and 18% of first-degree relatives of CLL patients.[52,53] MBL is most often discovered incidentally when peripheral blood is subjected to flow cytometry for other reasons. Like CLL, MBL has a male predominance. By definition, MBL patients lack symptoms related to bone marrow infiltration, palpable lymphadenopathy, or spleno-megaly and the patients should have no evidence of an autoimmune or infectious process that could produce a transiently skewed κ:λ light chain ratio.[54] Some investigators have suggested that a repeat flow cytometry assessment of blood be performed to confirm that the monoclonal B-cell population is stable over a 3-month period.[55] A paraprotein may be present in some patients and, in such cases, the possibility of a concurrent plasma cell neoplasm must be excluded.[55]

DIAGNOSIS: MICROSCOPIC FEATURES

The bone marrow findings of MBL patients have not been well -studied, but most patients have low-level bone marrow infiltration by CLL-type cells comprising 10% to 20% of the cellularity.[56] It is uncertain if patients with less than 5×10^9/L CLL cells in the blood but with more extensive bone marrow infiltrates should be classified as CLL or as MBL: the International Workshop on Chronic Lymphocytic Leukemia recommends that the marrow should contain at least 30% lymphoid cells to qualify for CLL, but this is an arbitrary figure.[57] Of note, 6.5% of MBL patients in one recent study had extensive (more than 70%) and/or diffuse pattern bone marrow involvement, yet these patients have not required therapy after 5 years of follow-up.[58] Cytopenias due to bone marrow infiltration and/or autoimmune cell destruction, however, qualify a patient for CLL, irrespective of the peripheral blood monoclonal B cell count. Currently, a bone marrow biopsy does not seem to be indicated to evaluate asymptomatic patients presenting with MBL.[54,55] There are no characteristic morphologic features of the clonal lymphocytes in the peripheral blood smear and these usually comprise the minority of the lymphocytes.

DIAGNOSIS: ANCILLARY STUDIES

The diagnosis of MBL is established by flow cytometry of peripheral blood demonstrating an abnormal monotypic B-cell population, below the threshold level of 5×10^9/L required to diagnose CLL. Monoclonality of the population should be established by clonal expression of surface κ or λ light chain or, in cases lacking surface immunoglobulin expression, an aberrant phenotype resembling that of CLL cells. PCR evaluation for clonal *IGH* rearrangement may also be used to support a monoclonal B-cell population.[55] Three main immunophenotypic variants of MBL are recognized: the most common is so-called CLL-like, with B cells expressing dim CD20 and dim surface light chain and coexpressing both CD5 and CD23 (**Fig. 8**). The two less common variants are cases with CD5-negative B cells and cases with a CD20 bright, CD5-positive, CD23-negative B-cell phenotype. The prevalence of CD5-negative MBL is approximately 1% in patients over 40 years of age with a median age of 78 years, whereas the prevalence of CD5-positive, CD23-negative MBL is unknown.[51,59] Some cases of CD5-negative clonal B-cell lymphocytosis may manifest with a peripheral blood cell count of greater than 5×10^9/L and cytogenetic abnormalities, yet exhibit a stable, nonprogressive clinical course akin to MBL[60]; the classification of such cases is uncertain.

Gene expression profiling of MBL cases with a CLL-like phenotype has shown close similarity to CLL, with no distinguishing specific protein expression.[61] Most cases of MBL (up to 90%) show a high level of somatic hypermutation, similar to the favorable prognosis category of mutated CLL.[62] MBL shares similar cytogenetic abnormalities with CLL, with del(13q) the most common abnormality and trisomy 12 occurring in about 20% of cases. The adverse prognostic markers del(11q) and del(17p) appear to be limited mainly to MBL patients with higher monoclonal lymphocyte counts.[2] Overall, the immunoglobulin gene mutation status, incidence of ZAP-70 and CD38 expression, and distribution of cytogenetic abnormalities of MBL are similar to low-stage (Rai stage 0) CLL,[62] with the possible exception of the high-risk cytogenetic lesions del(11q) and del(17p) that were found to be less frequent in MBL in one study.[56]

DIFFERENTIAL DIAGNOSIS

An important differential of CD5 negative MBL is hairy cell leukemia: hairy cells are usually infrequent in the blood and may be missed on cursory examination of the peripheral smear. HCL should, therefore, be excluded in any putative CD5-negative MBL case. Clues to the diagnosis of hairy cell leukemia, a progressive B-cell lymphoma that

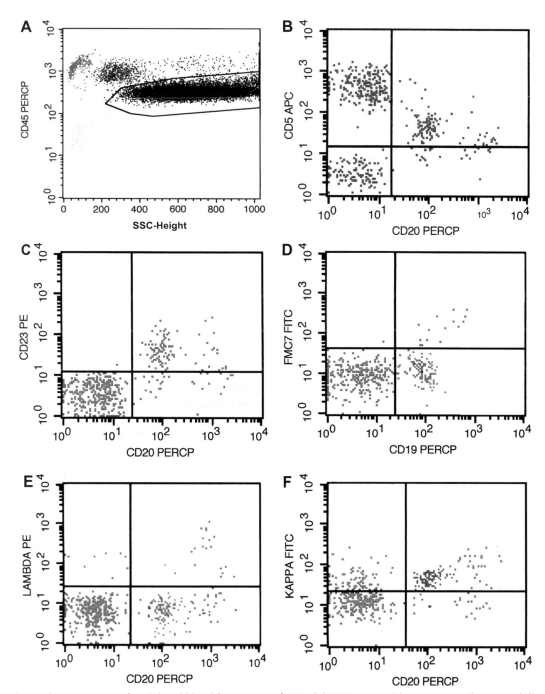

Fig. 8. Flow cytometry of peripheral blood from a case of MBL. (*A*) CD45 versus side scatter reveals a normal distribution of lymphocytes (*red*), monocytes (*green*), and granulocytes (*dark blue*). Within the lymphocyte gate, there is a subpopulation of B cells that is dimmer for CD20 than the less numerous normal B cells and is dimly positive for CD5 (*B*) and for CD23 (*C*). Unlike the polyclonal CD20 bright positive normal B cells (*red*), the abnormal CD20 dim positive B cells (*turquoise*) are negative for FMC7 (*D*) and are negative for λ light chain (*E*) but positive for κ light chain (*F*), indicating a small abnormal monoclonal B-cell population amid normal, polyclonal B cells and T cells.

usually requires therapy, are the presence of monocytopenia, identification of hairy cells on careful review of the peripheral smear, and splenomegaly. Expression of CD103, CD11c, and CD25 on the circulating neoplastic cells, even if few in number, is highly characteristic of hairy cell leukemia and a diagnosis of CD5-negative MBL should not be made if the clonal B cells display

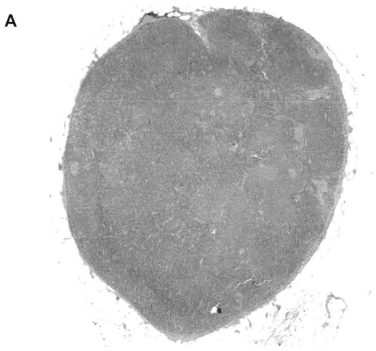

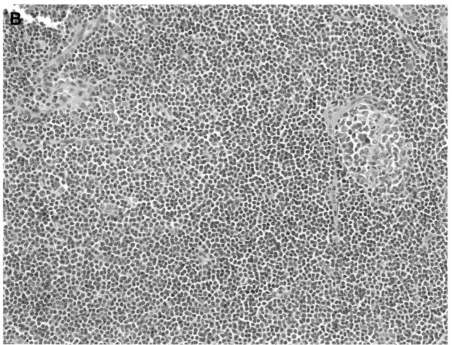

Fig. 9. A case of CLL-like cells involving a cervical lymph node taken incidentally to stage papillary thyroid carcinoma. (*A*) The lymph node is not enlarged, but its architecture appears partly effaced. (*B*) On high power, there are sheets of monotonous small lymphocytes.

this immunophenotype. Mantle cell lymphoma should be excluded by cyclin-D1 assessment and/or FISH study in all cases of circulating clonal CD5-positive, CD23-negative B cells. Although there is general agreement that bone marrow examination is not necessary to evaluate patients with CLL-type MBL, some investigators have advocated performing a bone marrow investigation to evaluate all putative MBL cases that lack CD5 and/or CD23 expression.[55]

Almost all patients with SLL have circulating monotypic CLL-type cells[44] and MBL is distinguished from such cases by absence of palpable lymphadenopathy or organomegaly on physical

Fig. 9. A case of CLL-like cells involving a cervical lymph node taken incidentally to stage papillary thyroid carcinoma. The monotonous small lymphocytes express PAX5 (*C*) and coexpress CD5 (*D*), amid scattered residual T cells staining for CD3 (*E*). Given that this patient did not have clinically evident lymphadenopathy or splenomegaly and had <5 ×10^9/L CLL cells in the peripheral blood, this may represent an example of MBL involving a lymph node. *(Images courtesy of* Dr Nancy Lee Harris, Massachusetts General Hospital, Boston, MA.)

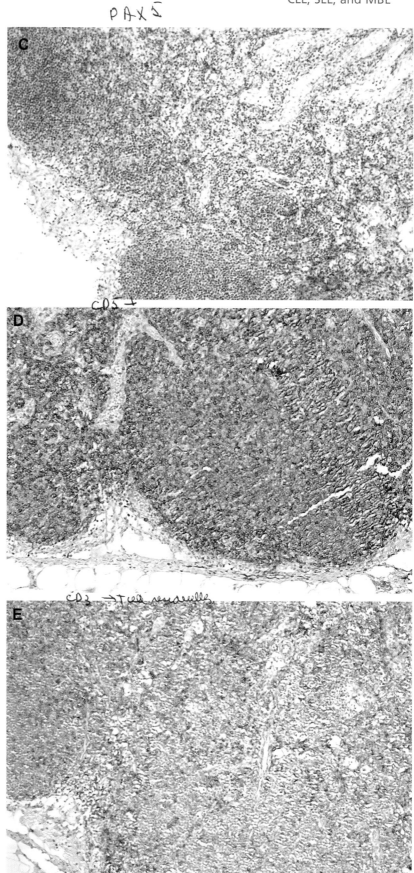

△△ Differential Diagnosis of MBL

MBL Versus	Helpful Distinguishing Features
CLL	• Monoclonal B-cell count is >5 × 10⁹/L and/or there are symptoms related to the neoplastic B-cell proliferation
Hairy cell leukemia	• Circulating neoplastic cells express CD103, CD25, and CD11c • Monocytopenia is almost always present • Bone marrow is infiltrated by hairy cells in an interstitial or diffuse pattern
Reactive lymphocytosis	• Transient (<3 months) • Usually polyclonal or oligoclonal rather than monoclonal • T cells usually predominate over B cells

---

examination.[54] One area of uncertainty is the classification of cases where lymph nodes taken out incidentally (such as for staging of a solid tumor) are found to be infiltrated by CLL-type cells (see **Fig. 9**). In one recent study of 36 patients with CLL-infiltrates in lymph nodes biopsied incidentally or to evaluate lymphadenopathy (and lacking defining criteria for CLL), only five patients developed progressive lymphadenopathy after a median follow-up time of 18 months. The presence of proliferation centers in the infiltrated lymph nodes, but not their size or whether or not the lymph nodes were biopsied incidentally or due to clinical enlargement, was associated with progressive lymphadenopathy.[44] These findings suggest that MBL may also present with tissue infiltration and lack palpable lymphadenopathy that would be diagnostic of SLL.

PROGNOSIS

Fifteen percent to 34% of patients with MBL (1%–2% per year) eventually progress to CLL.[2,57] Reported incidences vary based on the type of study: population based studies tend to detect patients with lower monoclonal B-cell counts who have lower likelihood of progression, whereas monoclonal B-cell counts and progression to CLL are higher in studies based on MBL detected in patients coming to medial attention due to leukocytosis or other abnormal blood counts (so-called clinical MBL). A higher monoclonal B-cell count is associated with a higher likelihood of progressing to CLL or SLL as well as eventually requiring treatment. Higher monoclonal B-cell counts are also correlated with adverse overall survival.[2,62,63] The presence of trisomy 12 or del(17p) detected by FISH are independently

Pitfalls
OF CHRONIC LYMPHOCYTIC LEUKEMIA, SMALL LYMPHOCYTIC LYMPHOMA, AND MONOCLONAL B-CELL LYMPHOCYTOSIS

! Other lymphomas, including follicular lymphoma, mantle cell lymphoma, and splenic marginal zone lymphoma, may present with lymphocytosis mimicking CLL.

! CLL cases may manifest an atypical immunophenotype, such as negativity for CD23, unusually bright expression of CD20 and/or unusually bright expression of surface light chain; such cases may still be diagnosed as CLL if other features support this diagnosis.

! Lymph nodes involved by SLL may exhibit many components of retained architecture, including many reactive germinal centers and patent sinuses.

! Some cases of CLL or SLL may express CD20 at such a low-level as to appear negative by flow cytometry or immunohistochemistry, necessitating the use of other B-cell markers; surface immunoglobulin may also appear negative, although monotypic cytoplasmic immunoglobulin expression can usually be demonstrated by flow cytometry in such cases.

! Cases of putative MBL with a non-CLL immunophenotype (negative for CD5 and/or CD23) should be investigated to exclude a non-Hodgkin's lymphoma/leukemia presenting with minimal blood involvement, such as mantle cell lymphoma, splenic marginal zone lymphoma, or hairy cell leukemia.

associated with progression to CLL or SLL requiring therapy.[56] Nevertheless, the current recommendation is to follow MBL patients with complete blood counts every 6 to 12 months to detect any progression of lymphocytosis, whereas FISH testing and assessment of immunoglobulin gene mutation status are not indicated.[54,64] Overall, patients with MBL have a low risk of dying from CLL and usually die of unrelated causes.

REFERENCES

1. Landgren O, Albitar M, Ma W, et al. B-cell clones as early markers for chronic lymphocytic leukemia. N Engl J Med 2009;360:659–67.

2. Rawstron AC, Bennett FL, O'Connor SJ, et al. Monoclonal B-cell lymphocytosis and chronic lymphocytic leukemia. N Engl J Med 2008;359:575–83.

3. Binet JL, Auquier A, Dighiero G, et al. A new prognostic classification of chronic lymphocytic leukemia derived from a multivariate survival analysis. Cancer 1981;48:198–206.

4. Muller-Hermelink HK, Montserrat E, Catovsky D, et al. Chronic lymphocytic leukaemia/small lymphocytic lymphoma. In: Swerdlow SH, Campo E, Harris NL, et al, editors. WHO classification of tumours of haematopoietic and lymphoid tissues. Lyon (France): World Health Organization Classification of Tumours; 2008. p. 180–2.

5. Frater JL, McCarron KF, Hammel JP, et al. Typical and atypical chronic lymphocytic leukemia differ clinically and immunophenotypically. Am J Clin Pathol 2001;116:655–64.

6. Montserrat E, Villamor N, Reverter JC, et al. Bone marrow assessment in B-cell chronic lymphocytic leukaemia: aspirate or biopsy? A comparative study in 258 patients. Br J Haematol 1996;93:111–6.

7. Thiele J, Zirbes TK, Kvasnicka HM, et al. Focal lymphoid aggregates (nodules) in bone marrow biopsies: differentiation between benign hyperplasia and malignant lymphoma—a practical guideline. J Clin Pathol 1999;52:294–300.

8. Chetty R, Echezarreta G, Comley M, et al. Immunohistochemistry in apparently normal bone marrow trephine specimens from patients with nodal follicular lymphoma. J Clin Pathol 1995;48:1035–8.

9. Thaler J, Greil R, Dietze O, et al. Immunohistology for quantification of normal bone marrow lymphocyte subsets. Br J Haematol 1989;73:576–7.

10. Rozman C, Montserrat E, Rodriguez-Fernandez JM, et al. Bone marrow histologic pattern—the best single prognostic parameter in chronic lymphocytic leukemia: a multivariate survival analysis of 329 cases. Blood 1984;64:642–8.

11. Bergmann MA, Eichhorst BF, Busch R, et al. Prospective evaluation of prognostic parameters in early stage Chronic Lymphocytic Leukemia (CLL):

results of the CLL1-Protocol of the German CLL Study Group (GCLLSG). Blood 2007;110:165.

12. Henrique R, Achten R, Maes B, et al. Guidelines for subtyping small B-cell lymphomas in bone marrow biopsies. Virchows Arch 1999;435:549–58.

13. Carulli G, Stacchini A, Marini A, et al. Aberrant expression of CD8 in B-cell non-Hodgkin lymphoma: a multicenter study of 951 bone marrow samples with lymphomatous infiltration. Am J Clin Pathol 2009;132:186–90 quiz 306.

14. Delgado J, Matutes E, Morilla AM, et al. Diagnostic significance of CD20 and FMC7 expression in B-cell disorders. Am J Clin Pathol 2003;120:754–9.

15. Matutes E, Owusu-Ankomah K, Morilla R, et al. The immunological profile of B-cell disorders and proposal of a scoring system for the diagnosis of CLL. Leukemia 1994;8:1640–5.

16. Morice WG, Kurtin PJ, Hodnefield JM, et al. Predictive value of blood and bone marrow flow cytometry in B-cell lymphoma classification: comparative analysis of flow cytometry and tissue biopsy in 252 patients. Mayo Clin Proc 2008;83:776–85.

17. O'Malley DP, Vance GH, Orazi A. Chronic lymphocytic leukemia/small lymphocytic lymphoma with trisomy 12 and focal cyclin d1 expression: a potential diagnostic pitfall. Arch Pathol Lab Med 2005;129: 92–5.

18. Matutes E, Morilla R, Owusu-Ankomah K, et al. The immunophenotype of splenic lymphoma with villous lymphocytes and its relevance to the differential diagnosis with other B-cell disorders. Blood 1994; 83:1558–62.

19. Morice WG, Chen D, Kurtin PJ, et al. Novel immunophenotypic features of marrow lymphoplasmacytic lymphoma and correlation with Waldenstrom's macroglobulinemia. Mod Pathol 2009;22:807–16.

20. Ferry JA, Yang WI, Zukerberg LR, et al. CD5+ extranodal marginal zone B-cell (MALT) lymphoma. A low grade neoplasm with a propensity for bone marrow involvement and relapse. Am J Clin Pathol 1996; 105:31–7.

21. Cervantes F, Pereira A, Marti JM, et al. Bone marrow lymphoid nodules in myeloproliferative disorders: association with the nonmyelosclerotic phases of idiopathic myelofibrosis and immunological significance. Br J Haematol 1988;70:279–82.

22. Horny HP, Wehrmann M, Griesser H, et al. Investigation of bone marrow lymphocyte subsets in normal, reactive, and neoplastic states using paraffin-embedded biopsy specimens. Am J Clin Pathol 1993;99:142–9.

23. Kremer M, Quintanilla-Martinez L, Nahrig J, et al. Immunohistochemistry in bone marrow pathology: a useful adjunct for morphologic diagnosis. Virchows Arch 2005;447:920–37.

24. Pezzella F, Munson PJ, Miller KD, et al. The diagnosis of low-grade peripheral B-cell neoplasms in

bone marrow trephines. Br J Haematol 2000;108: 369–:376.

25. Del Giudice I, Chiaretti S, Tavolaro S, et al. Spontaneous regression of chronic lymphocytic leukemia: clinical and biologic features of 9 cases. Blood 2009;114:638–46.

26. Dighiero G, Hamblin TJ. Chronic lymphocytic leukaemia. Lancet 2008;371:1017–29.

27. Rai KR, Han T. Prognostic factors and clinical staging in chronic lymphocytic leukemia. Hematol Oncol Clin North Am 1990;4:447–56.

28. Johansson P, Eisele L, Klein-Hitpass L, et al. Percentage of smudge cells determined on routine blood smears is a novel prognostic factor in chronic lymphocytic leukemia. Leuk Res 2010;34: 892–8.

29. Dohner H, Stilgenbauer S, Benner A, et al. Genomic aberrations and survival in chronic lymphocytic leukemia. N Engl J Med 2000;343:1910–6.

30. Yin CC, Lin KI, Ketterling RP, et al. Chronic lymphocytic leukemia With t(2;14)(p16;q32)involves the BCL11A and IgH genes and is associated with atypical morphologic features and unmutated IgVH genes. Am J Clin Pathol 2009;131:663–70.

31. Shanafelt TD, Witzig TE, Fink SR, et al. Prospective evaluation of clonal evolution during long-term follow-up of patients with untreated early-stage chronic lymphocytic leukemia. J Clin Oncol 2006; 24:4634–41.

32. Hamblin TJ, Davis Z, Gardiner A, et al. Unmutated Ig V(H) genes are associated with a more aggressive form of chronic lymphocytic leukemia. Blood 1999; 94:1848–54.

33. Tobin G, Soderberg O, Thunberg U, et al. V(H)3-21 gene usage in chronic lymphocytic leukemia–characterization of a new subgroup with distinct molecular features and poor survival. Leuk Lymphoma 2004;45:221–8.

34. Rassenti LZ, Huynh L, Toy TL, et al. ZAP-70 compared with immunoglobulin heavy-chain gene mutation status as a predictor of disease progression in chronic lymphocytic leukemia. N Engl J Med 2004;351:893–901.

35. Wiestner A, Rosenwald A, Barry TS, et al. ZAP-70 expression identifies a chronic lymphocytic leukemia subtype with unmutated immunoglobulin genes, inferior clinical outcome, and distinct gene expression profile. Blood 2003;101:4944–51.

36. Zanotti R, Ambrosetti A, Lestani M, et al. ZAP-70 expression, as detected by immunohistochemistry on bone marrow biopsies from early-phase CLL patients, is a strong adverse prognostic factor. Leukemia 2007;21:102–9.

37. Hamblin TJ, Orchard JA, Ibbotson RE, et al. CD38 expression and immunoglobulin variable region mutations are independent prognostic variables in chronic lymphocytic leukemia, but CD38 expression

may vary during the course of the disease. Blood 2002;99:1023–9.

38. Asslaber D, Pinon JD, Seyfried I, et al. microRNA-34a expression correlates with MDM2 SNP309 polymorphism and treatment-free survival in chronic lymphocytic leukemia. Blood 2010;115:4191–7.

39. Foucar K, Rydell RE. Richter's syndrome in chronic lymphocytic leukemia. Cancer 1980;46:118–34.

40. Tsimberidou AM, Keating MJ. Richter's transformation in chronic lymphocytic leukemia. Semin Oncol 2006;33:250–6.

41. Rossi D, Cerri M, Capello D, et al. Biological and clinical risk factors of chronic lymphocytic leukaemia transformation to Richter syndrome. Br J Haematol 2008;142:202–15.

42. Ben-Ezra J, Burke JS, Swartz WG, et al. Small lymphocytic lymphoma: a clinicopathologic analysis of 268 cases. Blood 1989;73:579–87.

43. Nola M, Pavletic SZ, Weisenburger DD, et al. Prognostic factors influencing survival in patients with B-cell small lymphocytic lymphoma. Am J Hematol 2004;77:31–5.

44. Gibson SE, Swerdlow SH, Ferry JA, et al. Reassessment of small ly mphocytic lymphoma (SLL) ni the era of monoclonal B lymphocytosis (MBL). Mod Pathol 2010;23:296A–7A.

45. Lampert IA, Wotherspoon A, Van Noorden S, et al. High expression of CD23 in the proliferation centers of chronic lymphocytic leukemia in lymph nodes and spleen. Hum Pathol 1999;30:648–54.

46. Bahler DW, Aguilera NS, Chen CC, et al. Histological and immunoglobulin VH gene analysis of interfollicular small lymphocytic lymphoma provides evidence for two types. Am J Pathol 2000;157: 1063–70.

47. Ellison DJ, Nathwani BN, Cho SY, et al. Interfollicular small lymphocytic lymphoma: the diagnostic significance of pseudofollicles. Hum Pathol 1989;20: 1108–18.

48. Garcia CF, Hunt KE, Kang H, et al. Most morphologic features in chronic lymphocytic leukemia/small lymphocytic lymphoma (CLL/SLL) do not reliably predict underlying FISH genetics or immunoglobulin heavy chain variable region somatic mutational status. Appl Immunohistochem Mol Morphol 2010; 18:119–27.

49. Asplund SL, McKenna RW, Howard MS, et al. Immunophenotype does not correlate with lymph node histology in chronic lymphocytic leukemia/small lymphocytic lymphoma. Am J Surg Pathol 2002;26: 624–9.

50. Soma LA, Craig FE, Swerdlow SH. The proliferation center microenvironment and prognostic markers in chronic lymphocytic leukemia/small lymphocytic lymphoma. Hum Pathol 2006;37:152–9.

51. Rawstron AC, Green MJ, Kuzmicki A, et al. Monoclonal B lymphocytes with the characteristics of

"indolent" chronic lymphocytic leukemia are present in 3.5% of adults with normal blood counts. Blood 2002;100:635–9.

52. Marti GE, Carter P, Abbasi F, et al. B-cell monoclonal lymphocytosis and B-cell abnormalities in the setting of familial B-cell chronic lymphocytic leukemia. Cytometry B Clin Cytom 2003;52:1–12.

53. Rawstron AC, Yuille MR, Fuller J, et al. Inherited predisposition to CLL is detectable as subclinical monoclonal B-lymphocyte expansion. Blood 2002; 100:2289–90.

54. Shanafelt TD, Ghia P, Lanasa MC, et al. Monoclonal B-cell lymphocytosis (MBL): biology, natural history and clinical management. Leukemia 2010;24: 512–20.

55. Marti GE, Rawstron AC, Ghia P, et al. Diagnostic criteria for monoclonal B-cell lymphocytosis. Br J Haematol 2005;130:325–32.

56. Rossi D, Sozzi E, Puma A, et al. The prognosis of clinical monoclonal B cell lymphocytosis differs from prognosis of Rai 0 chronic lymphocytic leukaemia and is recapitulated by biological risk factors. Br J Haematol 2009;146:64–75.

57. Hallek M, Cheson BD, Catovsky D, et al. Guidelines for the diagnosis and treatment of chronic lymphocytic leukemia: a report from the International Workshop on Chronic Lymphocytic Leukemia updating the National Cancer Institute-Working Group 1996 guidelines. Blood 2008;111:5446–56.

58. Herrick JL, Shanafelt TD, Kay NE, et al. Monoclonal B-cell lymphocytosis (MBL): a bone marrow study of an indolent form of chronic lymphocytic leukemia. Mod Pathol 2008;21:256A.

59. Ghia P, Prato G, Scielzo C, et al. Monoclonal CD5+ and CD5-B-lymphocyte expansions are frequent in the peripheral blood of the elderly. Blood 2004; 103:2337–42.

60. Amato D, Oscier DG, Davis Z, et al. Cytogenetic aberrations and immunoglobulin VH gene mutations in clinically benign CD5- monoclonal B-cell lymphocytosis. Am J Clin Pathol 2007;128:333–8.

61. Rawstron AC, Bennett F, Hillmen P. The biological and clinical relationship between CD5+23+ monoclonal B-cell lymphocytosis and chronic lymphocytic leukaemia. Br J Haematol 2007;139:724–9.

62. Shanafelt TD, Kay NE, Rabe KG, et al. Brief report: natural history of individuals with clinically recognized monoclonal B-cell lymphocytosis compared with patients with Rai 0 chronic lymphocytic leukemia. J Clin Oncol 2009;27:3959–63.

63. Shanafelt TD, Kay NE, Jenkins G, et al. B-cell count and survival: differentiating chronic lymphocytic leukemia from monoclonal B-cell lymphocytosis based on clinical outcome. Blood 2009;113: 4188–96.

64. Dighiero G. Monoclonal B-cell lymphocytosis—a frequent premalignant condition. N Engl J Med 2008;359:638–40.

SPLENIC B-CELL LYMPHOMAS/LEUKEMIAS

James R. Cook, MD, PhD

KEYWORDS

• Spleen • Lymphoma • Splenic marginal zone • Hairy cell leukemia

ABSTRACT

The diagnosis and classification of lymphoproliferative disorders in the spleen are frequently challenging. While some lymphomas, such as hairy cell leukemia and splenic marginal zone lymphoma, characteristically present with primarily splenic involvement, secondary involvement of the spleen may be seen with any lymphoma. Precise classification requires integration of the morphologic findings with clinical data, phenotypic studies, and often cytogenetic and/or molecular genetic analysis. Correlation with the findings in peripheral blood and bone marrow may also be required in some cases. This article discusses the diagnostic approach to splenic-based lymphoproliferative disorders in routine practice and describes the clinicopathologic features of lymphoid neoplasms that characteristically present in the spleen.

OVERVIEW

The diagnosis and classification of B-cell lymphomas involving the spleen are frequently challenging. Essentially any systemic B-cell lymphoproliferative disorder may show prominent secondary involvement of the spleen. Only a few B-cell lymphomas, however, typically present with isolated splenomegaly; this review is focused on this group of primary splenic lymphomas/leukemias.

In the 2008 World Health Organization (WHO) classification, there are two well-defined small B-cell neoplasms that characteristically present with prominent splenic involvement: splenic marginal zone lymphoma (SMZL) and hairy cell leukemia (HCL). In addition, it is now recognized that there are cases of splenic-based small B-cell lymphomas that do not meet current defined criteria for either of these entities. The WHO classification has therefore included a new category, splenic lymphoma/leukemia, unclassifiable, which includes two provisional entities: HCL variant (HCL-V) and splenic diffuse red pulp small B-cell lymphoma (SDRPSBL). As provisional entities, the criteria for these diagnoses remain tentative, and these diagnoses should be made only with caution. Finally, diffuse large B-cell lymphomas

Key Features
SPLENIC B-CELL LYMPHOMAS AND LEUKEMIAS

1. Secondary involvement of the spleen may be seen in essentially any systemic lymphoma. Knowledge of the clinical presentation and history is helpful to distinguish between primary and secondary splenic involvement.

2. Some splenic leukemias/lymphomas, such as hairy cell leukemia (HCL), may be definitively diagnosed on the basis of peripheral blood findings, whereas other cases may require knowledge of bone marrow or splenic histology for definitive classification.

3. Peripheral blood or bone marrow flow cytometric studies are an essential component of the diagnosis and classification of splenic lymphomas/leukemias.

4. Evaluation of the bone marrow growth pattern often aids in correct diagnosis.

Department of Clinical Pathology, Mail Stop L11, Cleveland Clinic, 9500 Euclid Avenue, Cleveland, OH 44195, USA
E-mail address: cookj2@ccf.org

Surgical Pathology 3 (2010) 933–954
doi:10.1016/j.path.2010.09.004

(DLBCLs) may also present with isolated splenic disease. Correct diagnosis and classification of these disorders require knowledge of the clinical findings; ancillary studies, such as flow cytometry; and knowledge of the peripheral blood, bone marrow, and, in some cases, spleen morphology.

SPLENIC MARGINAL ZONE LYMPHOMA

Splenic marginal zone lymphoma (SMZL) is a neoplasm of small B cells that typically presents with involvement of the peripheral blood, bone marrow, and spleen.[1,2] The lymphoma is thought to represent a neoplasm of memory B cells normally found in the marginal zones of the splenic white pulp.[3,4] Because a definitive diagnosis of SMZL is based on splenic histology, and because this lymphoma displays a nonspecific B-cell phenotype, recognizing cases of SMZL from examination of peripheral blood or bone marrow alone may be challenging. Nevertheless, the typical peripheral blood and bone marrow findings in the setting of isolated splenomegaly are generally sufficient to at least strongly favor this diagnosis, even in the absence of a splenectomy specimen.[5]

CLINICAL FEATURES

Splenic marginal zone lymphoma presents in adulthood, with a median age of approximately 65 years. Men and women are equally affected.[6,7] Symptoms include fatigue or abdominal pain due to splenomegaly. Systemic lymphadenopathy is uncommon. There is typically a peripheral blood lymphocytosis and there may be anemia and/or thrombocytopenia. A paraprotein, usually IgM, is found in approximately one-third of patients. Some studies have reported an association with hepatitis C virus.[8,9]

DIAGNOSIS: GROSS AND MICROSCOPIC FEATURES

The peripheral blood in SMZL typically displays an absolute lymphocytosis, and many of those without an absolute lymphocytosis will display low-level peripheral blood involvement by flow cytometry. The cells of SMZL characteristically are small with mature chromatin and a moderate amount of pale cytoplasm (Fig. 1). Some cases exhibit cytoplasmic projections, leading to the alternate name, splenic lymphoma with villous lymphocytes.[10] The presence of villous morphology, however, is not required for the diagnosis of SMZL, and villous lymphocyte cytology may also been seen in other lymphoproliferative disorders. In the bone marrow, there is a nodular and/or interstitial infiltrate of small lymphocytes. In some cases, the nodules may contain reactive germinal centers. There is also characteristically an intrasinusoidal infiltrate of neoplastic B cells, although this is often only apparent using immunohistochemical stains (Fig. 2).[2,11]

On gross examination, the spleen in SMZL is diffusely enlarged. Prominent, enlarged white pulp nodules are seen grossly on the cut surface of the spleen (Fig. 3) and histologically (Fig. 4). In most cases, the white pulp nodules display a biphasic pattern, characterized by a central core of mantle zone-like small lymphocytes with condensed chromatin and scant cytoplasm surrounded by a peripheral zone of monocytoid-appearing cells with slightly irregular nuclear contours and abundant pale cytoplasm.[2,6,12,13] Both components of the biphasic nodules have been shown to represent part of the same clonal proliferation. In up to half of cases, however, the white pulp nodules may consist entirely of monocytoid-appearing cells (so-called monophasic pattern) (Fig. 5). The significance of monophasic versus biphasic histology remains uncertain.[13] Most cases display a scant neoplastic lymphoid infiltrate within the red pulp as well, although this may only be apparent by using immunohistochemical stains. Plasmacytic differentiation, sometimes consisting of clonal plasma cells within residual, colonized germinal centers, may be seen in a minority of cases. Splenic hilar lymph nodes typically show a nodular proliferation of monocytoid-appearing cells, often with preserved and dilated sinuses (Fig. 6).

DIAGNOSIS: ANCILLARY STUDIES

By flow cytometry, SMZL exhibits a clonal B-cell population with a so-called nonspecific phenotype: positive for CD20 and CD79a and negative for CD5, CD10, CD23, and CD43. CD11c is frequently expressed, and CD103 may be seen in a subset of cases.[2,5,6,12] Cyclin D1 is negative by immunohistochemistry. The cytogenetic findings in SMZL are diverse. The most common recurring abnormality is deletion of chromosome 7q31-32.[14,15] This abnormality is found, however, in only approximately 15% to 40% of cases. Trisomy 3, which is also seen in other forms of marginal zone lymphoma, has been reported in approximately 20% to 30% of SMZL cases.[13,16] MALT1 translocations, characteristic of some extranodal marginal zone lymphomas, are absent.

The diagnosis of SMZL is generally made on the basis of morphology and immunophenotype.[2,5] In most cases, the peripheral blood and bone marrow findings alone are sufficient to establish

Fig. 1. SMZL cells in the peripheral blood (*A, B*). SMZL cells typically display condensed chromatin, round to slightly irregular nuclear contours, eccentrically placed nuclei, moderate to abundant cytoplasm, and variable cytoplasmic projections.

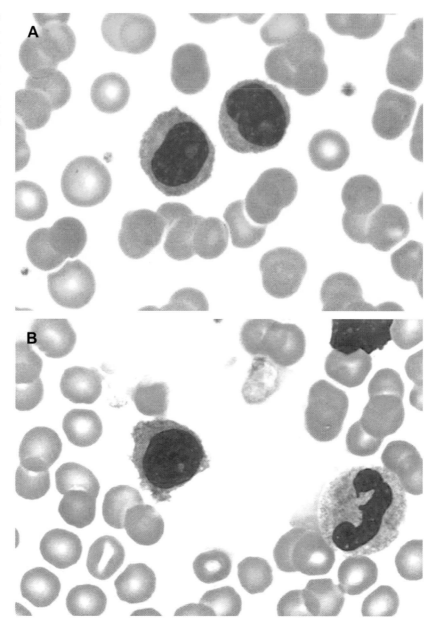

a presumptive diagnosis of SMZL and allow for appropriate clinical management.[5] The absence of CD25 and CD123 expression eliminates the possibility of HCL. By definition, however, a completely definitive diagnosis of SMZL (in particular distinguishing it from the recently described provisional entity SDRPSBL[17] discussed later), requires examination of a splenectomy specimen. A diagnosis of SMZL should not be rendered simply by default in cases of

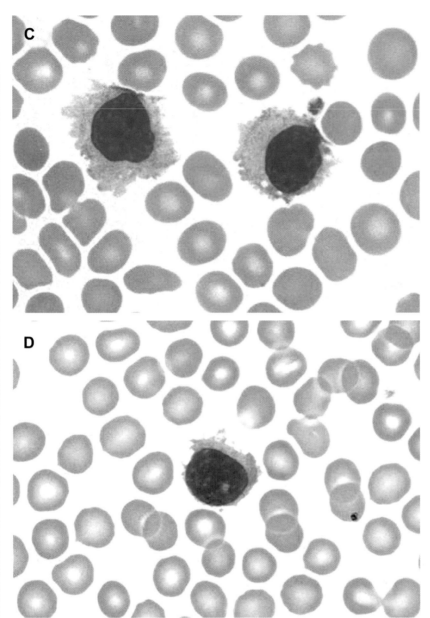

Fig. 1. SMZL cells in the peripheral blood (*C, D*).

splenic-based B-cell neoplasms with a nonspecific phenotype. Cases that do not meet the established morphologic and phenotypic criteria for any of the defined entities should be diagnosed instead as splenic B-cell lymphoma/leukemia, unclassifiable.

DIFFERENTIAL DIAGNOSIS

The differential diagnosis of SMZL in patients with isolated splenomegaly includes HCL, HCL-V, and SDRPSBL (**Table 1**). The features of each of these entities are discussed later. The possibility of secondary splenic involvement by a systemic

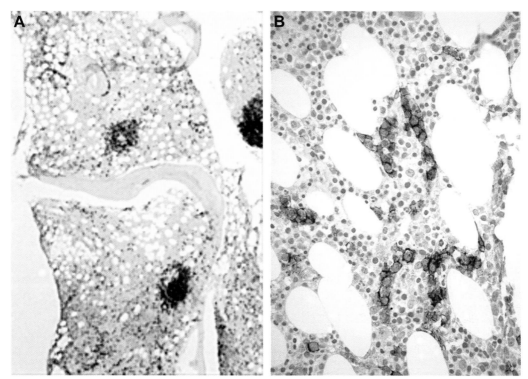

Fig. 2. SMZL involving the bone marrow. (*A*) At low power, there is a nodular nonparatrabecular and scattered interstitial infiltrate of small, neoplastic B cells. (*B*) At high power, the neoplastic cells are seen to display an intra-sinusoidal growth pattern in some areas, evidenced by linear arrays of closely opposed cells. (*A* and *B*, CD20 immunohistochemical staining).

Fig. 3. Spleen involved by SMZL. This spleen is massively enlarged (>5 kg) with many 1–2 mm white pulp nodules noted on cross-section.

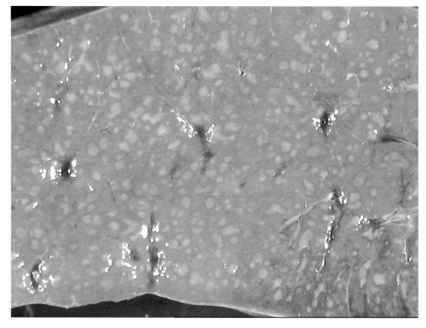

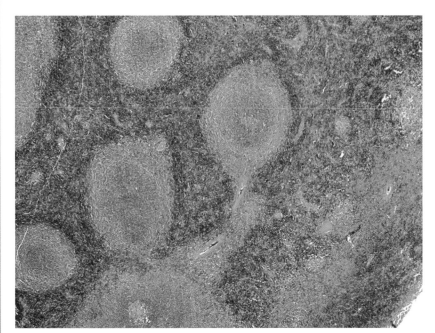

Fig. 4. Low-power image of SMZL involving the spleen, demonstrating an expansion of the white pulp.

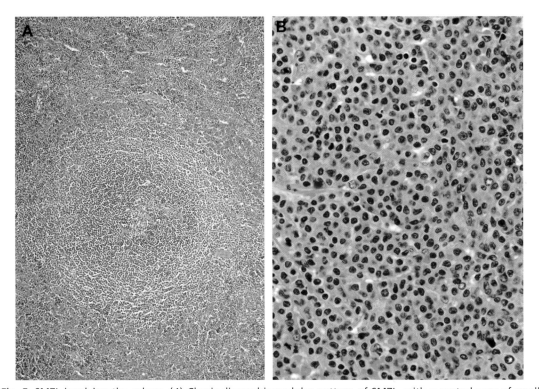

Fig. 5. SMZL involving the spleen. (*A*) Classic dimorphic nodular pattern of SMZL, with a central core of small, darkly staining, mantle zone-like lymphocytes surrounded by a rim of paler marginal zone-type cells. (*B*) Monomorphic pattern of SMZL, with nodules composed exclusively of small lymphocytes with monocytoid/marginal zone morphology.

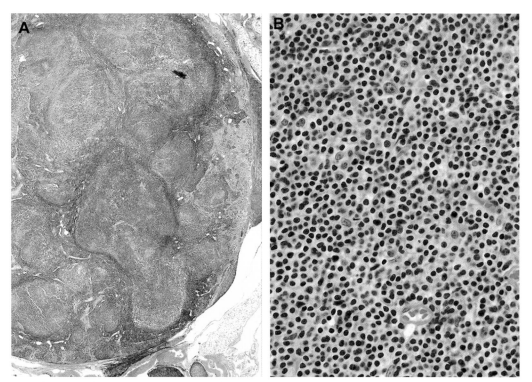

Fig. 6. Splenic hilar lymph node involvement by SMZL. (*A*) At low power, there is a nodular lymphoid proliferation with partial architectural preservation (note patent sinuses on right side of image). (*B*) At high power, the nodules are composed of small lymphocytes with monocytoid features (abundant pale cytoplasm and round to slightly irregular nuclei).

lymphoma must also be considered. In particular, follicular lymphoma (FL) and chronic lymphocytic leukemia/small lymphocytic lymphoma (CLL/SLL) may occasionally present with predominantly splenic involvement. FL presenting in the spleen may show a prominent nodular proliferation of neoplastic germinal centers that may be surrounded by a peripheral zone of marginal zone-like cells.[18,19] The diagnosis of FL can be established by identifying the presence of germinal center antigens (CD10 and/or BCL6) on the neoplastic cells. CLL/SLL involving the spleen displays a small lymphoid proliferation, including proliferation centers, in the white pulp nodules as well as a prominent red pulp infiltrate. The presence of CD5 expression, usually with CD23, helps to distinguish CLL/SLL from SMZL; however, a minority of cases of SMZL are reported to show coexpression of CD5.[20] In such cases, correlation with splenic histology is essential for definitive diagnosis.

PROGNOSIS

Splenic marginal zone lymphoma generally exhibits an indolent clinical course with more than 60% of patients alive after 5 years.[1,5] Due to the rarity of SMZL, the optimal treatment regimen remains unclear. Treatment options for symptomatic patients include single or multiagent chemotherapy; immunotherapy, such as rituximab; or splenectomy. Splenectomy alone may give prolonged clinical remissions for some patients. For asymptomatic patients, a "watch and wait" strategy may also be appropriate. Approximately 10% of patients undergo eventual transformation to DLBCL.

HAIRY CELL LEUKEMIA

Hairy cell leukemia (HCL) is a small B-cell neoplasm with distinctive morphology and immunophenotype that typically presents with involvement of the spleen, liver, and bone marrow but sparing of

Table 1
Differential diagnosis of splenic small B-cell lymphomas/leukemias: histologic and immunophenotypic features

Lymphoma/Leukemia	Cytology	White Pulp Pattern	Red Pulp Pattern	Bone Marrow Pattern	Immunophenotype
Splenic marginal zone lymphoma	Lymphocytosis, moderate pale cytoplasm, variable villous projections	Enlarged nodules, biphasic pattern	Scant lymphoid infiltrate	Nodular, interstitial, intrasinusoidal	CD20+ CD5− CD10− CD23− · CD11c+/− CD103−/+ CD25− DBA.44−/+
Chronic lymphocytic leukemia	Lymphocytosis, scant cytoplasm	Enlarged nodules	Prominent lymphoid infiltrate	Nodular, interstitial, diffuse	CD20dim+ CD5+ CD10− CD23+/− · CD11c+/− CD103− CD25− CD123−
Follicular lymphoma	Variable lymphocytosis, scant cytoplasm, clefted nuclei	Enlarged nodules, may have biphasic pattern	Minimal lymphoid infiltrate	Nodular, paratrabecular	CD20+ CD5− CD10+ · CD23−/+ BCL6+ BCL2+/−
Hairy cell leukemia	Minimal lymphocytosis, abundant cytoplasm, oval to reniform nuclei, surface hairy projections	Atrophic	Diffuse lymphoid infiltrate, blood lakes	Interstitial and diffuse	CD20+ CD5− CD10− CD23− CD11c+ · CD103+ CD25+ Annexin A1+ CD123+ DBA.44+
Hairy cell leukemia variant	Lymphocytosis, round to indented nuclei, often prominent nucleoli	Atrophic	Diffuse lymphoid infiltrate	Interstitial and diffuse	CD20+ CD5− CD10− CD23− CD11c+ · CD103+ CD25− Annexin A1− CD123− DBA.44+
Splenic diffuse red pulp small B-cell lymphoma	Lymphocytosis, moderate basophilic cytoplasm, condensed chromatin, variable cytoplasmic projections	Atrophic or replaced	Diffuse lymphoid infiltrate	Interstitial, intrasinusoidal, and nodular	CD20+ CD5−/+ CD10− CD23− CD11c+ · CD103−/+ CD25− Annexin A1− CD123− DBA.44+

Abbreviations: −, negative; +, positive.

lymph nodes.[21] The normal counterpart of HCL cells remains uncertain, but the neoplasm is thought to resemble activated memory B cells.[22,23]

CLINICAL FEATURES

Hairy cell leukemia presents in middle-aged to elderly patients, with a median age of approximately 50 years and a male predominance (male-to-female ratio approximately 5:1).[21,24] Presenting symptoms are typically secondary to splenomegaly and cytopenias and may include abdominal pain/fullness, fatigue, or bleeding. There is characteristically a peripheral blood monocytopenia, which may predispose to infection.

DIAGNOSIS: GROSS AND MICROSCOPIC FEATURES

Hairy cells display distinctive cytologic findings in the peripheral blood (**Fig. 7**).[21,24] The cells are small to medium in size, with somewhat eccentrically placed, oval to reniform nuclei. The cytoplasm is blue-gray with a characteristic flocculent appearance, and there are variably prominent cytoplasmic projections (hairs). In most cases, the peripheral blood shows pancytopenia with relatively few circulating neoplastic cells. Many of the neoplastic cells may not show all of the diagnostic cytologic findings. For this reason, a diligent search through the peripheral smear is often required in order to identify cells with classic HCL morphology.

In the bone marrow, there is often prominent reticulin fibrosis, leading to an inaspirable marrow ("dry tap"). When sufficient bone marrow cellularity is present in an aspirate smear, hairy cells are usually identifiable, although the characteristic cytologic features noted in the peripheral blood may be more difficult to appreciate in aspirate smears. In trephine biopsies, there is a variable, interstitial, or diffuse (but not nodular) infiltrate of small lymphocytes with abundant pale to clear cytoplasm (**Fig. 8**). The cytoplasmic borders of the neoplastic cells are often crisply defined, leading to a "fried-egg" appearance. In some cases with less prominent bone marrow involvement, the bone marrow may be hypocellular with few hematopoietic elements and a subtle interstitial lymphoid infiltrate that may lead to misdiagnosis

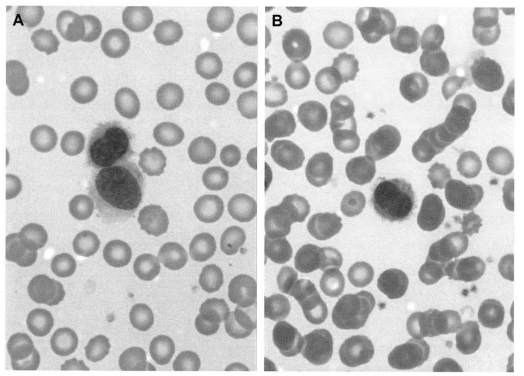

Fig. 7. HCL cells in the peripheral blood (*A* and *B*). Typical hairy cells are small to intermediate in size with eccentrically placed nuclei, indented to reniform nuclei, and prominent cytoplasmic hairy projections.

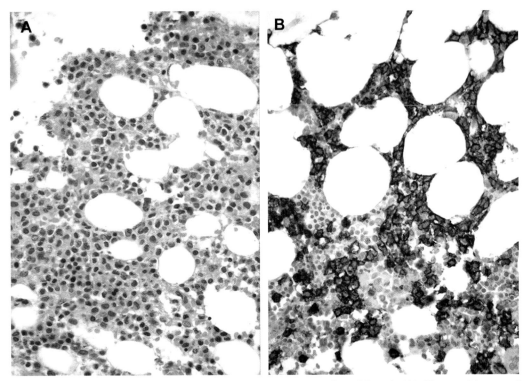

Fig. 8. HCL involving the bone marrow. (*A*) There is a subtle, interstitial small lymphoid infiltrate without nodular lymphoid aggregates. (*B*) A CD20 immunohistochemical stain highlights the extensive interstitial infiltrate of neoplastic B cells.

as aplastic anemia. In such cases, immunohisto-chemical staining for B cells may be necessary to confirm the presence of a neoplastic infiltrate.

On gross examination of splenectomy specimens from HCL patients, the spleen is diffusely enlarged with atrophic white pulp nodules and a prominent red pulp (**Fig. 9**). Due to the marked red pulp expansion, the spleen involved by HCL is often described as having a "beefy red" appearance. Microscopically, HCL involving the spleen exhibits a prominent diffuse red pulp infiltrate of neoplastic cells with atrophic white pulp nodules (**Fig. 10**). The hairy cell infiltrates are typically most prominent in the cords of Billroth, the splenic

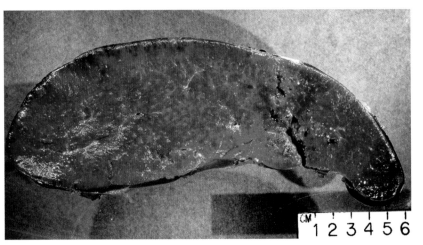

Fig. 9. Spleen involved by HCL. The cut surface displays a homogeneous, dark red appearance with little residual white pulp.

Fig. 10. HCL involving the spleen. There is a diffuse infiltrate of neoplastic cells throughout the red pulp.

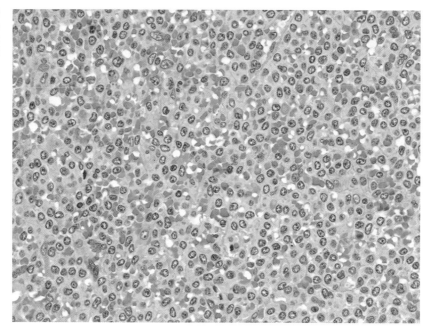

red pulp tissue between the vascular sinusoids. Focal disruption of the splenic sinusoids leads to formation of so-called blood lakes, representing collections of erythrocytes lined by hairy cells (**Fig. 11**). Although widespread lymphadenopathy is distinctly rare in HCL, splenic hilar nodes may be involved, where the hairy cell infiltrates typically grow in the paracortical regions and spare the sinuses; intra-abdominal lymphadenopathy may also occur.

Fig. 11. Blood lake in spleen involved by HCL. The red pulp contains aggregates of erythrocytes that are surrounded by the hairy cells.

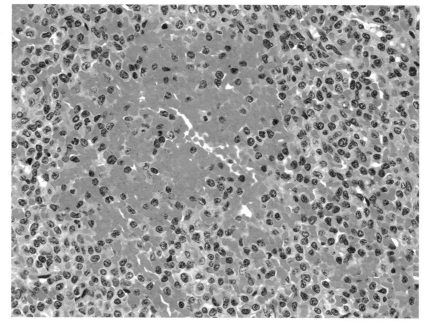

DIAGNOSIS: ANCILLARY STUDIES

Historically, cytochemical staining for tartrate-resistant acid phosphatase (TRAP) was considered an important marker for HCL.[21,24] Interpretation of TRAP stains can be difficult, however: there is often variable staining in the neoplastic cells and a positive result can include cases where only rare neoplastic cells show bright staining. Moreover, TRAP positivity is neither sensitive nor specific for HCL. For these reasons, TRAP cytochemical staining has now largely been replaced by flow cytometry or immunohistochemical staining in the diagnosis of HCL.

Flow cytometry is perhaps the most useful ancillary technique in the diagnosis of HCL. HCL shows bright expression of CD20 and CD22 and shows characteristic bright coexpression of CD11c, CD25, and CD103.[21,24] None of the latter three antigens is seen exclusively in HCL, but the combination of all three is highly sensitive and specific for this diagnosis. More recently, bright expression of CD123 has been also shown a highly sensitive and specific marker for HCL.[25,26] The majority of cases are negative for CD5 and CD10; however, a minority of cases, perhaps 10% overall, may coexpress CD10, and rare CD5-positive cases have also been reported.[27,28] By immunohistochemistry, most cases show positivity for DBA.44, TRAP, annexin A1, and CD123. Cyclin D1 staining, usually weak, is also seen in a majority of cases, although HCL lacks the *IGH-CCND1* translocation seen in mantle cell lymphoma and many cases of plasma cell myeloma.[29] Cytogenetic or fluorescence in situ hybridization studies are of limited value in the work-up of suspected HCL. There are no known characteristic cytogenetic abnormalities in HCL. Such studies, therefore, are useful only in helping exclude other entities from the differential diagnosis.

The diagnosis of HCL is established by demonstrating peripheral blood or bone marrow morphology consistent with hairy cells and an appropriate immunophenotype (as discussed previously). Because the vast majority of cases can be diagnosed by flow cytometry, splenectomy is now only rarely required for diagnosis.

DIFFERENTIAL DIAGNOSIS

The differential diagnosis of HCL includes other mature lymphoid leukemias, such as SMZL, and CLL (see **Table 1**). Immunophenotypic studies, especially flow cytometry of the peripheral blood, can address this differential diagnosis adequately in most cases. Evaluation of bone marrow growth pattern is also useful—the presence of a diffuse growth pattern favors HCL rather than SMZL and a nodular growth pattern essentially excludes a diagnosis of HCL. Cases with morphologic features consistent with HCL that show expression of CD11c and CD103 without CD25 have been considered in the past to represent HCL-V.[30] However, HCL-V is no longer considered biologically closely related to HCL; it remains a controversial diagnosis and is now considered a provisional entity in the 2008 WHO Classification (HCL-V is discussed later).

PROGNOSIS

Due to advances in therapy over the past several decades, the clinical course of HCL has greatly improved and death due to HCL is now uncommon. With current therapies using purine analogs, such as 2-chlorodeoxyadenosine (2-CDA), long-term disease-specific survival of HCL patients is over 95% at 13 years.[31] Late relapses (5 to 10 years after initial therapy and clinical remission) occur in 25% to 50% of patients, but the relapsed disease usually responds to retreatment with purine analogs.[32] Minimal residual disease in treated HCL can be detected using sensitive methods, such as flow cytometry and polymerase chain reaction, and may correlate with disease relapse.[33] However, patients with detectable minimal residual disease may remain in clinical remission for many years. Thus, minimal residual disease is not generally used as an indication for additional therapy in HCL patients in clinical remission.[24]

HAIRY CELL LEUKEMIA VARIANT (PROVISIONAL ENTITY, 2008 WHO CLASSIFICATION)

Hairy cell leukemia variant (HCL-V) is a splenic-based mature lymphoid leukemia with some cytologic and phenotypic resemblance to HCL.[30,34] Despite these similarities, HCL-V is now believed to be biologically unrelated to HCL. HCL-V does not typically respond to HCL-type therapies, such as 2-CDA.[35] HCL-V shares many features in common with another, more recently described mature lymphoid leukemia, known as SDRPSBL, and it is currently unclear whether or not HCL-V and SDRPSBL represent two distinct entities or ends of a spectrum of one biologic entity. For this reason, both HCL-V and SDRPSBL are currently defined as provisional entities in the 2008 WHO classification scheme.[30]

CLINICAL FEATURES

HCL-V presents predominantly in the middle-aged and elderly population, and is reported to occur with a slight male predominance.[30,34] HCL-V is approximately 10 times less common than typical HCL. Patients generally present with spleno-megaly and involvement of the bone marrow and peripheral blood.

DIAGNOSIS: GROSS AND MICROSCOPIC FEATURES

In the peripheral blood, there is usually an absolute lymphocytosis in contrast to the pancytopenia typically observed in HCL.[34,36] The lymphocytes of HCL-V generally resemble those of HCL, with an eccentrically placed, round to indented nucleus and variable cytoplasmic projections or hairs. Unlike HCL, however, the cells of HCL-V frequently display a prominent nucleolus (**Fig. 12**). In the bone marrow, HCL-V is reported to show an interstitial and diffuse growth pattern similar to that of HCL (**Fig. 13**), although there is little detailed data in the literature regarding its bone marrow morphology. In one study of 10 cases,[36] nine displayed a predominantly interstitial or intrasinusoidal growth pattern, whereas one showed a diffuse pattern. There may be mild retic-ulin fibrosis, although unlike HCL, the marrow is usually aspirable.

Similar to typical HCL, HCL-V diffusely involves the splenic red pulp. On gross examination, the spleen cut surface demonstrates a "beefy red" appearance with inconspicuous white pulp. Splenic histology has only rarely been reported in HCL-V and these cases generally show diffuse effacement of the red pulp (**Fig. 14**). In one report of three cases,[36] all cases displayed marked red pulp involvement with obliteration of the white pulp.

DIAGNOSIS: ANCILLARY STUDIES

Hairy cell leukemia variant is positive for pan-B-cell antigens, including CD19, CD20, and CD22, and is generally positive for CD11c and CD103. In contrast to HCL, CD25 and CD123 expression

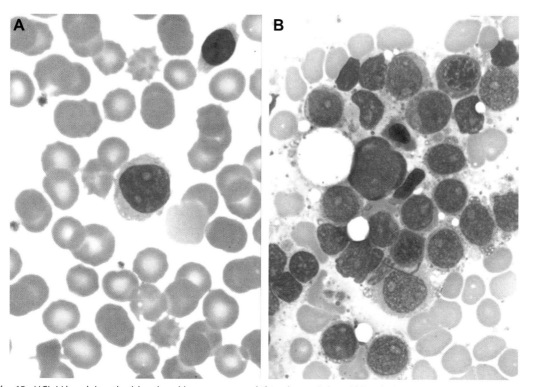

Fig. 12. HCL-V involving the blood and bone marrow. (*A*) In the peripheral blood, the neoplastic cells are small to intermediate in size with uniform, distinct nucleoli, and moderate amounts of cytoplasm. (*B*) Neoplastic cells in the bone marrow aspirate show similar features.

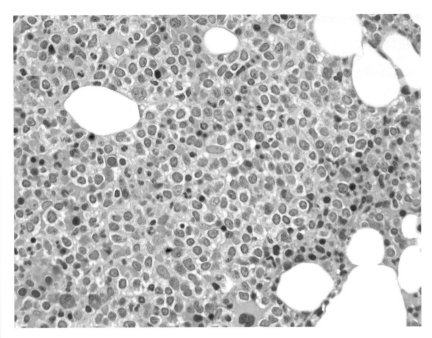

Fig. 13. HCL-V involving the bone marrow. The trephine biopsy (same case as illustrated in **Fig. 12**) shows a diffuse and interstitial infiltrate without nodular lymphoid aggregates. The neoplastic cells contain abundant pale cytoplasm.

are absent.[30,34,36] By cytochemical staining, HCL-V is only weakly positive or negative for TRAP. By immunohistochemistry, annexin A1 and TRAP immuno-histochemistry are negative. On cytogenetic studies, a subset of HCL-V cases is reported to show del(17p) involving the *TP53* locus. As with HCL, however, there are no known specific cytogenetic or molecular abnormalities associated with HCL-V. The diagnosis of HCL-V is best reserved for cases with uniformly nucleolated cells in the peripheral blood, a CD103+, CD11c+, CD25−, CD123− phenotype, and an interstitial, intrasinusoidal and/or diffuse pattern of bone marrow infiltration.

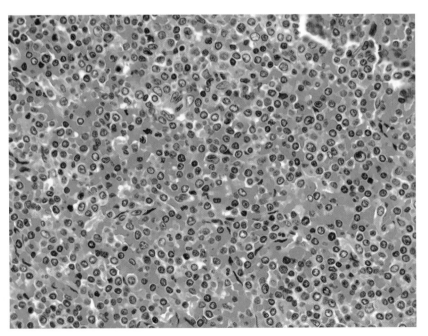

Fig. 14. HCL-V involving the spleen. The splenectomy specimen (same case as illustrated in **Fig. 12**) shows a diffuse infiltrate of neoplastic cells throughout the red pulp. White pulp nodules are absent.

DIFFERENTIAL DIAGNOSIS

The differential diagnosis of HCL-V includes typical HCL, SMZL, and CLL (see **Table 1**). Because of the presence of frequently prominent nucleoli in HCL-V, the diagnosis of prolymphocytic leukemia or blastoid variant of mantle cell lymphoma may also be considered. Flow cytometry is useful in the distinction from CLL, mantle cell lymphoma, and typical HCL. The CD11c+, CD103+, CD25− phenotype of HCL-V is also seen in a subset of cases of SMZL and thus the distinction between SMZL and HCL-V can be challenging. In bone marrow biopsy sections, the finding of reactive germinal centers within a nodular infiltrate is more suggestive of SMZL, whereas a dense, diffuse, sheet-like infiltrate favors a diagnosis of HCL-V. Interstitial and intrasinusoidal patterns of infiltration may be seen in both SMZL and HCL-V, however, and there may be overlapping cytology of the neoplastic cells in the peripheral blood. In such cases, splenic histology is required to make this distinction. The differential diagnosis with SDRPSBL is even more challenging (discussed later).

PROGNOSIS

Patients with HCL-V generally do not respond to purine nucleoside analogs, such as those used to treat typical HCL.[34,35] Nevertheless, HCL-V is reported to usually follow an indolent clinical course, with responses to single agent monoclonal antibody therapy or splenectomy.

SPLENIC DIFFUSE RED PULP SMALL B-CELL LYMPHOMA (PROVISIONAL ENTITY, 2008 WHO CLASSIFICATION)

Splenic diffuse red pulp small B-cell lymphoma (SDRPSBL) is a recently described, uncommon lymphoproliferative disorder currently recognized as a provisional entity in the 2008 WHO classification.[17,30,37] As discussed previously, SDRPSBL seems to show substantial overlap with cases of HCL-V and it is currently unclear whether or not the two truly represent separate diseases. Due to ongoing controversies about the boundaries of SDRPSBL and HCL-V, these diagnoses should be rendered cautiously.

CLINICAL FEATURES

Splenic diffuse red pulp small B-cell lymphoma (SDRPSBL) arises in middle-aged to elderly populations, with a median age of 77 reported in the largest series and with a male predominance (male-to-female ratio 1.6:1). Patients typically present with splenomegaly and peripheral blood lymphocytosis. A minority of cases may present with anemia and thrombocytopenia.

DIAGNOSIS: GROSS AND MICROSCOPIC FEATURES

The peripheral blood frequently shows an absolute lymphocytosis with distinctive cytology: the lymphoid cells are small with moderate amounts of somewhat basophilic cytoplasm, condensed chromatin, and cytoplasmic projections (**Fig. 15**).[17,30,37] The cytoplasmic projections may mimic the hairy cells of HCL, but the lymphocytes display a more condensed chromatin and more basophilic cytoplasm than is seen in HCL. Prominent nucleoli, a characteristic feature of HCL-V, are seen in only occasional cases of reported SDRPSBCL. The bone marrow is involved in all cases of SDRPSBL, with an interstitial or intrasinusoidal growth pattern (**Fig. 16**).[17,37,38] A marked or exclusively intrasinusoidal pattern frequently coincides with particularly prominent peripheral blood lymphocytosis. Nodules may be present, but germinal centers, as may be seen in the nodules of SMZL, are not identified. The spleen in SDRPSBL is grossly involved by a marked red pulp expansion, similar to that noted in gross specimens involved by HCL or HCL-V. By definition, the spleen contains a dense infiltrate within the red pulp that expands the red pulp (**Fig. 17**).[38] Little residual white pulp is identified. Blood lakes similar to those noted in HCL are described in a minority of cases.

DIAGNOSIS: ANCILLARY STUDIES

Splenic diffuse red pulp small B-cell lymphoma (SDRPSBL) is positive for pan-B-cell antigens and shows surface immunoglobulin light chain restriction by flow cytometry. CD11c is expressed in the great majority of cases (>90%), with a minority of cases showing coexpression of CD103 (38%), CD123 (16%), and/or CD5 (14%).[17] In distinction from HCL, annexin A1 is negative by immunohistochemistry. By conventional cytogenetic studies, most cases display a normal karyotype.[17] Recurrent abnormalities described in a minority of cases of SDRPSBL include del(7q), trisomy 18, and trisomy 3/3q. Translocation t(11;14)(q13;q32) that characterizes mantle cell lymphoma is absent.

The diagnosis of SDRPSBL currently requires the integration of peripheral blood cytologic features, phenotypic studies, bone marrow histology and splenic histology. This diagnosis should not be rendered on the basis of peripheral blood or bone

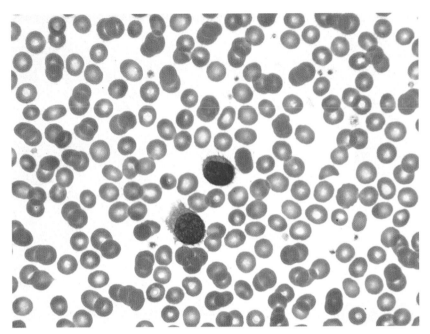

Fig. 15. SDRPSBCL cells in the peripheral blood. This case displays small lymphocytes resembling those of SMZL. Ancillary studies demonstrated a CD11c+, CD25−, CD103− phenotype by flow cytometry and an isolated del(7q) by conventional cytogenetic analysis.

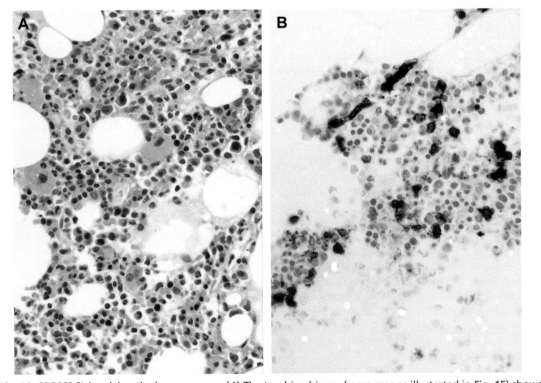

Fig. 16. SDRPSBCL involving the bone marrow. (*A*) The trephine biopsy (same case as illustrated in **Fig. 15**) shows a sparse, subtle interstitial lymphoid infiltrate. (*B*) A CD20 immunohistochemical stain highlights increased scattered neoplastic B cells with a partially intrasinusoidal growth pattern (two linear cell arrays in upper part of panel).

Fig. 17. SDRPSBCL involving the spleen. The splenectomy specimen (same case as illustrated in **Fig. 15**) shows a diffuse infiltrate of neoplastic cells throughout the red pulp. The white pulp is obliterated by the neoplastic infiltrate.

marrow studies alone. In the absence of splenic histology, an appropriate differential diagnosis should be provided. A definitive diagnosis may not be necessary for current therapeutic management: once a diagnosis of typical HCL is excluded, cases of SMZL, HCL-V, and SDRPSBL are typically managed in a similar fashion.

DIFFERENTIAL DIAGNOSIS

The differential diagnosis in SDRPSBL includes CLL, HCL, SMZL, and HCL-V (see **Table 1**). Cases of CLL should exhibit characteristic lymphocyte cytology, with heavily condensed chromatin and a CD5+, CD23+ phenotype in most cases. A minority of cases of SDRPSBL are reported to express either CD5 or CD23 or, in rare cases, both. In these cases, the lack of proliferation centers in histologic sections of spleen or lymph node argues against a diagnosis of CLL. The characteristic cytoplasmic projections observed in the lymphocytes of SDRPSBL may suggest the possibility of HCL, but flow cytometric studies distinguish between these two entities: all cases of HCL are positive for the combination of CD11c, CD103, CD25, and CD123, whereas SDRPSBL is

usually positive for CD11c but only occasionally positive for the other markers and never positive for all of the typical HCL markers. The differential diagnosis with SMZL is difficult because of overlapping cytologic features, similar bone marrow growth patterns, identical immunophenotypic profiles, and similar cytogenetic findings. These similarities have suggested that SDRPSBL might be considered a diffuse variant of SMZL. The distinction between SDRPSBL and SMZL is best established by the histologic features in the spleen, where SMZL displays a typical white pulp nodular growth pattern, whereas SDRPSBL by definition grows diffusely throughout the red pulp. The distinction between SDRPSBL and HCL-V is, as discussed previously, still controversial. Currently, a diagnosis of HCL-V is favored in cases that exhibit prominent nucleoli in peripheral blood lymphocytes, especially when CD11c and CD103 are coexpressed. The absence of prominent nucleoli may favor a diagnosis of SDRPSBL.

PROGNOSIS

There are few published data regarding long-term follow-up of patients with SDRPSBL, because this is a recently described entity.[17,30,37] From the available data, the clinical course seems indolent in most patients.

DIFFUSE LARGE B-CELL LYMPHOMA

Diffuse large B-cell lymphoma (DLBCL) is reported to be the most common form of lymphoma encountered in splenectomy specimens, representing up to half of splenic lymphomas in some series.[39,40] DLBCL identified in the spleen often represents secondary dissemination of a systemic lymphoma or transformation of an underlying low-grade B-cell lymphoma, analogous to a Richter transformation in CLL/SLL. DLBCL may also occur as a primary splenic lymphoma. The distinction between primary and secondary splenic DLBCL is made entirely on the basis of clinical presentation, because there are no known morphologic, phenotypic, or genetic findings specific for primary splenic DLBCL.

CLINICAL FEATURES

Primary splenic DLBCL presents in adulthood, with most cases arising in patients over 50 years of age.[41] Symptoms are related to hypersplenism, including abdominal pain and peripheral blood cytopenias. Some patients may present with B symptoms.

DIAGNOSIS: GROSS AND MICROSCOPIC FEATURES

On gross examination of the splenectomy specimen, most cases display a so-called macronodular pattern, with one or more gross mass lesions that disrupt and replace the splenic architecture (**Fig. 18**). In a subset of cases, a micronodular pattern is observed, where the neoplastic cells form enlarged white pulp nodules throughout the spleen in the absence of a gross confluent mass lesion. This micronodular pattern is similar to that seen in some primary splenic small B-cell lymphomas, such as SMZL.[41,42]

In cases with a macronodular growth pattern, the mass lesions are composed of diffuse sheets of large lymphoid cells that disrupt and replace the usual splenic architecture (**Fig. 19**).[41] The surrounding splenic parenchyma is typically uninvolved, with unremarkable microscopic morphology. Cases with this pattern generally resemble typical nodal DLBCLs. In cases with a micronodular pattern, there are many enlarged white pulp nodules that contain variable numbers of large, transformed B cells (**Fig. 20**).[41,42] Some of the micronodular cases contain relatively few large, atypical B cells surrounded by many small CD3+ cells forming the nodules. These cases are histologically similar to nodal cases of T-cell/ histiocyte-rich large B-cell lymphoma and have been reported as micronodular T-cell-rich large B-cell lymphoma of the spleen. Some investigators have proposed that these latter cases may

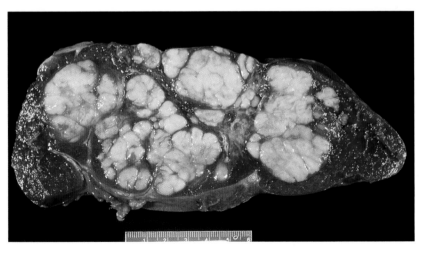

Fig. 18. DLBCL involving the spleen. Cross-sectioning identifies multiple distinct tumoral mass lesions. The surrounding, uninvolved splenic parenchyma is grossly unremarkable. (*Photo courtesy of* Dr R. Hasserjian.)

Fig. 19. DLBCL involving the spleen. Involved regions show diffuse sheets of large lymphocytes with vesicular nuclei and prominent nucleoli.

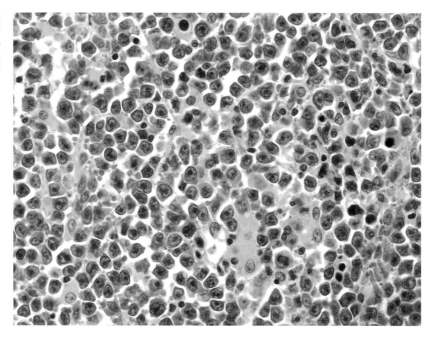

represent a distinct clinicopathologic entity.[42] Other cases contain micronodules composed predominantly of neoplastic CD20+ cells with few T cells. Rare cases of splenic DLBCLs with diffuse involvement of the splenic red pulp have also been reported.[43,44] It is currently unclear whether or not these may represent a variant of intravascular large B-cell lymphoma.

DIAGNOSIS: ANCILLARY STUDIES

Splenic DLBCLs, including both macronodular and micronodular types, are positive for pan-B-cell antigens, such as CD20 and CD79a. Clonality can generally be demonstrated by flow cytometry or by *IGH* gene rearrangement studies. As with primary nodal DLBCLs, the phenotypic profile of splenic large B-cell lymphomas is heterogeneous. Germinal center markers, including CD10 and BCL6, are expressed in a subset of cases. Most cases reported as micronodular T-cell-rich large B-cell lymphoma exhibit a CD20+, CD10−, BCL6+ phenotype. Micronodular cases show a lack of CD21+ follicular dendritic cells within

the tumor nodules.[41,42] There is little cytogenetic information available regarding splenic DLBCLs.

The diagnosis of splenic DLBCL is established by recognizing large, atypical B cells that grow in either macronodular, grossly apparent tumoral mass lesions or in a miliary fashion as many micronodules throughout the white pulp. A lack of follicular dendritic cells by CD21 immunohistochemistry confirms the diffuse growth pattern and excludes the possibility of FL.

DIFFERENTIAL DIAGNOSIS

In most macronodular cases, the diagnosis of splenic DLBCL is straightforward. Lack of cyclin D1 expression is helpful in excluding a blastoid mantle cell lymphoma, which may resemble DLBCL morphologically. In cases with a micronodular growth pattern, the differential diagnosis is usually broader. In cases with T-cell-rich micronodules, the differential diagnosis includes nodular lymphocyte-predominant Hodgkin lymphoma (NLPHL). The lack of CD21 staining within the nodules and the lack of characteristically lobulated "popcorn cell" morphology of the

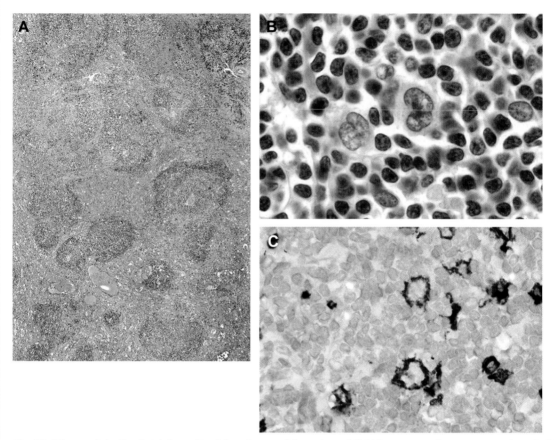

Fig. 20. Micronodular T-cell-rich large B-cell lymphoma of the spleen. (*A*) At low power, there are many lymphoid nodules within the white pulp. (*B*) At high power, the nodules contain small lymphocytes and occasional scattered large, atypical cells. (*C*) The large atypical cells, but not the surrounding small lymphocytes, are positive for CD20 by immunohistochemical staining.

large neoplastic cells help exclude a diagnosis of NLPHL. In cases with micronodules containing many large B cells, the possibility of FL or SMZL with increased large cells could be considered. The lack of CD21 staining within the nodules excludes FL, whereas a lack of distinct marginal zone cytologic differentiation or a biphasic nodular pattern argues against a diagnosis of SMZL.

PROGNOSIS

There are few data in the literature concerning survival of patients with primary splenic DLBCL treated with modern combination chemotherapy. Overall, the prognosis of splenic DLBCL seems similar to that reported for nodal DLBCL, with a majority of patients alive after 5 years.[41] Cases

Pitfalls

SPLENIC B-CELL LYMPHOMAS AND LEUKEMIAS

! Prominent marginal zones may be seen in reactive white pulp nodules, such as in some cases of idiopathic thrombocytopenic purpura: flow cytometry studies are useful to evaluate for B-cell clonality in any enlarged spleen.

! Cytochemical TRAP staining alone is insufficient for diagnosis of HCL and is not a substitute for immunophenotyping.

! Cells with classic hairy cell morphology may be rare in the peripheral blood of patients with HCL, even in the presence of extensive bone marrow and splenic disease.

! Micronodular T-cell-rich large B-cell lymphomas of the spleen may be easily confused with a reactive infiltrate: recognition of scattered, large neoplastic B cells on immunohistochemical stains facilitates diagnosis.

! The presence of an intrasinusoidal growth pattern is characteristic of SMZL but may also be seen in other B-cell lymphoproliferative disorders.

! Deletions of chromosome 7q are the most common cytogenetic abnormality in SMZL, but this abnormality is neither sensitive nor specific for SMZL.

! A minority of cases of SMZL can display an atypical phenotypic profile, with expression of CD5 or, rarely, CD10.

of micronodular T-cell-rich large B-cell lymphoma of the spleen may display a more aggressive clinical course.[41,42]

REFERENCES

1. Oscier D, Owen R, Johnson S. Splenic marginal zone lymphoma. Blood Rev 2005;19:39–51.

2. Isaacson PG, Piris MA, Berger F, et al. Splenic B-cell marginal zone lymphoma. In: Swerdlow SH, Campo E, Harris NL, et al, editors. WHO classification of tumours of haematopoietic and lymphoid tissues. Lyon (France): IARC Press; 2008. p. 185–7.

3. Bahler DW, Pindzola JA, Swerdlow SH. Splenic marginal zone lymphomas appear to originate from different B cell types. Am J Pathol 2002;161:81–8.

4. Morse HC 3rd, Kearney JF, Isaacson PG, et al. Cells of the marginal zone—origins, function and neoplasia. Leuk Res 2001;25:169–78.

5. Matutes E, Oscier D, Montalban C, et al. Splenic marginal zone lymphoma proposals for a revision of diagnostic, staging and therapeutic criteria. Leukemia 2008;22:487–95.

6. Mollejo M, Menarguez J, Lloret E, et al. Splenic marginal zone lymphoma: a distinctive type of low-grade B-cell lymphoma. A clinicopathological study of 13 cases. Am J Surg Pathol 1995;19:1146–57.

7. Berger F, Felman P, Thieblemont C, et al. Non-MALT marginal zone B-cell lymphomas: a description of clinical presentation and outcome in 124 patients. Blood 2000;95:1950–6.

8. Viswanatha DS, Dogan A. Hepatitis C virus and lymphoma. J Clin Pathol 2007;60:1378–83.

9. Matutes E. Splenic marginal zone lymphoma with and without villous lymphocytes. Curr Treat Options Oncol 2007;8:109–16.

10. Melo JV, Robinson DS, Gregory C, et al. Splenic B cell lymphoma with "villous" lymphocytes in the peripheral blood: a disorder distinct from hairy cell leukemia. Leukemia 1987;1:294–8.

11. Franco V, Florena AM, Campesi G. Intrasinusoidal bone marrow infiltration: a possible hallmark of splenic lymphoma. Histopathology 1996;29:571–5.

12. Papadaki T, Stamatopoulos K, Belessi C, et al. Splenic marginal-zone lymphoma: one or more entities? A histologic, immunohistochemical, and molecular study of 42 cases. Am J Surg Pathol 2007;31:438–46.

13. Dufresne SD, Felgar RE, Sargent RL, et al. Defining the borders of splenic marginal zone lymphoma: a multiparameter study. Hum Pathol 2010;41:540–51.

14. Watkins AJ, Huang Y, Ye H, et al. Splenic marginal zone lymphoma: characterization of 7q deletion and its value in diagnosis. J Pathol 2010;220:461–74.

15. Mateo M, Mollejo M, Villuendas R, et al. 7q31-32 allelic loss is a frequent finding in splenic marginal zone lymphoma. Am J Pathol 1999;154:1583–9.

16. Sole F, Salido M, Espinet B, et al. Splenic marginal zone B-cell lymphomas: two cytogenetic subtypes, one with gain of 3q and the other with loss of 7q. Haematologica 2001;86:71–7.

17. Traverse-Glehen A, Baseggio L, Bauchu EC, et al. Splenic red pulp lymphoma with numerous basophilic villous lymphocytes: a distinct clinicopathologic and molecular entity? Blood 2008;111:2253–60.

18. Howard MT, Dufresne S, Swerdlow SH, et al. Follicular lymphoma of the spleen: multiparameter analysis of 16 cases. Am J Clin Pathol 2009;131:656–62.

19. Mollejo M, Rodriquez MS, Montes S, et al. Splenic follicular lymphomas. A clinicopathologic study of 33 cases. Mod Pathol 2008;21:266A.

20. Baseggio L, Traverse-Glehen A, Petinataud F, et al. CD5 expression identifies a subset of splenic marginal

zone lymphomas with higher lymphocytosis: a clinico-pathological, cytogenetic and molecular study of 24 cases. Haematologica 2010;95:604–12.

21. Foucar K, Falini B, Catovsky D, et al. Hairy cell leukemia. In: Swerdlow SH, Campo E, Harris NL, et al, editors. WHO classification tumours of the haematopoietic and lymphoid tissues. Lyon (France): IARC Press; 2008. p. 188–90.

22. Weston-Bell N, Townsend M, Di Genova G, et al. Defining origins of malignant B cells: a new circulating normal human IgM(+)D(+) B-cell subset lacking CD27 expression and displaying somatically mutated IGHV genes as a relevant memory population. Leukemia 2009;23:2075–80.

23. Cawley JC, Hawkins SF. The biology of hairy-cell leukaemia. Curr Opin Hematol 2010;17(4):341–9.

24. Sharpe RW, Bethel KJ. Hairy cell leukemia: diagnostic pathology. Hematol Oncol Clin North Am 2006;20:1023–49.

25. Munoz L, Nomdedeu JF, Lopez O, et al. Interleukin-3 receptor alpha chain (CD123) is widely expressed in hematologic malignancies. Haematologica 2001;86:1261–9.

26. Del Giudice I, Matutes E, Morilla R, et al. The diagnostic value of CD123 in B-cell disorders with hairy or villous lymphocytes. Haematologica 2004;89:303–8.

27. Jasionowski TM, Hartung L, Greenwood JH, et al. Analysis of CD10+ hairy cell leukemia. Am J Clin Pathol 2003;120:228–35.

28. Chen YH, Tallman MS, Goolsby C, et al. Immunophenotypic variations in hairy cell leukemia. Am J Clin Pathol 2006;125:251–9.

29. Miranda RN, Briggs RC, Kinney MC, et al. Immunohistochemical detection of cyclin D1 using optimized conditions is highly specific for mantle cell lymphoma and hairy cell leukemia. Mod Pathol 2000;13:1308–14.

30. Piris MA, Foucar K, Mollejo M, et al. Splenic B-cell lymphoma/leukemia, unclassifiable. In: Swerdlow SH, Campo E, Harris NL, et al, editors. WHO classification of tumours of haematopoietic and lymphoid tissues. Lyon (France): IARC Press; 2008. p. 191–3.

31. Zinzani PL, Tani M, Marchi E, et al. Long-term follow-up of front-line treatment of hairy cell leukemia with 2-chlorodeoxyadenosine. Haematologica 2004;89:309–13.

32. Else M, Ruchlemer R, Osuji N, et al. Long remissions in hairy cell leukemia with purine analogs: a report of 219 patients with a median follow-up of 12.5 years. Cancer 2005;104:2442–8.

33. Sausville JE, Salloum RG, Sorbara L, et al. Minimal residual disease detection in hairy cell leukemia. Comparison of flow cytometric immunophenotyping with clonal analysis using consensus primer polymerase chain reaction for the heavy chain gene. Am J Clin Pathol 2003;119:213–7.

34. Matutes E, Wotherspoon A, Catovsky D. The variant form of hairy-cell leukaemia. Best Pract Res Clin Haematol 2003;16:41–56.

35. Robak T. Current treatment options in hairy cell leukemia and hairy cell leukemia variant. Cancer Treat Rev 2006;32:365–76.

36. Cessna MH, Hartung L, Tripp S, et al. Hairy cell leukemia variant: fact or fiction. Am J Clin Pathol 2005;123:132–8.

37. Mollejo M, Algara P, Mateo MS, et al. Splenic small B-cell lymphoma with predominant red pulp involvement: a diffuse variant of splenic marginal zone lymphoma? Histopathology 2002;40:22–30.

38. Kanellis G, Mollejo M, Montes-Moreno S, et al. Splenic diffuse red pulp small B-cell lymphoma: revision of a series of cases reveals characteristic clinico-pathological features. Haematologica 2010;95(7):1122–9.

39. Kraemer BB, Osborne BM, Butler JJ. Primary splenic presentation of malignant lymphoma and related disorders. A study of 49 cases. Cancer 1984;54:1606–19.

40. Arber DA, Rappaport H, Weiss LM. Non-Hodgkin's lymphoproliferative disorders involving the spleen. Mod Pathol 1997;10:18–32.

41. Mollejo M, Algara P, Mateo MS, et al. Large B-cell lymphoma presenting in the spleen: identification of different clinicopathologic conditions. Am J Surg Pathol 2003;27:895–902.

42. Dogan A, Burke JS, Goteri G, et al. Micronodular T-cell/histiocyte-rich large B-cell lymphoma of the spleen: histology, immunophenotype, and differential diagnosis. Am J Surg Pathol 2003;27:903–11.

43. Kashimura M, Noro M, Akikusa B, et al. Primary splenic diffuse large B-cell lymphoma manifesting in red pulp. Virchows Arch 2008;453:501–9.

44. Morice WG, Rodriguez FJ, Hoyer JD, et al. Diffuse large B-cell lymphoma with distinctive patterns of splenic and bone marrow involvement: clinicopathologic features of two cases. Mod Pathol 2005;18:495–502.

DIAGNOSIS OF NODAL PERIPHERAL T-CELL LYMPHOMAS

Matthew Howard, MD[a],*, Ahmet Dogan, MD, PhD[b]

KEYWORDS

- T-cell lymphoma • Angioimmunoblastic • Anaplastic large cell lymphoma
- Lymph node hyperplasia

ABSTRACT

Lymph node-based peripheral T-cell lymphomas are rare and exhibit a morphologic spectrum that overlaps with reactive lymphoid hyperplasia, B-cell lymphomas, and Hodgkin lymphoma, presenting a diagnostic challenge. This review focuses on the major categories of lymph node-based peripheral T-cell lymphomas recognized by the 2008 World Health Organization Classification of Tumours of Haematopoietic and Lymphoid Tissues. Diagnostic strategies for approaching T-cell neoplasms using a combined clinical, morphologic, immunophenotypic, and genetic approach are presented. Practical information to aid in distinguishing peripheral T-cell lymphomas from other hematologic malignancies and benign conditions is provided.

ANGIOIMMUNOBLASTIC T-CELL LYMPHOMA

OVERVIEW

The disease currently recognized as angioimmunoblastic T-cell lymphoma (AITL) was first described in the 1970s as a clinical syndrome characterized by generalized lymphadenopathy, hepatosplenomegaly, anemia, and hypergammaglobulinemia.[1–3] It was initially described using a variety of terms, including immunoblastic lymphadenopathy, lymphogranulomatosis X, and angioimmunoblastic lymphadenopathy with dysproteinemia; the latter term has now come to define the clinical syndrome found in patients with AITL.

Key Features
ANGIOIMMUNOBLASTIC T-CELL LYMPHOMA

1. Three possible architectural patterns

   Pattern I: Partial preservation of the lymph node architecture

   Pattern II: Loss of normal architecture except for the presence of occasional depleted follicles with concentrically arranged follicular dendritic cells.

   Pattern III: Normal architecture completely effaced; no B-cell follicles are identified

2. Paracortical polymorphic infiltrate of lymphocytes, transformed large lymphoid cells, plasma cells, macrophages, and eosinophils within a prominent vascular network

3. Neoplastic T cells typically intermediate in size with round centroblast-like nuclei and abundant pale cytoplasm

CLINICAL FEATURES

AITL is one of the most common types of peripheral T-cell lymphoma (PTCL). It accounts for 15% to 20% of all T-cell lymphomas and 1% to 2% of all non-Hodgkin lymphomas. No geographic predilection or race bias has been identified. AITL affects men more than women (male-to-female ratio 1.5:1).[4] The patients typically present in the seventh decade (median age of presentation is 52 years) but rarely it may affect

[a] Division of Hematopathology, Department of Laboratory Medicine and Pathology, Mayo Clinic, 200 First Street SW, Rochester, MN 55905, USA

[b] Division of Anatomic Pathology, Department of Laboratory Medicine and Pathology, Mayo Clinic, 200 First Street SW, Rochester, MN 55905, USA

* Corresponding author.
E-mail address: Howard.Matthew@mayo.edu

Surgical Pathology 3 (2010) 955–988
doi:10.1016/j.path.2010.09.001

surgpath.theclinics.com

patients as young as 20 years. Patients commonly present with generalized lymphadenopathy and involvement of extranodal sites, such as the lungs, skin, or bone marrow. More than half of patients present with a systemic syndrome characterized by elevated lactate dehydrogenase, anemia with a positive direct antiglobulin test, and hypergammaglobulinemia.

DIAGNOSIS: MICROSCOPIC FEATURES

On microscopic examination, AITL demonstrates partial effacement of the lymph node architecture by a polymorphic infiltrate, which is found predominantly within the paracortical areas. The architectural changes in AITL fall into three overlapping patterns, which may reflect temporal progression of the disease.[5]

In pattern I (15% of the cases), there is partial preservation of the lymph node architecture. Hyperplastic B-cell follicles with poorly developed mantle zones and ill-defined borders are easily identified within the cortex of the lymph node and merge into the expanded paracortex that contains a polymorphic infiltrate of lymphocytes, large immunoblasts, plasma cells, macrophages, and eosinophils within a prominent vascular network.

Pattern II (25% of the cases) demonstrates loss of normal architecture except for the presence of occasional depleted follicles with concentrically arranged follicular dendritic cells (FDCs) (Fig. 1). FDC proliferation extending beyond the follicles can sometimes be identified and may be highlighted by CD21 and/or CD23 immunostains (Fig. 2). The remainder of the lymph node shows a polymorphic infiltrate with increased numbers of immunoblasts and vascular proliferation similar to that found in pattern I.

In pattern III (60% of the cases), the normal architecture is completely effaced by neoplastic T cells; B-cell follicles are absent (Fig. 3). As with pattern I, prominent irregular proliferation of FDCs can be seen in routine sections in some cases. Generally, extensive vascular proliferation and a polymorphic infiltrate similar to that seen in patterns I and II can also be identified. There may seem to be a transition from pattern I to pattern III in serial biopsies as the neoplastic process progresses, although any pattern may be present in a given biopsy.

The neoplastic T-cell infiltrate in AITL is typically composed of intermediate-sized T cells with round centroblast-like nuclei and abundant pale to clear cytoplasm. In approximately half of the cases, the neoplastic cells occur as perivascular or perifollicular collections of atypical medium to large-sized lymphocytes with pale cytoplasm.[6] Cytologic features of malignancy may not be obvious, however, and are easily overlooked. In approximately one-third of cases, the neoplastic T cells are accompanied by a B-cell component. The B-cell component may have a wide range of morphologic features, including reactive immunoblastic hyperplasia and plasmacytosis, or may mimic classical Hodgkin lymphoma by acquiring Reed-Sternberg (RS)-like morphology.

Generalized lymphadenopathy is often the main presenting sign in patients with AITL, and the diagnosis rests on histologic examination of an involved lymph node; however, many patients also have extranodal and/or bone marrow involvement at the time of diagnosis. The histologic appearances in these extranodal sites are usually nonspecific but can share features with the nodal disease, such as increased vascularity and a polymorphous inflammatory infiltrate. Cytologic features of malignancy in such extranodal sites of AITL are rarely identified and tumor involvement often can only be shown by immunohistochemistry and molecular clonality analysis.[7,8]

DIAGNOSIS: ANCILLARY STUDIES

Immunohistochemistry shows the expansion of the interfollicular areas by a diffuse infiltrate of CD3+ T cells, which predominantly coexpress CD4 (see Fig. 2A, B). A subpopulation of benign, reactive CD8+ cells may also be intermixed. B-cell markers, such as CD20 and CD79a, highlight the residual follicle center and mantle zone B cells as well as many of the large transformed immunoblasts in the interfollicular areas (see Fig. 2E and Fig. 3D). These B cells can be numerous, to the extent of mimicking a large B-cell lymphoma or classical Hodgkin lymphoma, although they usually are polytypic in their expression of surface immunoglobulin light chains. An important immunophenotypic feature in AITL is the expansion of the FDC meshworks, which typically surround the paracortical small vessels. This occasionally may be observed on hematoxylin-eosin sections but often requires staining for FDC markers, such as CD21, by immunohistochemistry (see Fig. 2F and Fig. 3E).

Immunophenotyping of the neoplastic T cells in AITL is difficult, because in many cases the neoplastic cells are not readily identifiable. Gene expression profiling studies have recently shown that the neoplastic cells of AITL express several markers characteristic of follicular helper T cells (T_{FH} cells), such as CD10, CXCL13, and PD1 (CD279) (see Fig. 2C, D and Fig. 3C).[9–11] CD10 is not expressed by normal peripheral T cells except for T_{FH} cells, which represent a small subset of all T cells. Expression of CD10 is highly specific for AITL, because other nodal PTCLs

Fig. 1. Microscopic features of AITL, pattern II. The lymph node architecture is largely effaced by an infiltrate of intermediate-sized cells with abundant pale cytoplasm (*A, B*) (*A,* H&E, ×40, *B,* H&E, ×400).

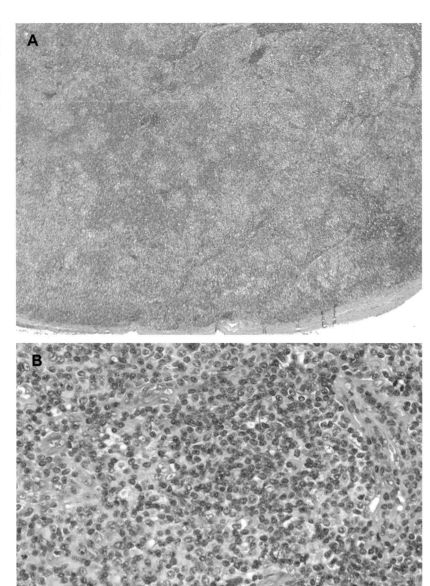

rarely express this antigen.[6,12] CXCL13 and PD1 have a more broad expression profile. CXCL13 is expressed not only by T$_{FH}$ cells but also by FDCs.[9] PD1 is strongly expressed by most T$_{FH}$ cells but also weakly by paracortical T cells.[13] CD10 may provide the highest specificity but has a lower sensitivity; PD1 provides higher sensitivity but lower specificity for identifying the neoplastic cells of AITL.[14] Therefore, using at least two of these T$_{FH}$ markers is prudent.

The neoplastic cells in AITL account for a relatively small portion of the infiltrate in the earliest cases (pattern I). The neoplastic T cells in these early cases are intimately related to the residual reactive B-cell follicles and the expanded FDC meshworks. Some of the neoplastic cells are located within the follicle centers, whereas others surround the follicles. As the neoplastic process progresses (patterns II and III), the tumor cells spill into the interfollicular area but still remain

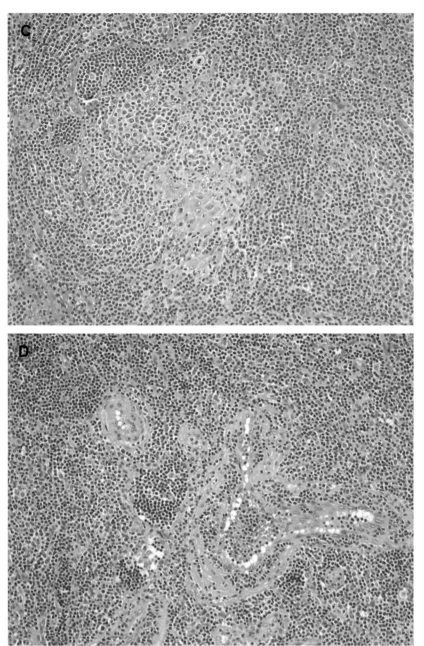

Fig. 1. Microscopic features of AITL, pattern II. Occasional depleted follicles are noted (*C*) (H&E, ×200), along with a proliferation of high endothelial venules (*D*) (H&E, ×200).

associated with the FDC meshworks. This suggests that the FDC microenvironment may be important in neoplastic growth and progression.

Virtually all cases of AITL contain increased numbers of Epstein-Barr virus (EBV)-infected cells with immunoblastic or RS-like morphology (see **Fig. 3**F). Double immunolabeling suggests that these EBV-infected cells are B cells; there is no convincing evidence for EBV infection in the neoplastic T cells.[15] The presence of morphologic and immunophenotypic characteristics of AITL, such as vascular proliferation, atypical cellular infiltrates, FDC proliferation, an EBV-positive B-cell component, and expression of T_{FH} differentiation markers (CD10, CXCL13, and/or PD1), favor a diagnosis of AITL. Nevertheless, approximately 10% of all nodal T-cell neoplasms exhibit overlapping features between PTCL, not otherwise specified (PTCL, NOS) and AITL. In such cases, a definitive diagnosis may not be possible.[16,17]

Fig. 2. Typical immuno-histochemical findings in AITL, pattern II. The neoplastic cells express CD3 (*A*) (×200), CD4 (*B*) (×200), and the T_{FH} markers, CD10 (*C*) (×200) and CXCL13 (*D*, next page) (×200).

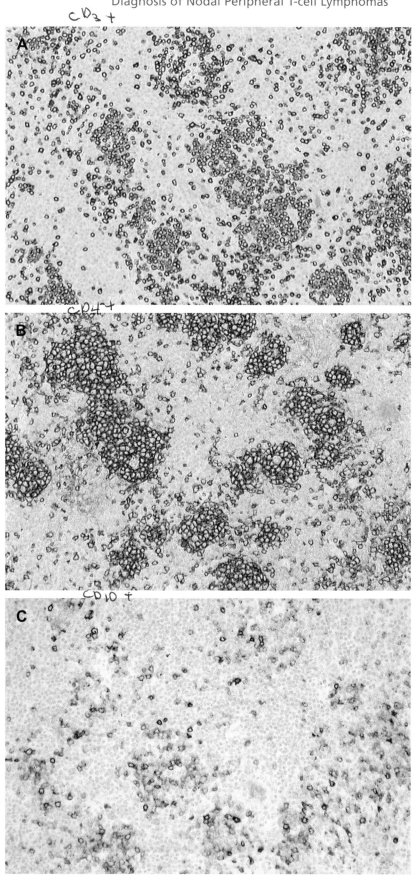

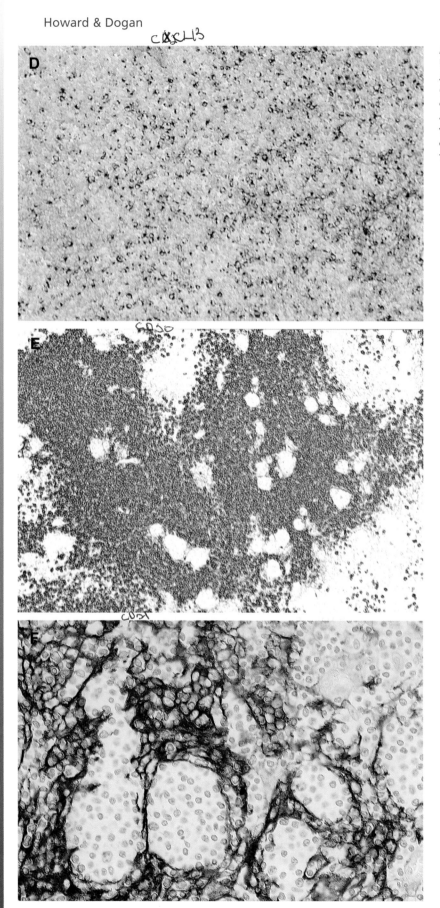

Fig. 2. Typical immuno-histochemical findings in AITL, pattern II. CD20 (*E*) (×100) highlights aggregates of B cells, which are expanded along with follicular dendric cell networks that stain for CD21 (*F*) (×400).

Fig. 3. AITL, pattern III. The lymph node architecture is entirely effaced; no residual follicles are present (*A*) (H&E, ×100). By immunohistochemistry, the infiltrate is composed of CD3 positive T cells (*B*) (×100), which coexpress CD10 (*C*) (×400).

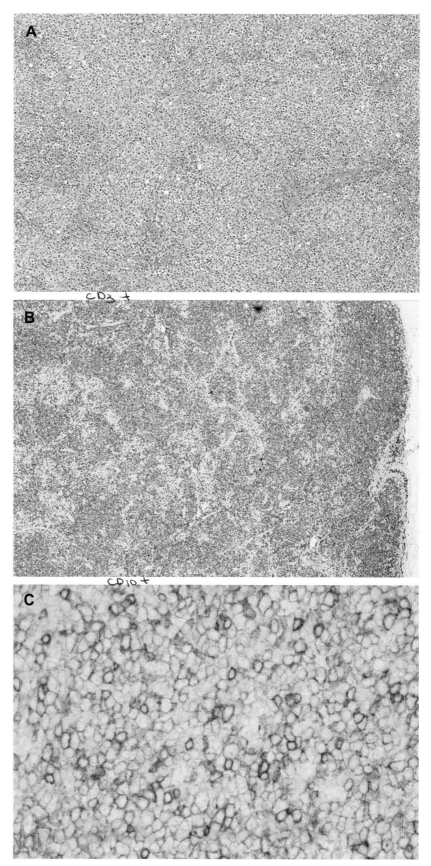

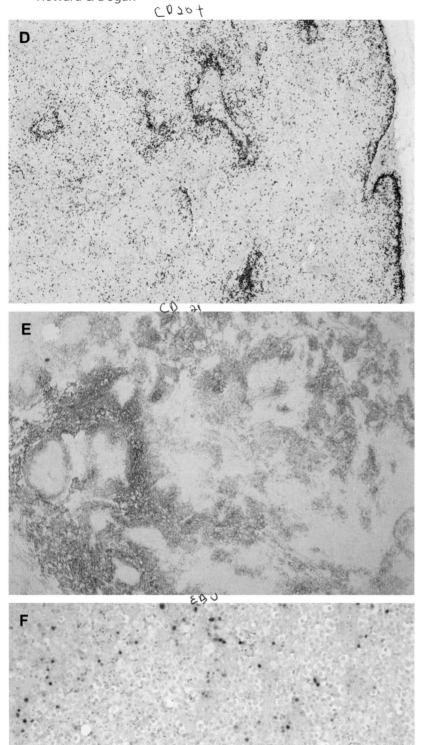

Fig. 3. AITL, pattern III. (*D*) CD20 highlights residual non-neoplastic B cells, which have been largely obliterated by the infiltrate (×40). (*E*) CD21 stains expanded FDC networks throughout the lymph node (×40). (*F*) EBV positive cells are also present on an in situ hybridization stain for EBER (×200).

DIFFERENTIAL DIAGNOSIS

AITL can mimic several reactive and neoplastic conditions, including reactive follicular and para-cortical hyperplasia, Castleman disease, classical Hodgkin lymphoma, diffuse large B-cell lymphoma (DLBCL), and other PTCLs. Early cases showing pattern I histology appear similar to reactive lymphoid hyperplasia with a marked paracortical component and may be difficult to recognize as neoplastic. Diagnostic clues that suggest AITL include markedly increased vascularity in para-cortical areas, the presence of aggregates of atyp-ical lymphoid cells with clear cytoplasm in perifollicular areas, the presence of a mixture of hyperplastic and depleted follicles, and the presence of CD10, PD1, and/or CXCL13-positive T cells in perifollicular areas. The final diagnosis may be reached only after molecular clonality analysis and additional biopsies, particularly if the first biopsy is limited in size. In the plasma cell variant of Castleman disease, depleted follicles with FDC whorls are seen. Similarly, depleted follicles are also frequently found in AITL. The appearance of the interfollicular zone is dissimilar, however, with a monotonous infiltrate of plasma cells and small lymphoid cells without atypia in Castleman disease. Increased vascularity is also generally not as prominent in Castleman disease as in AITL.

A pitfall in the diagnosis of AITL is classical Hodg-kin lymphoma. A significant subset of AITL cases contains EBV-mediated B-cell proliferations, which sometimes exhibit the morphologic appearance of RS cells. The background may also contain a clas-sical Hodgkin lymphoma inflammatory milieu, including eosinophils, histiocytes and plasma cells. Diagnostic clues that might indicate an underlying T-cell lymphoma include the presence of not only EBV+ RS-like cells but also a wider range of EBV+ cells that includes immunoblasts and plasma cells, marked cytologic atypia of the small background cells, an aberrant T-cell phenotype, and expansion of FDC meshworks. The EBV-positive B-cell proliferation arising in the back-ground of AITL may have a monomorphic immunoblastic morphology mimicking an EBV+ DLBCL; additionally, AITL cases of EBV-negative large B cells may resemble T-cell/histiocyte-rich large B-cell lymphoma. Distinction of these neoplasms from AITL may be difficult in some cases and may depend on demonstrating an abnormal T-cell immunophenotype and a T-cell gene rearrangement. Finally, in some cases of AITL, the FDC proliferation can be prominent and may raise the possibility of a spindle-cell neoplasm, such as FDC sarcoma. Awareness of the cytologic abnormalities of the background lymphocytes, immunophenotyping for T-cell markers, and molecular testing are all important in establishing the diagnosis in such a situation.

Differential Diagnosis ANGIOIMMUNOBLASTIC T-CELL LYMPHOMA	
AITL Versus	**Helpful Distinguishing Features**
Reactive follicular and paracortical hyperplasia	• Absence of markedly increased paracortical vascularity • Absence of atypical perifollicular cells with clear cytoplasm • Lack of T-cell clone
Castleman disease (plasma cell variant)	• Monotonous plasma cell infiltrate • Small lymphocytes lacking significant atypia • Less prominent increase in vascularity
Classical Hodgkin lymphoma	• Lack of cytologic atypia • Lack of immunophenotypic aberrancy of background T cells • Lack of expanded follicular dendritic meshworks
DLBCL	• Lack of aberrant T-cell immunophenotype • Lack of T-cell receptor (TCR) gene rearrangement
Other PTCLs	• Lack of characteristic increased vascularity • Lack of expanded follicular dendritic meshworks • Lack of T_{FH} phenotype

Pitfalls ANGIOIMMUNOBLASTIC T-CELL LYMPHOMA
! Early AITL cases showing pattern I histology appear similar to reactive lymphoid hyper-plasia with a marked paracortical component.
! EBV-mediated B-cell proliferations in AITL can morphologically mimic Hodgkin lymphoma, with EBV-positive B-cells that resemble RS cells as well as a background milieu of eosin-ophils, plasma cells, and histiocytes.
! There can be morphologic overlap with other PTCLs involving the lymph node.

PROGNOSIS

The clinical course of AITL is aggressive with a median survival of approximately 3 years. No AITL-specific therapy is currently available. Most patients are initially treated with cyclophosphamide, doxorubicin, vincristine, and prednisone (CHOP)-based regimens with variable responses. Some sustained responses have been achieved by high-dose therapy with peripheral blood stem cell transplantation. There also may be a role for immunoregulatory drugs, such as cyclosporine.

ALK-POSITIVE ANAPLASTIC LARGE CELL LYMPHOMA

OVERVIEW

Anaplastic large cell lymphoma (ALCL) is a neoplasm of mature T cells that expresses CD30 and can be divided into anaplastic lymphoma kinase (ALK)-positive and ALK-negative subtypes. These two subtypes are morphologically indistinguishable from each other and are subcategorized based on the presence of a translocation of the *ALK* gene located on chromosome 2p23. ALK-positive ALCL has been categorized by the World Health Organization (WHO) as a separate entity from ALK-negative ALCL due to differences in demographics and prognosis.[18] Because they are distinct entities by WHO classification, ALK-positive and ALK-negative ALCL are discussed separately in this review, although there is significant morphologic and immunophenotypic overlap.

CLINICAL FEATURES

ALCL is the second most common subtype of PTCL in the Western world, with just over half of cases classified as ALK-positive ALCL.[19–22] ALK-positive ALCL is a disease that affects mostly children and young adults and has a male predominance (male-to-female ratio approximately 2:1).[20,21,23] Both 5-year overall survival and failure-free survival are significantly better in patients with ALK-positive ALCL as compared with ALK-negative ALCL.[24] ALK-positive ALCL is one of the most common PTCLs involving lymph nodes, but it frequently involves extranodal sites as well: lung skin, bone, liver, and soft tissue are commonly involved.[23] Bone marrow is found to be involved in the staging bone marrow biopsies of approximately 30% of patients at presentation.[25] B symptoms, in particular fever, are common.[19,20,23] Peripheral blood involvement is rare but can suggest the small cell pattern when present (discussed later).[26]

> ### Key Features
> ### ALK-POSITIVE ANAPLASTIC LARGE CELL LYMPHOMA
>
> 1. Architectural effacement of the lymph node with occasional residual lymphoid follicles
>
> 2. Presence of hallmark cells: a large cell with a pleomorphic, often horseshoe-shaped nucleus and abundant cytoplasm
>
> 3. Different morphologic patterns with fewer hallmark cells are possible, although hallmark cells are nearly always present

DIAGNOSIS: MICROSCOPIC FEATURES

ALK-positive ALCL is characterized by neoplastic cells that efface the lymph node architecture (**Fig. 4**). Residual lymphoid follicles may be present in the background and may appear as non-neoplastic rests, which are surrounded by neoplastic infiltrates. Infiltration of the sinuses may also be present; particularly prominent involvement of the sinuses can mimic nonhematologic neoplasms, such as metastatic solid tumors. There are several histologic variants of ALCL, which, although they may have little prognostic or therapeutic usefulness, are important to recognize so that an appropriate diagnosis of ALCL can be made. Regardless of the histologic variant, ALCL is characterized the presence of large, atypical hallmark cells: large cells with a pleomorphic, horseshoe, or wreath-shaped nucleus and abundant cytoplasm (see **Fig. 4**B).[27] Hallmark cells are often the predominant cell type in the common pattern, which is seen in 60% of cases. Markedly lobated or multiple nuclei may be present and hallmark cells may resemble the RS cells of classical Hodgkin lymphoma.

Several morphologic patterns in addition to the common pattern are identified by the WHO.[18] The lymphohistiocytic pattern is seen in approximately 10% of cases and shows many reactive histiocytes in the background (**Fig. 5**). This non-neoplastic histiocytic infiltrate may be dramatic and may obscure the neoplastic cells.[28] The neoplastic hallmark cells may be smaller than is typical with the common pattern and often cluster around vessels, a helpful clue when attempting to find the hallmark cells. The small cell pattern, or small cell variant, is seen in 5% to 10% of cases and is characterized by mostly small to medium-sized neoplastic cells with nuclear pleomorphism.[29] Typical hallmark cells are present on careful examination and may also be clustered around vessels. The Hodgkin-like pattern is seen

Fig. 4. ALK-positive ALCL. There are large neoplastic cells in a background of small reactive T cells (*A*) (H&E, ×200). Typical cytologic features of hallmark cells are an irregularly contoured nucleus, occasionally with a wreath shape, and distinct eosinophilic cytoplasmic condensations (*B*) (H&E, ×400). By immunohistochemistry, the hallmark cells express the ALK protein (*C*) (×200).

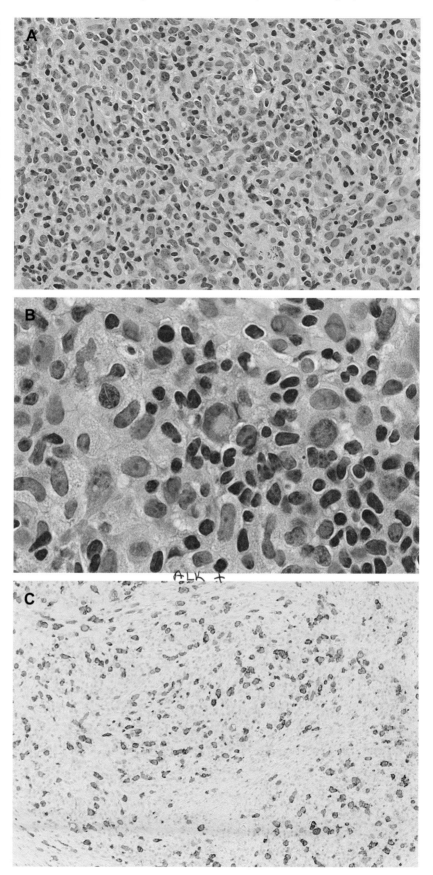

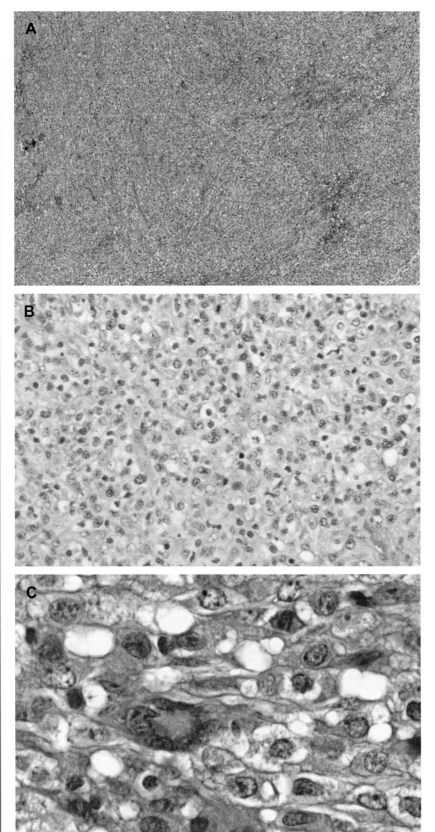

Fig. 5. ALK-positive ALCL, lymphohistiocytic variant. There is a dense infiltrate of non-neoplastic lymphocytes and histiocytes, which efface the lymph node architecture (*A, B*) (*A*, H&E, ×40, *B*, H&E, x200). Careful examination, however, reveals hallmark cells with wreath-shaped nuclei (*C*) (H&E, ×400).

Fig. 5. ALK-positive ALCL, lymphohistiocytic variant. By immunohistochemistry, CD68 highlights the numerous background histiocytes (*D*) (×200), whereas CD30 (*E*) (×400) and ALK (*F*) (×400) highlight the neoplastic cells.

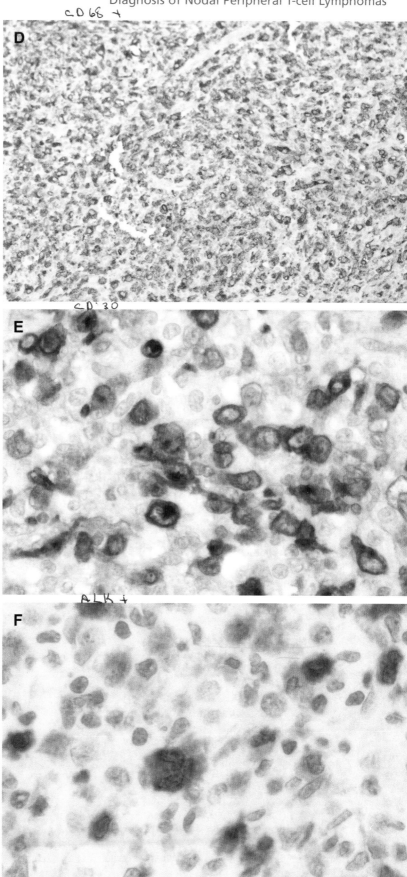

in approximately 3% of cases and shows features mimicking those seen in nodular sclerosis Hodgkin lymphoma (**Fig. 6**).[39] Approximately 15% of cases of ALK-positive ALCL consist of a heterogeneous mixture of the above morphologic patterns. This composite pattern is most often composed of a mixture of the lymphohistiocytic and small cell patterns. Rarer variants include cases in which tumor cells are predominantly multinucleated giant cells, smaller cells with round nuclei, or spindled cells (sarcomatoid pattern).[31] Some cases are hypocellular, with an edematous or myxoid background. The wide variation of morphologic features that can be found in ALCL may lead to misdiagnosis, especially when few hallmark cells are present.

DIAGNOSIS: ANCILLARY STUDIES

Immunohistochemistry is essential for diagnosis of ALK-positive ALCL, including demonstration of expression of CD30 and ALK (or demonstration of an *ALK* gene translocation) (see **Fig. 4**C and **Fig. 5**E, F). The cellular localization of ALK staining correlates with the partner gene involved in the *ALK* translocation, but the clinical significance of the translocation partner is unknown.[22] Most cases show loss of some T-cell antigens, and some cases show loss of all T-cell antigens (so-called null-cell type).[24,27] CD2 and CD4 are the T-cell antigens that are most commonly preserved, although CD4 staining can be observed in a wide range of hematologic malignancies, including other T-cell lymphomas, histiocyte or dendritic cell neoplasms, and acute myeloid leukemia. Rare cases of ALCL are CD8 positive, while cytotoxic proteins, such as perforin, T-cell intracellular antigen-1 (TIA1), and granzyme B, are often present irrespective of CD8 positivity.[24] Antibodies against β chain of α/β TCR, such as β-F1, and stains for the γ/δ TCR typically are negative. Most cases express epithelial membrane antigen (EMA).[27] Clusterin and CD56 also may be expressed.[32,33] Occasional expression of myeloid antigens CD13 and CD33 by ALK-positive ALCL can occur and should not be misinterpreted as evidence of extramedullary acute myeloid leukemia.[34] EBV is negative by both immunohistochemistry and in situ hybridization.[35] Although typically negative, occasional cases may express CD15 and this marker alone should not be used to differentiate between ALCL and classical Hodgkin lymphoma.[36] Flow cytometry is not used routinely for evaluation of ALCL. *TCR* genes are clonally rearranged in the majority of cases, regardless of whether or not T-cell antigens are expressed,[24] while

immunoglobulin heavy chain (*IGH*) genes are germline. Genetic studies, such as karyotyping or fluorescence in situ hybridization, can be used to confirm presence of *ALK* translocations; however, this is not necessary for diagnosis if ALK protein expression is demonstrated by IHC.

All cases of ALK-positive ALCL have translocations involving *ALK* on 2p23 and one of several various partner genes, most commonly the nucleophosmin gene *NPM* on 5q35.[37] Presence of the *NPM-ALK* translocation leads to both nuclear and cytoplasmic staining for ALK by IHC. Less common partners lead to diffuse cytoplasmic staining only (*TPM3, ATIC, TFG, TPM4, MYH9, ALO17*), granular cytoplasmic staining (*CLTC*), or membranous staining (*MSN*). Identification of the *ALK* partner gene in a given case is currently not necessary for diagnosis or management.

DIFFERENTIAL DIAGNOSIS

The common pattern of ALK-positive ALCL usually has characteristic morphologic features, in which the major differential diagnosis is between ALK-positive and ALK-negative ALCL. This differential lies solely on the demonstration of ALK protein expression by immunohistochemistry or by a translocation involving the *ALK* gene. The variant histologic patterns of ALK-positive ALCL may be confused with a variety of conditions. The Hodgkin-like pattern mimics its namesake, and the distinction between the two may be difficult. PAX5 staining may be helpful, because it is nearly always positive in Hodgkin lymphoma but is negative in ALCL (see **Fig. 6**E and F). The sarcomatoid pattern mimics soft tissue sarcomas. The small cell pattern may be misdiagnosed as PTCL, NOS

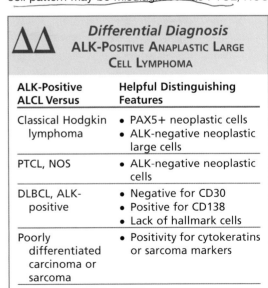

ΔΔ Differential Diagnosis ALK-Positive Anaplastic Large Cell Lymphoma	
ALK-Positive ALCL Versus	**Helpful Distinguishing Features**
Classical Hodgkin lymphoma	• PAX5+ neoplastic cells • ALK-negative neoplastic large cells
PTCL, NOS	• ALK-negative neoplastic cells
DLBCL, ALK-positive	• Negative for CD30 • Positive for CD138 • Lack of hallmark cells
Poorly differentiated carcinoma or sarcoma	• Positivity for cytokeratins or sarcoma markers

Fig. 6. ALK-positive ALCL, Hodgkin-like variant. Sclerotic bands surround a neoplastic infiltrate (*A*) (H&E, ×40). The neoplastic cells with prominent nucleoli demonstrate a RS-like morphology, which mimics classical Hodgkin lymphoma, nodular sclerosis type (*B*) (H&E, ×400). By immunohistochemistry, the neoplastic cells are CD3 negative (*C*) (×400).

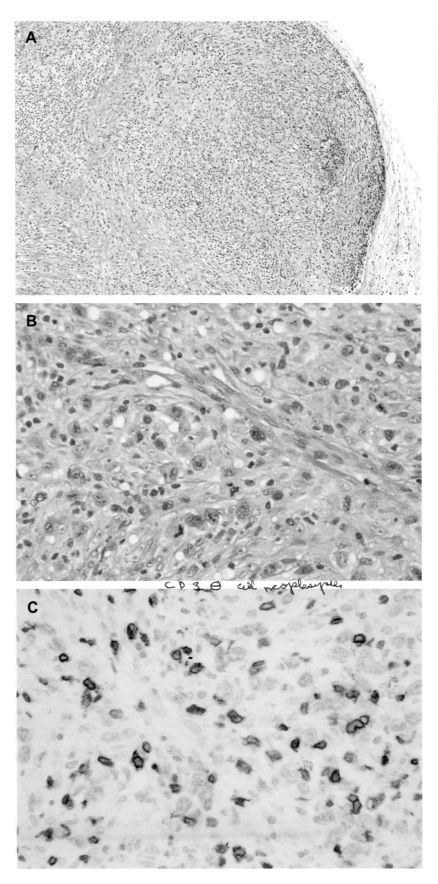

CD30 +

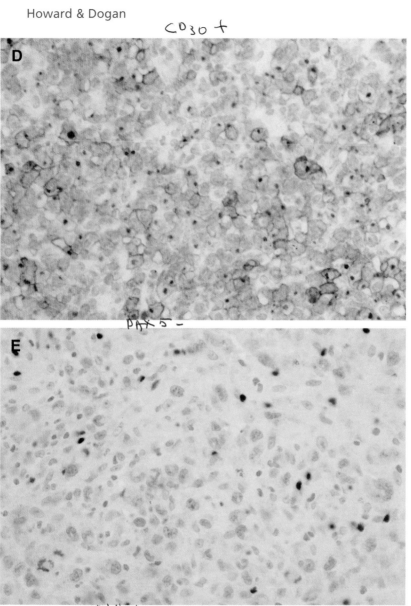

PAX 5 -

ALK +

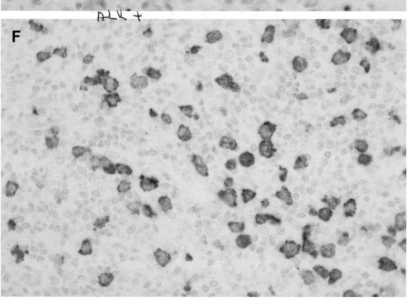

Fig. 6. ALK-positive ALCL, Hodgkin-like variant. The neoplastic cells are CD30 positive (*D*) (×400). Pax-5 is negative (*E*) (×400), whereas ALK is positive (*F*) (×400), excluding a diagnosis of classical Hodgkin lymphoma.

if testing for ALK is not performed. The lymphohistiocytic pattern occasionally may have sufficient inflammatory cells so as to obscure the tumor cells and mimic a reactive process and may also be confused with histiocytic sarcomas. A key to these pitfalls is the recognition of characteristic hallmark cells, often around blood vessels, which are a constant feature in ALCL. A subset of DLBCLs expresses ALK (as well as EMA) and has *ALK* translocations. Hallmark cells are absent in these cases, and the tumor cells are negative for CD30 and typically positive for CD138 and IgA.[38] ALK-positive DLBCL often lacks CD20 expression and may coexpress CD4, which may cause further confusion with ALK-positive ALCL.[38] Cases of ALK-positive ALCL with infiltration of the sinusoids and minimal nodal effacement can resemble metastatic neoplasms (**Fig. 7**), but cytologic and immunophenotypic features are distinct. In the differential diagnosis between ALK-positive ALCL and carcinoma, immunohistochemistry for keratins should always performed rather than EMA. Finally, a variety of other nonhematopoietic tumors can express ALK, including neuroblastoma,[39] inflammatory myofibroblastic tumors,[40] and a subset of lung carcinomas.[41] These tumors do not show significant morphologic overlap with ALCL and can easily be differentiated by immunohistochemistry

PROGNOSIS

Most adult patients with ALK-positive ALCL are treated with CHOP-like chemotherapy regimens;

Pitfalls
ALK-Positive Anaplastic Large Cell Lymphoma

! Neuroblastoma, inflammatory myofibroblastic tumors, and a subset of lung carcinomas may express ALK.

! Hodgkin lymphoma and certain sarcomas show morphologic overlap but are immunophenotypically distinct.

! Failure to recognize hallmark cells may result in erroneous diagnosis of PTCL or reactive lymphoid hyperplasia.

! ALK-positive DLBCL may be CD20 negative.

pediatric patients have responded to short-pulse chemotherapy regimens modeled after high-grade B-cell lymphoma protocols.[22] Retreatment often is effective for relapses and refractory cases also may respond to allogeneic bone marrow transplantation.[42] Several targeted therapies have been explored in clinical trials, including therapies using monoclonal antibodies against the CD30 molecule and small-molecule inhibitors of the ALK tyrosine kinase.[43,44] The prognosis of ALK-positive ALCL is one of the most favorable among PTCLs, with a 5-year overall survival rate of 70% to 80%. Generally, complete remission in ALK-positive ALK is associated with long-term overall survival. These outcomes are significantly better than those for either ALK-negative ALCL or PTCL, NOS.

Fig. 7. ALCL mimicking a metastatic nonhematologic tumor. In this case, an ALK-positive ALCL infiltrates the subcapsular lymph node sinus, producing a pattern difficult to distinguish from metastatic carcinoma or melanoma (H&E, ×200).

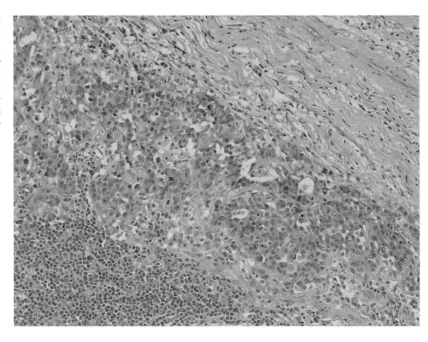

ALK-NEGATIVE ANAPLASTIC LARGE CELL LYMPHOMA

OVERVIEW

ALK-negative ALCL is a neoplasm of mature T cells that express CD30 and is morphologically indistinguishable from ALK-positive ALCL. However, it lacks expression of ALK protein and translocations of the *ALK* gene. Differences in demographics, biology, and outcome have led to listing ALK-negative ALCL as a separate entity in the WHO classification. ALK-negative ALCL must be distinguished from ALK-positive ALCL and CD30-positive PTCL, NOS.[18]

CLINICAL FEATURES

ALK-negative ALCL is a primarily a disease of adults, with a peak incidence in the sixth decade.[19] In this regard, it differs from ALK-positive ALCL, which is primarily a disease of the young. The male-to-female ratio of ALK-negative ALCL is approximately 1.5:1. Although ALK-negative ALCL is primarily a nodal disease, extranodal sites may be involved in up to half of patients: the most common extranodal sites are skin, lung, and liver.[19] Most patients present with advanced (stage III or IV) disease and most have B symptoms.[19]

DIAGNOSIS: MICROSCOPIC FEATURES

ALK-negative ALCL has similar morphologic features to the common pattern of ALK-positive ALCL. It typically effaces the lymph node architecture, although some cases may predominantly involve the node sinuses and mimic metastatic neoplasms. Hallmark cells usually are seen, and multinucleated cells with wreath-like nuclei are common (**Fig. 8**). The cells in ALK-negative ALCL tend to be larger and more pleomorphic than in

---

Key Features
ALK-Negative Anaplastic Large Cell Lymphoma

1. Architectural effacement of the lymph node with occasional residual lymphoid follicles.

2. Presence of hallmark cells: a large cell with a pleomorphic, often horseshoe or wreath-shaped nucleus and abundant cytoplasm.

3. Different morphologic patterns with fewer hallmark cells are possible, although hallmark cells are, by definition, always present.

ALK-positive ALCL.[45] The WHO classification does not include distinct variants or patterns of ALK-negative ALCL as it does for ALK-positive ALCL.[18] RS-like cells and a variable inflammatory background milieu may be seen, leading to a differential diagnosis with CHL. A small-cell variant of ALK-negative is not recognized, because it would be difficult or impossible to distinguish from cases of PTCL, NOS that express CD30.

DIAGNOSIS: ANCILLARY STUDIES

Immunohistochemistry for CD30 and ALK are the cornerstones of the diagnosis of ALK-negative ALCL. CD30 staining should be strong and uniform, with membranous, Golgi, and sometimes cytoplasmic staining. CD30 expression can occur in PTCL, NOS but it is usually weaker and less uniform than in ALCL. The tumor's T-cell lineage may not initially be apparent, because ALK-negative ALCL may lack expression of multiple T-cell antigens. Extensive immunophenotypic testing for multiple antigens generally reveals the T-cell lineage, even though commonly performed stains, such as CD3, may be negative. Positive staining for EMA and/or clusterin may be helpful in the distinction from PTCL, NOS; however, these markers are present less often than in ALK-positive ALCL.[19] If positive, EMA, clusterin, CD56, and cytotoxic markers, such as TIA-1 and granzyme B, may be helpful in the differential diagnosis with classical Hodgkin lymphoma. CD43 is often expressed in ALK-negative ALCL but is not expressed in classical Hodgkin lymphoma. Occasionally, classical Hodgkin lymphoma may express cytotoxic markers and/or T-cell antigens, which can lead to incorrect diagnosis of classical Hodgkin lymphoma as ALCL.[46] Conversely, ALK-negative ALCL may express CD15 and lack expression of CD45. EBV is typically absent in ALK-negative ALCLs; its presence would suggest the possibility of either classical Hodgkin lymphoma or AITL. As with ALK-positive ALCL, flow cytometry does not have a major role in diagnosis. *TCR* genes are clonally rearranged in the majority of cases; *IGH* is germline. PCR for *TCR* and *IGH* gene rearrangements may help distinguish ALK-negative ALCL from classical Hodgkin lymphoma, particularly if a sensitive PCR technique is used. Rare cases of ALK-negative ALCL may lack clonal *TCR* gene rearrangements, however, and *IGH* gene rearrangement is not always detected by PCR in classical Hodgkin lymphoma. Genetic studies to exclude *ALK* translocations generally are not necessary if reliable immunohistochemistry for ALK protein is available.

Fig. 8. ALK-negative ALCL. (*A, B*) Horseshoe-shaped hallmark cells with eosinophilic nucleoli are present in a background of smaller reactive T cells, features indistinguishable from those of ALK-positive ALCL on routine histology (*A*, H&E, ×200, *B*, H&E, ×400).

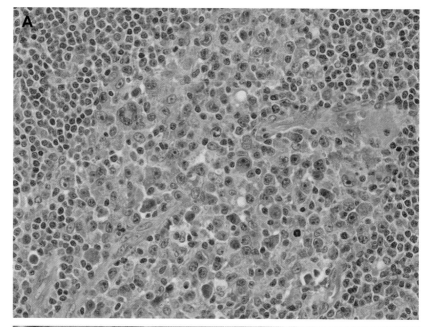

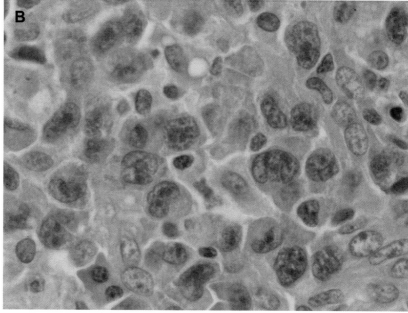

DIFFERENTIAL DIAGNOSIS

The differential diagnosis of ALK-negative ALCL is primarily with <u>ALK-positive ALCL</u>. ALK-negative ALCL must be distinguished from ALK-positive ALCL by either immunohistochemistry for the ALK protein or genetic analysis for *ALK* translocations. Again, genetic analysis is not required if reliable ALK immunohistochemistry is available. Once ALK negativity is established, ALK-negative ALCL must

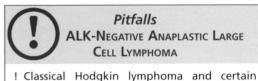

be differentiated from CD30-positive PTCL, NOS, particularly in light of recent data suggesting prognostic significance to this distinction.[19] This distinction is primarily morphologic and is based on the cytologic features consistent with hallmark cells in a majority of tumor cells. Immunohistochemistry is also helpful, because ALK-negative ALCL is often TIA-1, EMA, or clusterin positive. The WHO recommends an approach that preserves the homogeneity of ALK-negative ALCL, reserving that term for cases with morphology and phenotype indistinguishable from ALK-positive ALCL, except for the absence of ALK expression.[18]

Another entity in the differential diagnosis of ALCL is secondary lymph node involvement by cutaneous ALCL. This distinction is not possible without clinical staging data. If staging data are not available, the possibility of secondary involvement by a cutaneous lymphoma should be mentioned in the pathology report. In abdominal lymph nodes, secondary nodal involvement by CD30-positive enteropathy-associated T-cell lymphoma may be considered. Again, clinical data are useful in making such a distinction. It is critical to differentiate Hodgkin-like ALK-negative ALCL from classical Hodgkin lymphoma due to differing treatments. Immunohistochemistry for PAX5 is helpful in this differential diagnosis, because it is weakly positive in most cases of classical Hodgkin lymphoma and is negative in virtually all ALK-negative ALCLs.[47] Other B-cell lymphomas, such as DLBCL, more rarely mimic ALK-negative ALCL but can be distinguished by their expression of B-cell markers. Like ALK-positive ALCL, ALK-negative ALCL may show a primarily sinusoidal pattern with minimal architectural effacement, mimicking metastatic tumors.

PROGNOSIS

CHOP chemotherapy or similar cytotoxic regimens are generally the mainstay of treatment for patients with ALK-negative ALCL. Relapsed or refractory cases may be treated with stem cell transplantation. Therapeutic modalities specific for this entity have not been identified; however, patients with ALK-negative ALCL have been included in various experimental approaches for treatment of PTCL in general, including those targeting CD30. The prognosis of ALK-negative ALCL is distinctly poorer than that of its ALK-positive counterpart, with a 5-year overall survival rate of 49% (vs 80%).[19] This difference seems independent of the older median age of patients with ALK-negative ALCL. Conversely, compared with PTCL, NOS, ALK-negative ALCL has a more favorable 5-year overall survival rate (49% vs 32%, respectively), a difference that is more pronounced when ALK-negative ALCL is compared with the subset of PTCL, NOS that is CD30 positive (49% vs 19%).[19] The differences in survival between ALK-negative ALCL, ALK-positive ALCL, and PTCL, NOS provide a rationale for considering ALK-negative ALCL as a separate disease entity, distinct from both ALK-positive ALCL and PTCL, NOS.

PERIPHERAL T-CELL LYMPHOMA, NOT OTHERWISE SPECIFIED

OVERVIEW

PTCL, NOS is a group of mature T-cell lymphomas that do not meet criteria for any of the other specific PTCL entities defined in the WHO classification system.[18] This heterogeneous category includes both nodal and extranodal lymphomas and encompasses a wide variety of morphologic and phenotypic findings. PTCL, NOS is more than just a "wastebasket category", because it can be considered to represent the prototype of PTCL in general, based on its high prevalence among T-cell lymphomas as well as the current lack of clinically meaningful approaches to further subclassify these neoplasms.[48]

CLINICAL FEATURES

In Western countries, PTCL, NOS is the most common PTCL subtype, representing from 30% to 60% of PTCLs.[20,21,49,50] Data from Surveillance, Epidemiology and End Results (SEER) registries show an apparent recent increase in the incidence of PTCL, NOS in the United States, although the influence of advancing diagnostic modalities and changes in lymphoma classification on these registry data is unclear.[49] It is primarily a disease of adults, with a median age of approximately 60 years and a male-to-female ratio of approximately 2:1.[20,21,49,50] Often PTCL, NOS presents with lymphadenopathy, with or without involvement of extranodal sites.[50] Most cases are disseminated, with 40% to 60% of patients presenting with stage IV disease.[20,49,50] Bone marrow and skin are the most commonly involved extranodal sites.[20] Peripheral blood may be involved but is rarely the presenting site. B symptoms are seen in approximately 40% of patients, elevated lactate dehydrogenase levels in approximately 60%, and a nonambulatory performance status in approximately 30%.[20,50] Unfavorable International Prognostic Index scores are seen in 60% of patients at presentation.[50]

DIAGNOSIS: MICROSCOPIC FEATURES

PTCL, NOS is a heterogeneous category of PTCLs that do not meet criteria for any other of the specifically defined lymphoma entities within the WHO classification.[18] Because of this broad definition, there is a wide range of morphologic findings. As with most T-cell lymphomas, the lymph node typically shows effacement of the normal architecture, commonly with either a diffuse or paracortical pattern (**Fig. 9**). The tumor cells in PTCL, NOS are medium to large-sized as a rule, although some cases may have an infiltrate which is composed of smaller neoplastic T cells.[51] Marked nuclear pleomorphism may also be present, and cases with RS-like morphology may be seen.[52] PTCL, NOS is not graded. The cellular background is variable but may contain small lymphocytes, plasma cells, eosinophils, histiocytes, large B cells, and/or vascular proliferation. The WHO classification recognizes three variants[18]:

1. Lymphoepithelioid
2. Follicular
3. T-zone.

The lymphoepithelioid variant (Lennert lymphoma) is characterized by small neoplastic cells with extensive clusters of epithelioid histiocytes.[51] This variant also may show scattered larger cells that may demonstrate RS morphology.[53] The follicular variant of PTCL, NOS typically shows an intrafollicular population of atypical cells with pale cytoplasm.[54] Some cases may show features resembling progressive transformation of germinal centers or a perifollicular growth pattern.[55] The T-zone variant of PTCL, NOS shows an extensively perifollicular pattern and is composed of small cells that may lack significant cytologic atypia (**Fig. 10**).[55] Although the clinical significance of these variants is not certain, it is important to avoid their misdiagnosis as Hodgkin lymphoma or, in the case of the T-zone variant, reactive lymphoid hyperplasia.

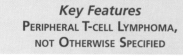

Key Features
PERIPHERAL T-CELL LYMPHOMA, NOT OTHERWISE SPECIFIED

1. Heterogeneous group of T-cell lymphomas that do not meet criteria for another WHO-defined lymphoma

2. Often show effacement of normal lymph node architecture

3. Often have medium to large-sized cytologically atypical cells

4. Often have aberrant loss of one or more T-cell antigens

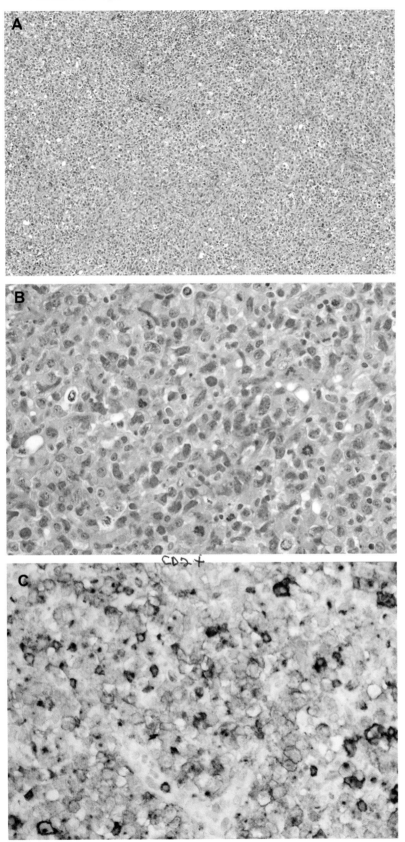

CD2+

Fig. 9. PTCL, NOS. The lymph node architecture is effaced by an infiltrate of intermediate-sized cells with irregular nuclear contours and small nucleoli (*A, B*) (*A*, H&E, ×100, *B*, H&E, ×200). By immunohistochemistry, the neoplastic infiltrate in this case is positive for CD2 (*C*) (×200).

CD 30+

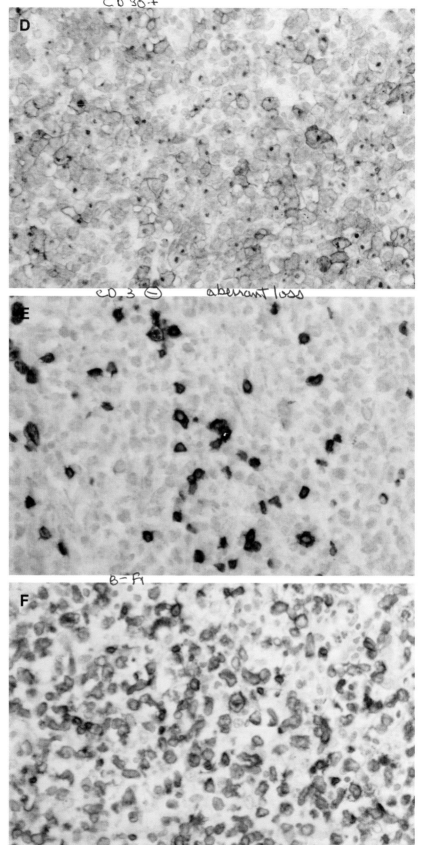

Fig. 9. PTCL, NOS. The neoplastic infiltrate is positive for CD30 (_D_) (×200), but shows aberrant loss of CD3 (_E_) (×200). β-F1 is positive (_F_) (×200), helping confirm a T-cell phenotype. ALK staining was negative (not shown), excluding a small cell variant of ALK-positive ALCL.

CD 3 ⊖   aberrant loss

β-F1

ALK ⊖

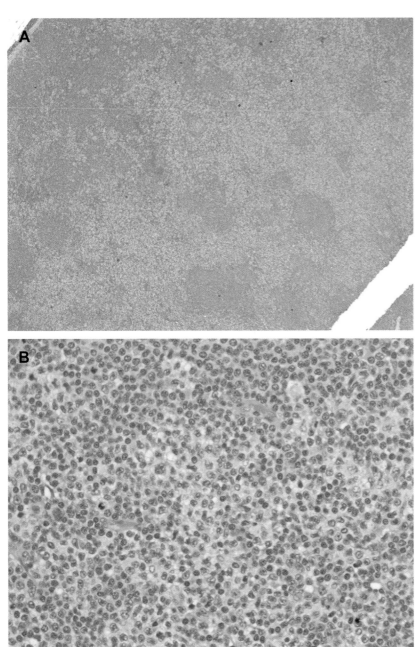

Fig. 10. PTCL, NOS, T zone variant. The infiltrate shows a perifollicular growth pattern (*A*) (H&E, ×20) and on high power is composed of small- to medium-sized lymphocytes with subtle nuclear atypia (*B*) (H&E, ×200).

DIAGNOSIS: ANCILLARY STUDIES

Immunohistochemistry is essential for proper diagnosis and subclassification of all PTCLs. Cases of PTCL, NOS generally show an aberrant immunophenotype with down-regulation of at least one T-cell antigen, frequently CD3, CD5, and/or CD7. These antigens may show dim staining by both paraffin section immunohistochemistry and flow cytometric immunophenotyping (see Fig. 9E). Generally, PTCL, NOS is CD4 positive although some may express CD8, in particular the lymphoepithelioid variant.[53,56] Cases may be double positive or double negative for CD4 and

CD8, although double-negative PTCL, NOS is less common. Most cases are positive for the TCR β chain (see **Fig. 9F**). All cases of PTCL, NOS should be negative for ALK. Cytotoxic markers and/or CD56 may occasionally be expressed. A subset of PTCLs, NOS expresses CD30, but morphology and immunohistochemical markers for TIA-1, clusterin, and EMA serve to distinguish these cases from ALK-negative ALCLs (**Fig. 11**). Cases of PTCL, NOS that express CD30 and CD15 may be confused with classical Hodgkin lymphoma but morphology is usually sufficient to differentiate between the two. In ambiguous cases, PAX5 staining shows characteristic weak positivity in most CHLs, whereas expression in PTCLs is rare. Negative PAX5 staining is also is helpful in occasional cases of PTCL, NOS that aberrantly coexpress other B-cell markers, such as CD20 or CD79a. While the absence of T_{FH} markers is helpful in ruling out the diagnosis of AITL, a T_{FH} phenotype, including expression of CD10, Bcl6, CXCL13, and/or PD1 may be seen in the follicular variant of PTCL, NOS. Regulatory T-cell (T_{REG}) markers, such as CD25 and FoxP3, may be seen in adult T-cell leukemia/lymphoma or mycosis fungoides. Morphologic evaluation for a blastic appearance of the neoplastic cells, as well as immunohistochemistry for terminal deoxynucleotidyl transferase (TdT), CD99, CD34, and CD1a, is helpful in excluding a T lymphoblastic leukemia/lymphoma.

Aberrant expression of T-cell antigens is common in various B-cell neoplasms. CD5 expression by mantle cell lymphoma or chronic lymphocytic leukemia/small lymphocytic lymphoma is rarely a diagnostic pitfall when comprehensive antibody panels are used. The common expression of CD5 in such B-cell neoplasms, however, underscores the importance of using a T-cell marker with high-lineage fidelity, such as CD3. CD5 should not be used as a lone T-cell marker because it may also be expressed in some cases of follicular lymphoma, marginal zone lymphoma, and DLBCL. DLBCL rarely may express CD3 and a variety of other T-cell markers. Staining for PAX5 and additional B-cell markers generally allows for precise lineage assignment, especially when combined with molecular studies, such as T-cell and B-cell gene rearrangement. The RS cells of classical Hodgkin lymphoma may express a variety of T-cell antigens, including cytotoxic markers. Negativity for CD43 and weak positivity for PAX5 are fairly consistent features of classical Hodgkin lymphoma that aid in the differential diagnosis from PTCL. T-cell antigens also may be expressed by non-lymphoid hematopoietic tumors. The neoplastic cells in systemic mast cell

disease typically express CD43 and often express CD2 and CD25; stains for mast cell tryptase and CD117 are helpful when mast cell disease is in the morphologic differential diagnosis. Extramedullary acute myeloid leukemia (myeloid sarcoma) involving the lymph node typically expresses CD43 and may express CD2, CD4, CD7, and CD56. Stains for myeloperoxidase, CD33, and CD34 as well as stains for lysozyme and CD68 aid in establishing this diagnosis. Blastic plasmacytoid dendritic cell neoplasms typically express CD4, CD43, and CD56 and may express CD2 and CD7.[57] The plasmacytoid dendritic cell marker CD123 is positive in these neoplasms; most cases also express TCL1 and approximately one-third express TdT.

Flow cytometry may be helpful in the evaluation of lymph nodes for PTCL by demonstrating aberrant antigenic loss. This is particularly true in cases with subtle involvement and may be particularly useful when combined with gene rearrangement studies. Flow cytometry also may be a more rigorous method for determining subtle antigen loss of a population of T cells with normal T cells in the background, because measurement of fluorescent intensity has greater analytic sensitivity than subjective interpretation of immunohistochemistry staining. Marked alterations in the CD4:CD8 ratio can be seen in reactive conditions and are nonspecific. Because of the importance of morphology and newer immunohistochemical markers, flow cytometry alone is rarely sufficient for definitive diagnosis and subclassification of PTCLs.

Evaluation for EBV by IHC using latent membrane protein 1 (LMP1) or by in situ hybridization using EBER should be considered. Most cases of PTCL, NOS are negative for EBV and diffuse EBV positivity in neoplastic cells may raise the possibility of rare nodal involvement by extranodal natural killer (NK)/T-cell lymphoma, nasal type. Scattered EBV+ B cells may be seen both in PTCL, NOS and AITL. Clonal rearrangements of *TCR* genes are seen in the majority of PTCL, NOS, and PCR for *TCR* and *IGH* gene rearrangement can be helpful in the distinction from atypical reactive hyperplasias and B-cell lymphomas. Cases of AITL may bear clonal B-cell proliferations and a positive *IGH* gene rearrangement, however.

PTCL, NOS does not show a specific diagnostic genetic abnormality, and complex karyotypes are common. A subset of cases with a follicular growth pattern has a t(5;9)(q33;q22) translocation that fuses the tyrosine kinase genes *ITK* and *SYK*[58] The resultant fusion protein has transforming properties in vitro, suggesting the translocation may be important in the pathogenesis of these

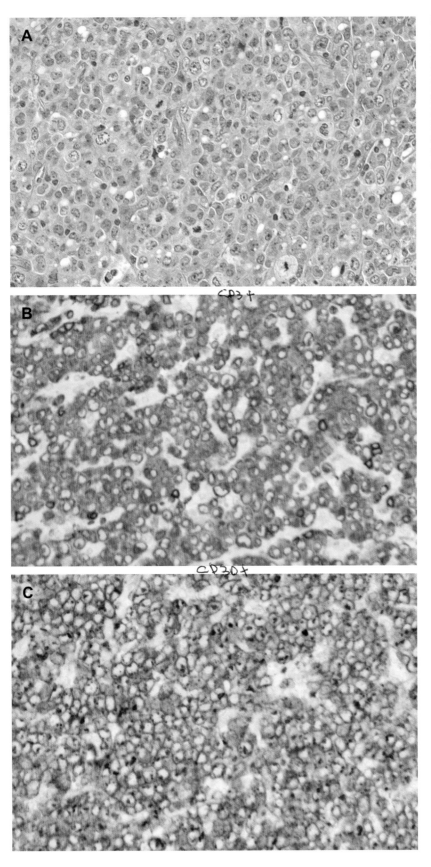

Fig. 11. PTCL, NOS, CD30 positive. (*A*) The neoplastic infiltrate is composed of large atypical lymphoid cells; classic hallmark cells are not identified (H&E, ×400). By immunohistochemistry, the neoplastic cells are positive for CD3 (*B*) (×400) and CD30 (*C*) (×400).

Fig. 11. PTCL, NOS, CD30 positive. ALK staining is negative (*D*) (×400). CD8 shows darkly staining non-neoplastic lymphocytes scattered amongst the CD8 dimly staining neoplastic T cells (*E*) (×400). TIA1 stains only the background non-neoplastic lymphocytes, with no staining of neoplastic cells (*F*) (×400).

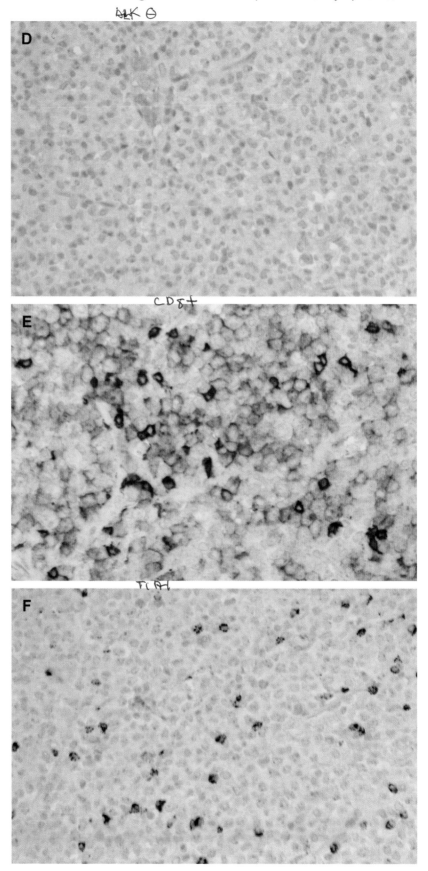

cases.[59] The overall incidence, however, of these *ITK-SYK* translocations in PTCL, NOS is low.[60]

DIFFERENTIAL DIAGNOSIS

Because PTCL, NOS encompasses cases of PTCL that do not meet criteria for any other specific subtype, the differential diagnosis is broad. There is significant overlap between the other two most common PTCLs that primarily involve lymph nodes: AITL and ALCL. Specifically, the follicular variant of PTCL, NOS and pattern I of AITL may show overlapping features. PTCL, NOS also must be differentiated from secondary involvement of the lymph node by extranodal PTCLs, in particular mycosis fungoides, adult T-cell leukemia/lymphoma, and T-cell prolymphocytic leukemia.[17,61] Blast-like morphology of the neoplastic cells can raise the possibility of T lymphoblastic leukemia/lymphoma, which may present in peripheral lymph nodes (although presentation in the thymus as a mediastinal mass is more common). Immunohistochemical staining for TdT is almost always positive in T-lymphoblastic leukemia/lymphoma but is negative in PTCL, NOS.

B-cell lymphomas are a significant part of the differential diagnosis of PTCL, NOS. T-cell/histiocyte-rich large B-cell lymphomas demonstrate scattered neoplastic B cells in a background of non-neoplastic T cells. Immunohistochemical staining of the large CD20+ neoplastic B cells and lack of cytologic atypia or phenotypic aberrancy in the background reactive T-cell infiltrate are the key to distinction of this entity from PTCL, NOS. The follicular variant of PTCL, NOS may morphologically mimic follicular lymphoma or marginal zone lymphoma.[54,55] Cases of PTCL, NOS with a nodular pattern and progressive transformation of germinal centers may resemble nodular lymphocyte-predominant (LP) Hodgkin lymphoma, but this entity contains both CD20-positive LP cells and background small B cells in most cases; rare cases of nodular LP Hodgkin lymphoma may exhibit a T-cell-rich nodular pattern that can be more problematic, however.[62] PTCL, NOS with RS-like cells may morphologically mimic classical Hodgkin lymphoma, although the immunophenotypes of these entities is usually distinct.

Nonlymphoid hematopoietic neoplasms, such as acute myeloid leukemia (myeloid sarcoma), systemic mast cell disease, and blastic plasmacytoid dendritic cell neoplasm, may masquerade as PTCL, NOS. Systemic mast cell disease is typically characterized by a paracortical infiltrate of

△△ **Differential Diagnosis**
PERIPHERAL T-CELL LYMPHOMA,
NOT OTHERWISE SPECIFIED

PTCL, NOS Versus	Helpful Distinguishing Features
AITL	• Prominent vascular proliferation • Expanded FDC meshworks • T_{FH} phenotype of neoplastic cells
T-cell/histiocyte-rich DLBCL	• CD20+ neoplastic B cells • Lack of cytologic or phenotypic aberrancy of background small cells
Nodular LP Hodgkin lymphoma	• CD20+ large LP cells • Background small B cells
Acute myeloid leukemia/ myeloid sarcoma	• Blastic cytologic features • Expression of myeloid markers
Blastic plasmacytoid dendritic cell neoplasm	• Blastic cytologic features • CD123+
Autoimmune lymphoproliferative syndrome	• Double negative (CD4−/CD8−) T cells lacking significant cytologic atypia • Lack of clonal *TCR* rearrangement
Chronic EBV infection	• Clinical features
Paracortical immunoblast proliferation due to anticonvulsant therapy	• Resolution of infiltrate after discontinuing drug
Kikuchi lymphadenitis	• CD8+ immunoblasts surrounding necrosis • CD123+ plasmacytoid dendritic cells • Myeloperoxidase (MPO+) histiocytes

neoplastic cells with pale cytoplasm; admixed eosinophils are often frequent, potentially mimicking the morphology of PTCL. Immunostains for the mast cells markers CD117 and tryptase are helpful in excluding this possibility.[61] Myeloid sarcoma typically has blastic cytologic features

Fig. 12. Lymphoepithelioid variant of PTCL, NOS (Lennert lymphoma). There is an infiltrate of small T cells with subtle cytologic atypia in a background of epithelioid histiocytes (*A, B*) (*A*, H&E, ×40, *B*, H&E, ×400). By immunohistochemistry, the neoplastic cells are CD3 positive (*C*) (×100).

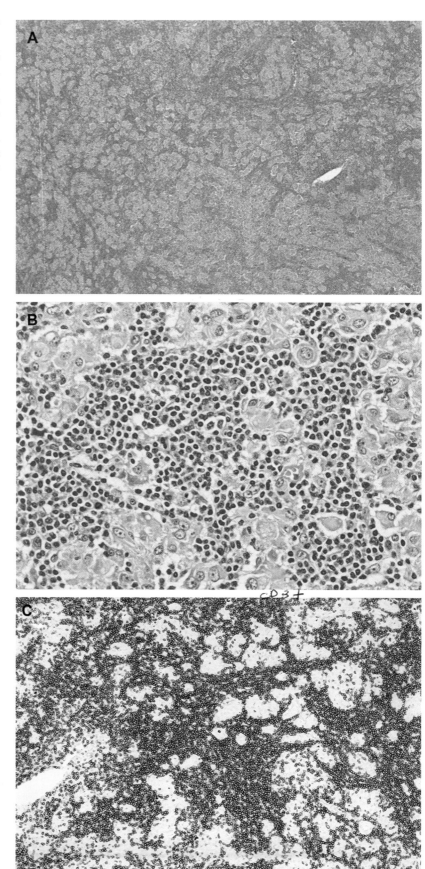

CD8+

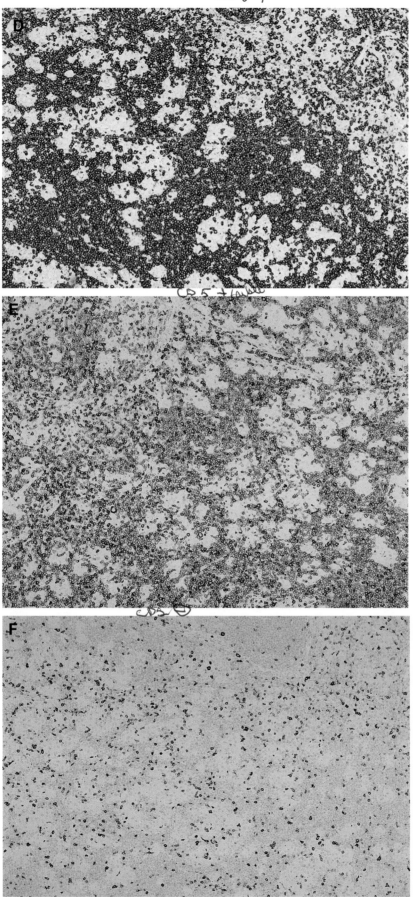

CD5 +/weak

CD7 (-)

Fig. 12. Lymphoepithelioid variant of PTCL, NOS (Lennert lymphoma). The neoplastic cells are CD8 positive (*D*) (×100) and there is aberrantly weak staining for CD5 (*E*) (×100) and aberrant loss of CD7 (*F*) (×100).

and a subtle infiltration pattern that does not replace or efface the lymph node architecture as with PTCL, NOS. Myeloid sarcoma cases that show complete architectural effacement, however, may be morphologically indistinguishable from PTCL, NOS. In addition, the expression of T-cell antigens, such as CD7 and CD4, is not uncommon in acute myeloid leukemia. Blastic plasmacytoid dendritic cell neoplasms also have blastic cytologic features and express the T-cell antigen CD4. Skin and bone marrow are the most commonly involved sites, but lymph node involvement is seen in approximately 25% of cases.[57] Immunohistochemistry is useful, because blastic plasmacytoid dendritic cell neoplasm typically expresses CD123 and often TdT, markers that should be absent from PTCL, NOS.

PTCL, NOS also may mimic benign or reactive processes. The T-zone variant of PTCL, NOS may resemble florid reactive paracortical hyperplasia (see **Fig. 10**). In some cases of PTCL, NOS, the reactive inflammatory background may be so pronounced as to obscure the neoplastic cell population; this can occur particularly in the lymphoepithelioid variant of PTCL, NOS (Lennert lymphoma), where the many epithelioid histiocytes resemble reactive granulomatous inflammation (**Fig. 12**). A marked immunoblastic proliferation in the paracortex may be seen in response to phenytoin and other anticonvulsants and a clonal *TCR* gene rearrangement may be found in such cases.[63] These atypical T-cell infiltrates resolve on cessation of the offending drug. Kikuchi lymphadenitis is characterized by marked paracortical expansion due to a prominent atypical lymphohistiocytic infiltrate with areas of geographic necrosis lacking neutrophils. Although there may be atypical-appearing enlarged CD8+ immunoblasts surrounding the necrotizing nodules in Kikuchi lymphadenitis, these are usually admixed with frequent CD123+ mature plasmacytoid dendritic cells and myeloperoxidase (MPO+) histiocytes and do not efface the lymph node architecture.

Special caution should be exercised in diagnosing PTCL, NOS in children: these lymphomas uncommon in the pediatric population and younger patients may have previously undiagnosed underlying immune dysfunctions leading to an unusual lymphoid proliferation. Autoimmune lymphoproliferative syndrome is a primary immune disorder is characterized by an apoptotic defect, often secondary to *FAS* or *FASL* mutations, that causes a marked paracortical expansion by double-negative (CD4−/CD8−) T cells.[64] Other types of immune dysregulation may also mimic PTCL, NOS, including common variable immunodeficiency, chronic active EBV infection,

Pitfalls
PERIPHERAL T-CELL LYMPHOMA, NOT OTHERWISE SPECIFIED

! B-cell lymphomas, such as T-cell/histiocyte-rich DLBCL, may show extensive T-cell infiltrates that mask the neoplastic B cells.

! Extramedullary acute myeloid leukemia (myeloid sarcoma) may aberrantly express T-cell markers and efface the lymph node.

! Morphologic and immunophenotypic overlap with AITL may create diagnostic challenges.

and systemic EBV-positive T-cell lymphoproliferative disease of childhood.[61] The latter is a clonal cytotoxic T-cell lymphoproliferative characterized by fulminant presentation and hemophagocytic syndrome.[65]

PROGNOSIS

As with other T-cell lymphomas, patients with PTCL, NOS are often treated with combination chemotherapy regimens, such as CHOP. Response rates of 50% to 60% have been reported.[66,67] High-intensity chemotherapy regimens have not been found to be superior to these combination chemotherapy regimens. The long-term prognosis of PTCL, NOS is poor and 5-year overall survival rates are only 20% to 30%. Clinical staging and the International Prognostic Index score are the main prognostic determinants.[20,21,49,50] A slightly more favorable clinical course has been reported in follicular and T-zone variants of PTCL, NOS as well as in cases showing deletions of 5q, 10q, and 12q.[68] Pathologic features reported to have an adverse influence on prognosis include high proliferation index, expression of cytotoxic markers, and association with EBV.[19,66]

REFERENCES

1. Lennert K. [Nature, prognosis and nomenclature of angioimmunoblastic lymphadenopathy (lymphogranulomatosis X or T-zone lymphoma)]. Dtsch Med Wochenschr 1979;104:1246–7 [in German].

2. Frizzera G, Moran EM, Rappaport H. Angio-immunoblastic lymphadenopathy with dysproteinaemia. Lancet 1974;1:1070–3.

3. Lukes RJ, Tindle BH. Immunoblastic lymphadenopathy. A hyperimmune entity resembling Hodgkin's disease. N Engl J Med 1975;292:1–8.

4. Mourad N, Mounier N, Briere J, et al. Clinical, biologic, and pathologic features in 157 patients with angioimmunoblastic T-cell lymphoma treated within the Groupe d'Etude des Lymphomes de l'Adulte (GELA) trials. Blood 2008;111:4463–70.

5. Dogan A, Gaulard P, Jaffe ES, et al. Angioimmunoblastic T-cell lymphoma. In: Swerdlow SH, editor. WHO classification of tumours of haematopoietic and lymphoid tissues. Lyon (France): International Agency for Research on Cancer (IARC); 2008. p. 309–11.

6. Attygalle AD, Chuang SS, Diss TC, et al. Distinguishing angioimmunoblastic T-cell lymphoma from peripheral T-cell lymphoma, unspecified, using morphology, immunophenotype and molecular genetics. Histopathology 2007;50:498–508.

7. Attygalle AD, Diss TC, Munson P, et al. CD10 expression in extranodal dissemination of angioimmunoblastic T-cell lymphoma. Am J Surg Pathol 2004;28:54–61.

8. Ortonne N, Dupuis J, Plonquet A, et al. Characterization of CXCL13+ neoplastic t cells in cutaneous lesions of angioimmunoblastic T-cell lymphoma (AITL). Am J Surg Pathol 2007;31:1068–76.

9. Grogg KL, Attygalle AD, Macon WR, et al. Angioimmunoblastic T-cell lymphoma: a neoplasm of germinal-center T-helper cells? Blood 2005;106:1501–2.

10. Attygalle A, Al-Jehani R, Diss TC, et al. Neoplastic T cells in angioimmunoblastic T-cell lymphoma express CD10. Blood 2002;99:627–33.

11. de Leval L, Rickman DS, Thielen C, et al. The gene expression profile of nodal peripheral T-cell lymphoma demonstrates a molecular link between angioimmunoblastic T-cell lymphoma (AITL) and follicular helper T (TFH) cells. Blood 2007;109:4952–63.

12. Grogg KL, Attygalle AD, Macon WR, et al. Expression of CXCL13, a chemokine highly upregulated in germinal center T-helper cells, distinguishes angioimmunoblastic T-cell lymphoma from peripheral T-cell lymphoma, unspecified. Mod Pathol 2006;19:1101–7.

13. Dorfman DM, Brown JA, Shahsafaei A, et al. Programmed death-1 (PD-1) is a marker of germinal center-associated T cells and angioimmunoblastic T-cell lymphoma. Am J Surg Pathol 2006;30:802–10.

14. Krishnan C, Warnke RA, Arber DA, et al. PD-1 expression in T-cell lymphomas and reactive lymphoid entities: potential overlap in staining patterns between lymphoma and viral lymphadenitis. Am J Surg Pathol 2010;34:178–89.

15. Ohshima K, Takeo H, Kikuchi M, et al. Heterogeneity of Epstein-Barr virus infection in angioimmunoblastic lymphadenopathy type T-cell lymphoma. Histopathology 1994;25:569–79.

16. Attygalle AD, Kyriakou C, Dupuis J, et al. Histologic evolution of angioimmunoblastic T-cell lymphoma in consecutive biopsies: clinical correlation and insights into natural history and disease progression. Am J Surg Pathol 2007;31:1077–88.

17. Huang Y, Moreau A, Dupuis J, et al. Peripheral T-cell lymphomas with a follicular growth pattern are derived from follicular helper T cells (TFH) and may show overlapping features with angioimmunoblastic T-cell lymphomas. Am J Surg Pathol 2009;33:682–90.

18. Swerdlow S, Campo E, Harris N, et al, editors. WHO classification of tumours of haematopoietic and lymphoid tissues. 4th edition. Lyon (France): International Agency for Research on Cancer; 2008. p. 306–19.

19. Savage KJ, Harris NL, Vose JM, et al. ALK-anaplastic large-cell lymphoma is clinically and immunophenotypically different from both ALK+ ALCL and peripheral T-cell lymphoma, not otherwise specified: report from the international peripheral T-cell lymphoma project. Blood 2008;111:5496–504.

20. Savage KJ, Chhanabhai M, Gascoyne RD, et al. Characterization of peripheral T-cell lymphomas in a single North American institution by the WHO classification. Ann Oncol 2004;15:1467–75.

21. Vose J, Armitage J, Weisenburger D. International peripheral T-cell and natural killer/T-cell lymphoma study: pathology findings and clinical outcomes. J Clin Oncol 2008;26:4124–30.

22. Rizvi MA, Evens AM, Tallman MS, et al. T-cell non-Hodgkin lymphoma. Blood 2006;107:1255–64.

23. Falini B, Pileri S, Zinzani PL, et al. ALK+ lymphoma: clinico-pathological findings and outcome. Blood 1999;93:2697–706.

24. Foss HD, Anagnostopoulos I, Araujo I, et al. Anaplastic large-cell lymphomas of T-cell and null-cell phenotype express cytotoxic molecules. Blood 1996;88:4005–11.

25. Fraga M, Brousset P, Schlaifer D, et al. Bone marrow involvement in anaplastic large cell lymphoma. Immunohistochemical detection of minimal disease and its prognostic significance. Am J Clin Pathol 1995;103:82–9.

26. Bayle C, Charpentier A, Duchayne E, et al. Leukaemic presentation of small cell variant anaplastic large cell lymphoma: report of four cases. Br J Haematol 1999;104:680–8.

27. Benharroch D, Meguerian-Bedoyan Z, Lamant L, et al. ALK-positive lymphoma: a single disease with a broad spectrum of morphology. Blood 1998;91:2076–84.

28. Pileri S, Falini B, Delsol G, et al. Lymphohistiocytic T-cell lymphoma (anaplastic large cell lymphoma CD30+/Ki-1 + with a high content of reactive histiocytes). Histopathology 1990;16:383–91.

29. Kinney M, Collins R, Greer J, et al. A small-cell-predominant variant of primary Ki-1 (CD30)+ T-cell lymphoma. Am J Surg Pathol 1993;17:859–68.

30. Vassallo J, Lamant L, Brugieres L, et al. ALK-positive anaplastic large cell lymphoma mimicking nodular sclerosis Hodgkin's lymphoma: report of 10 cases. Am J Surg Pathol 2006;30:223–9.

31. Chan JK, Buchanan R, Fletcher CD. Sarcomatoid variant of anaplastic large-cell Ki-1 lymphoma. Am J Surg Pathol 1990;14:983–8.

32. Wellmann A, Thieblemont C, Pittaluga S, et al. Detection of differentially expressed genes in lymphomas using cDNA arrays: identification of clusterin as a new diagnostic marker for anaplastic large cell lymphomas (ALCL). Blood 2000;96:398–404.

33. Dunphy CH, DeMello DE, Gale GB. Pediatric CD56+ anaplastic large cell lymphoma: a review of the literature. Arch Pathol Lab Med 2006;130:1859–64.

34. Juco J, Holden JT, Mann KP, et al. Immunophenotypic analysis of anaplastic large cell lymphoma by flow cytometry. Am J Clin Pathol 2003;119:205–12.

35. Brousset P, Rochaix P, Chittal S, et al. High incidence of Epstein-Barr virus detection in Hodgkin's disease and absence of detection in anaplastic large-cell lymphoma in children. Histopathology 1993;23:189–91.

36. Rosso R, Paulli M, Magrini U, et al. Anaplastic large cell lymphoma, CD30/Ki-1 positive, expressing the CD15/Leu-M1 antigen. Immunohistochemical and morphological relationships to Hodgkin's disease. Virchows Arch A Pathol Anat Histopathol 1990;416:229–35.

37. de Leval L, Bisig B, Thielen C, et al. Molecular classification of T-cell lymphomas. Crit Rev Oncol Hematol 2009;72(2):125–43.

38. Delsol G, Lamant L, Mariame B, et al. A new subtype of large B-cell lymphoma expressing the ALK kinase and lacking the 2; 5 translocation. Blood 1997;89:1483–90.

39. Chen Y, Takita J, Choi YL, et al. Oncogenic mutations of ALK kinase in neuroblastoma. Nature 2008;455:971–4.

40. Griffin CA, Hawkins AL, Dvorak C, et al. Recurrent involvement of 2p23 in inflammatory myofibroblastic tumors. Cancer Res 1999;59:2776–80.

41. Soda M, Choi YL, Enomoto M, et al. Identification of the transforming EML4-ALK fusion gene in non-small-cell lung cancer. Nature 2007;448:561–6.

42. Liso A, Tiacci E, Binazzi R, et al. Haploidentical peripheral-blood stem-cell transplantation for ALK-positive anaplastic large-cell lymphoma. Lancet Oncol 2004;5:127–8.

43. Savage KJ. Peripheral T-cell lymphomas. Blood Rev 2007;21:201–16.

44. Li R, Morris SW. Development of anaplastic lymphoma kinase (ALK) small-molecule inhibitors for cancer therapy. Med Res Rev 2008;28:372–412.

45. Pittaluga S, Wiodarska I, Pulford K, et al. The monoclonal antibody ALK1 identifies a distinct morphological subtype of anaplastic large cell lymphoma associated with 2p23/ALK rearrangements. Am J Pathol 1997;151:343–51.

46. Asano N, Oshiro A, Matsuo K, et al. Prognostic significance of T-cell or cytotoxic molecules phenotype in classical Hodgkin's lymphoma: a clinicopathologic study. J Clin Oncol 2006;24:4626–33.

47. Feldman AL, Dogan A. Diagnostic uses of Pax5 immunohistochemistry. Adv Anat Pathol 2007;14:323–34.

48. Macon WR. Peripheral T-cell lymphomas. Hematol Oncol Clin North Am 2009;23:829–42.

49. Abouyabis AN, Shenoy PJ, Lechowicz MJ, et al. Incidence and outcomes of the peripheral T-cell lymphoma subtypes in the United States. Leuk Lymphoma 2008;49:2099–107.

50. Rudiger T, Weisenburger DD, Anderson JR, et al. Peripheral T-cell lymphoma (excluding anaplastic large-cell lymphoma): results from the non-Hodgkin's lymphoma classification project. Ann Oncol 2002;13:140–9.

51. Suchi T, Lennert K, Tu LY. Histopathology and immunohistochemistry of peripheral T-cell lymphomas: a proposal for their classification. J Clin Pathol 1987;40:995–1015.

52. Barry TS, Jaffe ES, Sorbara L, et al. Peripheral T-cell lymphomas expressing CD30 and CD15. Am J Surg Pathol 2003;27:1513–22.

53. Yamashita Y, Nakamura S, Kagami Y, et al. Lennert's lymphoma: a variant of cytotoxic T-cell lymphoma? Am J Surg Pathol 2000;24:1627–33.

54. de Leval L, Savilo E, Longtine J, et al. Peripheral T-cell lymphoma with follicular involvement and a CD4+/bcl-6+ phenotype. Am J Surg Pathol 2001;25:395–400.

55. Rudiger T, Ichinohasama R, Ott MM, et al. Peripheral T-cell lymphoma with distinct perifollicular growth pattern: a distinct subtype of T-cell lymphoma? Am J Surg Pathol 2000;24:117–22.

56. Geissinger E, Odenwald T, Lee SS, et al. Nodal peripheral T-cell lymphomas and, in particular, their lymphoepithelioid (Lennert's) variant are often derived from CD8(+) cytotoxic T-cells. Virchows Arch 2004;445:334–43.

57. Petrella T, Bagot M, Willemze R, et al. Blastic NK-cell lymphomas (agranular CD4+CD56+ hematodermic neoplasms): a review. Am J Clin Pathol 2005;123:662–75.

58. Streubel B, Vinatzer U, Willheim M, et al. Novel t(5;9)(q33;q22) fuses ITK to SYK in unspecified

peripheral T-cell lymphoma. Leukemia 2006;20: 313–8.

59. Rigby S, Huang Y, Streubel B, et al. The lymphoma-associated fusion tyrosine kinase ITK-SYK requires pleckstrin homology domain - mediated membrane localisation for activation and cellular transformation. J Biol Chem 2009;284:26871–81.

60. Feldman AL, Sun DX, Law ME, et al. Overexpression of Syk tyrosine kinase in peripheral T-cell lymphomas. Leukemia 2008;22:1139–43.

61. Warnke RA, Jones D, Hsi ED. Morphologic and immunophenotypic variants of nodal T-cell lymphomas and T-cell lymphoma mimics. Am J Clin Pathol 2007; 127:511–27.

62. Fan Z, Natkunam Y, Bair E, et al. Characterization of variant patterns of nodular lymphocyte predominant Hodgkin lymphoma with immunohistologic and clinical correlation. Am J Surg Pathol 2003;27: 1346–56.

63. Abbondazo SL, Irey NS, Frizzera G. Dilantin-associated lymphadenopathy. Spectrum of histopathologic patterns. Am J Surg Pathol 1995;19:675–86.

64. Lim M, Straus SE, Dale J, et al. Pathologic findings in human autoimmune lymphoproliferative syndrome. Am J Pathol 1998;153:1541–50.

65. Quintanilla-Martinez L, Kumar S, Fend F, et al. Fulminant EBV(+) T-cell lymphoproliferative disorder following acute/chronic EBV infection: a distinct clinicopathologic syndrome. Blood 2000; 96:443–51.

66. Savage KJ. Prognosis and primary therapy in peripheral T-cell lymphomas. Hematology Am Soc Hematol Educ Program 2008;280–8.

67. Vose JM. Peripheral T-cell non-Hodgkin's lymphoma. Hematol Oncol Clin North Am 2008;22: 997–1005, x.

68. Zettl A, Rudiger T, Konrad MA, et al. Genomic profiling of peripheral T-cell lymphoma, unspecified, and anaplastic large T-cell lymphoma delineates novel recurrent chromosomal alterations. Am J Pathol 2004;164:1837–48.

HERPESVIRUS-ASSOCIATED B-CELL PROLIFERATIONS

Laurence de Leval, MD, PhD

KEYWORDS

- Epstein-Barr virus • Kaposi sarcoma herpesvirus • HHV-8 • HIV • Immunodeficiency
- Plasmablastic • Burkitt • Hodgkin • Castleman disease

ABSTRACT

This article reviews the spectrum of Epstein-Barr virus and Kaposi sarcoma herpesvirus (KSHV/HHV-8)-associated B-cell lymphoid proliferations, their pathologic features and clinical presentation, diagnostic criteria, and pathogenetic aspects. Emphasis is on the differential diagnosis issues and difficulties that the pathologist may face for the correct identification and interpretation of these lesions.

OVERVIEW

Herpesviruses are large double-stranded DNA viruses enclosed in an icosahedral capsid and surrounded by an outer envelope. They are highly disseminated among animals. There are 8 known human herpesviruses (HHV), which are further classified into alpha-, beta-, and gamma-herpesvirus subfamilies (Table 1). The alpha-herpesvirus subfamily comprises the herpesvirus types 1 and 2 (HSV-1 and HSV-2), which are typically associated with mucocutaneous lesions, and varicella-zoster virus (VZV), which causes chicken-pox and herpes zoster.[1] Members of the beta-herpesviridae include cytomegalovirus (CMV, also known as HHV-5), HHV-6 variants A and B, and HHV-7. Members of the gamma-herpesviridae include Epstein-Barr virus (EBV, also known as HHV-4) and Kaposi sarcoma herpesvirus (KSHV/HHV-8).

Common to all herpesviruses is their ability to evade host immune responses and to establish lifelong latent infections; members of the gamma-herpesviridae are strongly associated with malignancies. Both EBV and KSHV are B lymphotropic and a pathogenetic role for both viruses has been recognized in a wide variety of B-cell lymphomas arising in immunocompromised and/or immunocompetent individuals, ranging from commonly encountered entities to rare or exceptional forms of lymphoid proliferations.[2,3] This article reviews the spectrum of EBV- and KSHV/HHV-8-associated B-cell lymphoid proliferations, their pathologic features and clinical presentation, diagnostic criteria, and some pathogenetic aspects, with an emphasis on the differential diagnosis and difficulties that the pathologist may face for the correct identification and interpretation of these lesions.

EBV-ASSOCIATED B-CELL PROLIFERATIONS

EBV was identified as the first human tumor virus in cultures from a biopsy of a Burkitt lymphoma in 1964,[4] and was identified as the causative agent of infectious mononucleosis in 1968.[5] Since then, EBV has been implicated in the development of a large range of B-cell lymphoproliferative disorders, including, in addition to Burkitt lymphoma, classical Hodgkin lymphoma, immunodeficiency-associated lymphoid proliferations and lymphomas, and several diffuse large B-cell lymphoma

Institute of Pathology, Centre Hospitalier Universitaire Vaudois, 25 rue du Bugnon, 1011 Lausanne, Switzerland
E-mail address: Laurence.deLeval@chuv.ch

Surgical Pathology 3 (2010) 989–1033
doi:10.1016/j.path.2010.09.002

Table 1
Overview of human herpesviruses (HHV)

Herpesvirus	Subfamily	Clinical Manifestations	Oncogenicity
HHV-1/HSV-1	Alpha	Herpes	No
HHV-2/HSV-2	Alpha	Herpes	No
HHV-3/VZV	Alpha	Chickenpox, herpes zoster	No
HHV-4/EBV	Gamma	Infectious mononucleosis, carcinomas, mesenchymal malignancies, lymphomas, and lymphoproliferative disorders	Yes
HHV-5/CMV	Beta	Acute infection and reactivation	No
HHV-6 (A and B)	Beta	Exanthem subitum	No
HHV-7	Beta	Similar to HHV-6	No
HHV-8/KSHV	Gamma	Kaposi sarcoma, B-cell lymphoproliferative disorders and lymphomas	Yes

Abbreviations: CMV, cytomegalovirus; EBV, Epstein-Barr virus; HHV, human herpesviruses; HSV, herpes simplex virus; KSHV, Kaposi sarcoma herpesvirus; VZV, varicella-zoster virus.

entities or subtypes (**Table 2**). EBV infects more than 90% of the adult population worldwide and usually establishes a clinically silent lifelong infection (persistent infection). A disruption of the balance between the host antiviral immunity and the virus, usually resulting from decreased immune function, may lead to the development of an EBV-associated disease.[6,7]

EBV-infected cells not undergoing lytic replication display a restricted pattern of expression of the EBV genome. Based on the expression patterns of Epstein-Barr nuclear antigen (EBNA) and latent membrane protein (LMP) gene families, and Epstein-Barr small-coding RNAs (EBER), 3 types of latency programs have been described (**Table 3**). Latency I is limited to EBER and EBNA-1 expression, latency II in addition includes LMP-1 and LMP-2 expression, and latency III involves the unrestricted expression of all EBNAs, LMPs, and EBER. Latency I is associated with EBV-related Burkitt lymphoma, latency II is associated with EBV-positive classical Hodgkin lymphoma, and latency III is characteristic of post-transplant and HIV-associated lymphoid proliferations.[6,8,9] EBV-encoded latent genes induce B-cell transformation in vitro by altering cellular gene transcription and constitutively activating key cell-signaling pathways.[6] LMP-1 is the main transforming protein of EBV and is essential for EBV-induced B-cell transformation in vitro.[6]

Ascertaining the relationship of a lymphoid proliferation to EBV infection requires the detection of EBV products in the tumor cells. Because EBER is expressed at high levels in infected cells in all 3 latency programs, EBER detection by in situ hybridization (ISH) is the gold standard for EBV detection in tissue sections. There are commercially available antibodies against different EBV-encoded proteins (EBNA-1, EBNA-2, and LMP-1) suitable for immunohistochemistry assays, but these are usually less sensitive than EBER ISH.

KSHV/HHV-8-ASSOCIATED B-CELL PROLIFERATIONS

KSHV/HHV-8, originally identified in 1994 from a Kaposi sarcoma of an AIDS patient,[10] was subsequently found to be directly associated with various B-cell lymphoproliferative disorders most commonly arising in HIV-infected individuals. These include HHV-8-positive multicentric Castleman disease (MCD), large B-cell lymphoma arising in HHV-8-positive MCD, and primary effusion lymphoma and its extracavitary variant.[11,12] Less common forms of HHV-8-associated lymphoid proliferations have been reported in immunocompetent or immunocompromised patients, including germinotropic lymphoproliferative disorder (**Table 4**).[13–15] Importantly, some of these entities are characterized by coinfection with EBV.

Similar to EBV, primary HHV-8 infection, probably transmitted through saliva, is asymptomatic in most instances. In contrast to EBV, however,

Table 2
EBV-associated B-cell lymphoid proliferations

Disease	Population at Risk	EBV Association
Acute infection		
Infectious mononucleosis	Late adolescents or young adults	100%
Fatal infectious mononucleosis	Primary immune disorders (X-linked lymphoproliferative disorder and severe combined immunodeficiency)	100%
Burkitt lymphoma subtypes		
Endemic	African children	>90%
Sporadic	Children in non-endemic areas	15%–20%
HIV-associated	HIV-infected individuals	30%–40%
Classical Hodgkin lymphoma	Immunocompetent and immunocompromised individuals, young adults	40%
Immunodeficiency-associated lymphoproliferative disorders		
Primary immune disorders	Congenital immunodeficiencies	>80%
Post-transplant lymphoproliferative disorders	Solid organ transplant and bone marrow allograft recipients	>80%
Iatrogenic immunodeficiency-associated lymphoproliferative disorders	Patients with autoimmune diseases treated with methotrexate, antagonists of TNF-alpha or other immunomodulatory drugs	Varies according to histologic subtypes, overall <50%
Diffuse large B-cell lymphoma subtypes/entities		
Plasmablastic lymphoma	HIV-infected individuals	90%
DLBCL associated with HIV infection	HIV-infected individuals	>75%
Lymphomatoid granulomatosis	Congenital immunodeficiencies, posttransplant, HIV-infected individuals	100%
DLBCL associated with chronic inflammation	Chronic pyothorax or chronic suppuration	90%
EBV+ DLBCL of the elderly	Elderly patients (older than 50 years)	100%

Abbreviations: DLBCL, diffuse large B-cell lymphoma; EBV, Epstein-Barr virus; TNF, tumor necrosis factor.

HHV-8 is not ubiquitous and its seroprevalence in adults varies from 1% to 5% in Northern Europe and North America to 50% or more in Africa.[16] In HHV-8-associated lymphoproliferative disorders, most cells are latently infected and express several latency-associated viral products, including LANA-1 (latency-associated nuclear antigen 1, essential for maintenance of viral latency and interacting with several intracellular oncogenic pathways), v-cyclin (an analog of D-type cyclins, promoting cell-cycle progression), v-FLIP (viral Fas-ligand interleukin-1B-converting enzyme inhibitory protein, a potent activator of NF-κB), and LANA-2 (an antagonist of p53-mediated apoptosis in vitro).[12,17] Viral interleukin (IL)-6, which is abundantly produced in lytically infected

Table 3
Latent EBV-encoded genes

EBV-Encoded Genes	Main Function	Location	Expression in Latency I	Expression in Latency II	Expression in Latency III
EBNA-1	Genome maintenance	Nucleus	+	+	+
EBNA-2	Viral transactivator	Nucleus	−	−	+
EBNA-3	EBNA-2 antagonist	Nucleus	−	−	+
LMP-1	Viral oncogene	Membrane	−	+	+
LMP-2	Survival factor	Membrane	−	+	+
EBER-1 and EBER-2	Viral persistence	Nucleus	+	+	+

Abbreviations: EBER, Epstein-Barr small coding RNAs; EBNA, Epstein-Barr nuclear antigen; EBV, Epstein-Barr virus; LMP, latent membrane protein.

cells, is also variably expressed in latently infected cells and acts as a multifunctional cytokine analogous to human IL-6, promoting increased plasma cells and angiogenesis. Several lines of evidence indicate the role of the IL-6 signaling pathway in HHV-8-mediated lymphomagenesis.[12] For diagnostic purposes, immunohistochemistry with antibodies directed against LANA-1 represents the most widely used method to demonstrate HHV-8 in tissue sections for the diagnosis of the HHV-8-associated disorders.[18]

INFECTIOUS MONONUCLEOSIS

Primary EBV infection (transmitted by salivary contact) is usually asymptomatic, but if delayed until adolescence or adulthood may present symptomatically as infectious mononucleosis (IM). IM is usually characterized by expansion of EBV-infected B cells, eliciting the simultaneous expansion of activated CD8+ cytotoxic T lymphocytes, thought to both control the infection by lysing proliferating EBV-positive B cells as well as cause the symptoms of IM by excessive cytokine release. Although IM is normally a transient and self-limited benign disease, it can be an important source of diagnostic pitfalls with other reactive or neoplastic conditions, as will be discussed below.

Clinical Features

Patients most commonly present with fever, tonsillar enlargement and/or cervical lymphadenopathy, atypical CD8+ lymphocytosis in the peripheral blood, high EBV viral DNA levels, and positive heterophile antibody test (monospot).[19] Generalized lymphadenopathy and hepatosplenomegaly can be seen in severe cases.

Microscopic Features

In biopsied tonsils and affected lymph nodes, IM exhibits an interfollicular or paracortical hyperplasia which distorts the architecture, but preserves follicles and sinus patency (**Fig. 1**).[20] The lymphoid expansion comprises a polymorphic infiltrate of small lymphocytes, large lymphoid cells, immunoblasts (often showing plasmacytoid differentiation forming a spectrum to plasmablasts and plasma cells), cells resembling Reed-Sternberg cells, and occasionally bizarre giant forms. Focally, the immunoblasts may form sheets with a brisk mitotic and apoptotic rate and with clusters of apoptotic cells.[2–4] Geographic necrosis may be prominent.[6,21] Recognition of the spectrum of cell types encompassing small lymphocytes, large immunoblasts, and plasma cells is key to avoiding a misdiagnosis of malignancy.

Ancillary Studies

The large lymphoid cells in involved tissues are mostly EBV-infected B cells at a relatively late differentiation stage (CD20+ MUM1+ BCL-6−). Coexpression of CD30 is frequent, whereas CD15 is usually negative. Small cells dispersed within tissues are mostly T cells (with CD8+ cells predominating over CD4+ cells), and a subset of

Table 4
KSHV/HHV-8-associated B-cell lymphoproliferative disorders

Lymphoma Type	Morphology	Phenotype	HIV	EBV	Location	IGH Status	Clinical Course
HHV-8+ MCD disease	Plasmablasts in mantle zones	CD20−/+ CD79a− MUM1+ CD138− CD30− monotypic cIgM lambda+	+	−	Lymph nodes, spleen	Polyclonal, unmutated	Aggressive
Large B-cell lymphoma arising in HHV-8+ MCD	Clusters ("microlymphoma") or sheets (lymphoma) of plasmablasts in mantle zones, interfollicular areas, or diffusely infiltrating	CD20−/+ CD79a− MUM1+ CD138+ CD30− monotypic cIgM lambda+	+	−	Lymph nodes, spleen	Polyclonal and monoclonal, unmutated	Aggressive
Primary effusion lymphoma (PEL)	Large immunoblast-like cells, pleomorphic or anaplastic	CD45+ CD20− CD79a− MUM1+ CD138+ CD30+ immunoglobulin−	+	+ (most)	Body cavities (pleural, pericardial, peritoneal)	Monoclonal, mutated	Aggressive
Extracavitary PEL	Large immunoblast-like cells, pleomorphic or anaplastic	CD45± CD20−/+ MUM1+ CD138± CD30+ immunoglobulin−/+	+	+ (most)	Extranodal sites (gastrointestinal, skin, lung), rarely lymph nodes	Monoclonal, mutated	Variable
Germinotropic lymphoproliferative disorder	Plasmablasts in germinal centers	CD45− CD20− CD138− CD30+, cytoplasmic immunoglobulin+	−	+	Lymph nodes	Polyclonal or oligoclonal, mutated	Indolent

Abbreviations: EBV, Epstein-Barr virus; HHV, human herpesviruses; KSHV, Kaposi sarcoma herpesvirus; MCD, multicentric Castleman disease.

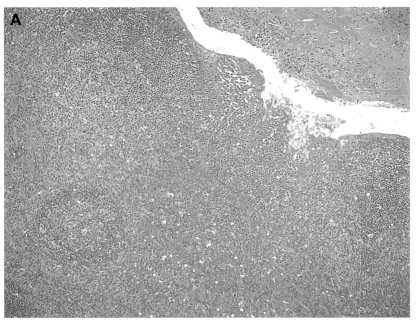

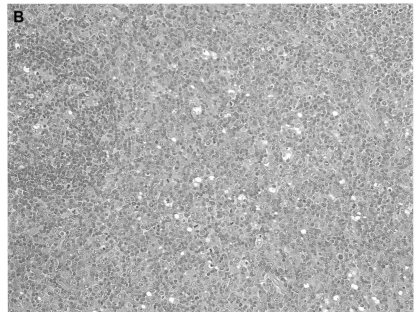

Fig. 1. Histology of IM involving the tonsil of a 13-year-old boy. (A) There is marked lymphoid hyperplasia affecting the perifollicular and interfollicular areas with associated ulceration; architecture is partially preserved as indicated by the persistence of a small lymphoid follicle (in lower left of image) (hematoxylin-eosin [H&E], ×100). (B) The perifollicular areas contain a proliferation comprising mostly large lymphoid cells, with abundant mitotic activity (H&E, ×200).

the CD8+ T cells can be enlarged, resembling immunoblasts (Fig. 2). EBV-infected B cells express a type III latency program and EBER ISH typically shows widespread staining of the large B cells and often plasma cells as well. Polymerase chain reaction (PCR) studies on IM cases fail to reveal monotypic B- or T-cell populations and the EBV is polyclonal, indicating infection of multiple individual cells rather than clonal expansion of a single EBV-infected cell.[22] However, cases of fatal or fulminant sporadic IM can show clonal EBV as well as clonal immunoglobulin heavy chain (*IGH*) or T-cell receptor (*TCR*) gene rearrangements (**Fig. 3**).[23]

Fig. 1. Histology of IM involving the tonsil of a 13-year-old boy. (*C*) The large lymphoid cells are highly atypical and comprise forms with Reed-Sternberg-like features (H&E, ×400). (*D*) Sheets of large lymphoid cells adjacent to areas of necrosis are very worrisome for malignancy (H&E, ×400).

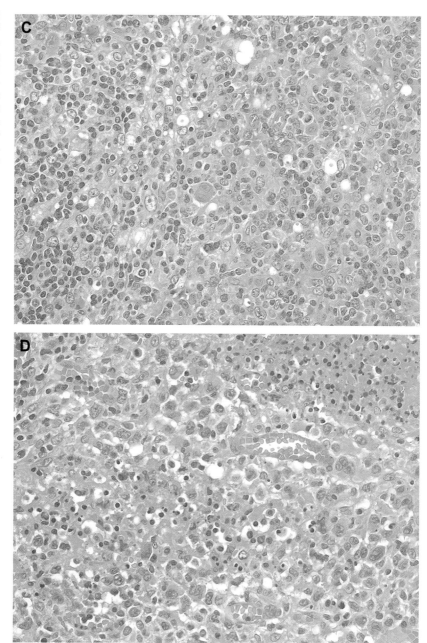

Differential Diagnosis

The differential diagnosis is with malignant lymphoma (non-Hodgkin or Hodgkin lymphomas) as well as with other reactive conditions. From the pathologist's point of view, IM can so strongly mimic malignant lymphoma histologically that it has been said that lymph node biopsy—resulting in an erroneous lymphoma diagnosis and inappropriate administration of chemotherapy—is one of the "complications" of the disease. Important

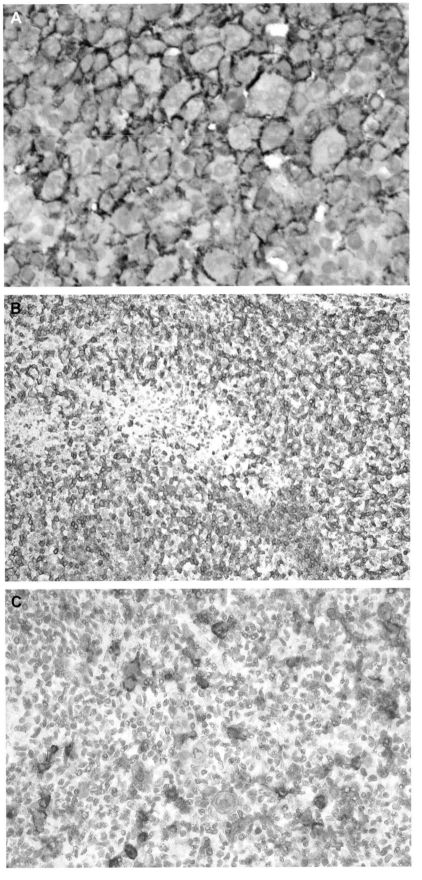

Fig. *2.* Immunohistochemical stains of IM case from **Fig.** **1.** (*A*) CD20 highlights the numerous large B cells (immunoperoxidase, ×400). (*B*) There is also an abundant infiltrate of CD8+ T cells, including some of the large cells (immunoperoxidase, ×200). (*C*) Some of the large atypical cells are strongly positive for CD30 (immunoperoxidase, ×400).

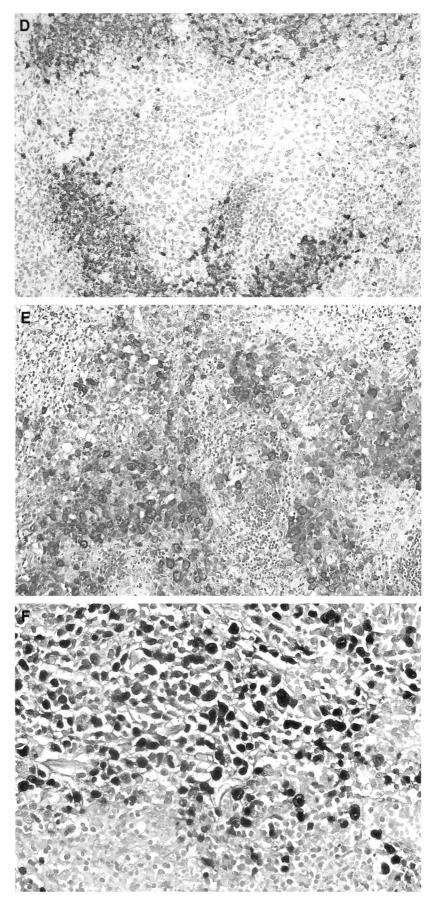

Fig. 2. Immunohistochemical stains of IM case from **Fig. 1**. (*D*) CD15 is negative in the large cells and only stains neutrophils in necrotic areas (immunoperoxidase, ×200). (*E*) EBV infection is demonstrated by strong positivity for EBNA-2, (immunoperoxidase, ×200) as well as positive EBER in situ hybridization (*F*) (×400).

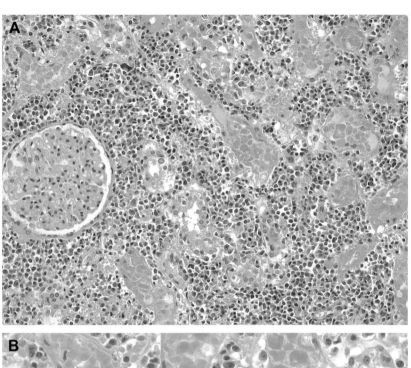

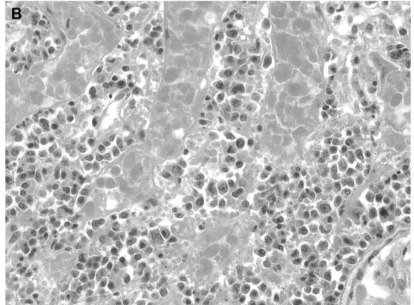

Fig. 3. Fatal IM at autopsy. (*A*) The kidney contains an infiltrate of large atypical lymphoid cells (H&E, ×200). (*B*) On high magnification, the cells have plasmacytoid features (H&E, ×400).

clues to the correct diagnosis include the following:

1. Obtaining adequate clinical information including peripheral blood findings, age of the patient, anatomic location of the lesions, and immune status.

2. Recognition of the preserved architecture and the morphologic spectrum of the proliferation.
3. Demonstration of EBV infection by EBER ISH or immunohistochemistry for EBV antigens.

When large cells are numerous, the differential diagnosis is with diffuse large B-cell lymphoma,

Fig. 3. Fatal IM at autopsy. (*C*) By immunohisto-chemistry, the cells are strongly positive for CD20 (immunoperoxi-dase, ×400). (*D*) In situ hybridization for EBER is positive (×400); molec-ular studies showed a monoclonal *IGH* gene rearrangement.

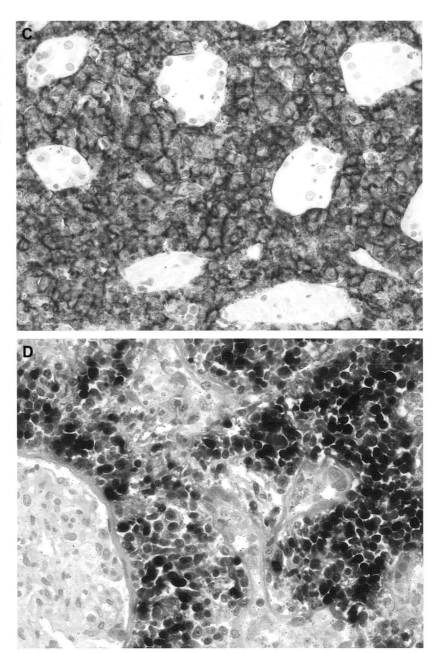

or sometimes with peripheral T-cell lymphoma in cases harboring numerous large T immunoblasts. The latter are only rarely EBV-positive and are usually associated with circulating atypical lymphocytes. In fact, examination of a peripheral blood smear can help "save the day" for the pathologist confronted with an IM tonsil or lymph node biopsy that mimics a malignant lymphoma, as the circulating atypical lymphocytes can be a clue to the diagnosis. Unlike the cells of most leukemic-phase lymphomas, the atypical lympho-cytes in IM (which are mostly CD8+ T cells) have a heterogeneous appearance, with abundant pale to deeply basophilic cytoplasm that often molds to adjacent red cells and oval to irregular nuclei with variable nucleoli. In tissue sections, the large B cells in IM usually do not form large, confluent sheets and although distorted, the tissue architecture is never completely effaced.[24] In problematic cases, genotyping studies may be useful, as *TCR* and *IGH* gene rearrangement studies are negative in IM cases.

Although the presence of very large numbers of EBER-positive cells in an immunocompetent patient should strongly suggest IM rather than lymphoma, EBV-positive lymphoid proliferations occurring in immunosuppressed patients can have similar histologic features as IM; IM is in fact a subtype of posttransplant lymphoproliferative disease. Thus, it is important to elicit a history of an immunosuppressed state in cases of suspected IM. EBV-positive diffuse large B-cell lymphoma (DLBCL) cases can occur in older patients without a documented history of specific immunosuppression (EBV-positive DLBCL of the elderly, discussed in more detail later in this article).[25,26] These cases are more commonly encountered in Asia, frequently occur in extranodal sites such as the tonsil, and can have numerous interspersed reactive T cells, mimicking IM. However, the age distribution is markedly different from IM and, unlike cases of IM, EBV-positive DBLCL of the elderly usually demonstrates clonal *IGH* rearrangements.

Recently, Dojcinov and colleagues[27] reported a series of EBV-positive mucocutaneous ulcerative lesions in patients with age-related immunosenescence or iatrogenic immunosuppression. These lesions, which frequently involved the oropharyngeal mucosa, comprise EBV-positive Reed-Sternberg-like cells in a polymorphous background and may mimic IM histologically. In contrast to IM, the atypical cells often expressed CD15 and the lesions were associated with clonal *IGH* and/or *TCR* gene rearrangements. Lymphomatoid granulomatosis may enter into the differential diagnosis, as this disease can have numerous EBV-positive large B cells in a T-cell rich background and positive EBV serology. However, the distribution of disease (lung and upper aerodigestive tract) and clinical presentation are different from IM.[18]

IM often contains enlarged immunoblasts resembling Reed-Sternberg cells, which may raise the differential diagnosis of Hodgkin lymphoma. However, the background cells are different and in IM, the immunoblasts are CD15 negative.[20] The predominance of CD8+ T cells in IM (as well as in other viral lymphadenopathies) also aids in the distinction from classical Hodgkin lymphoma, in which the T cells are predominantly CD4+.

Prognosis

IM is usually self-limited, but the disease may be fatal in cases with fulminant evolution when associated with hemophagocytic syndrome and pancytopenia or with X-linked or other immunodeficiency states.[23]

BURKITT LYMPHOMA

Clinical Features

Burkitt lymphoma (BL) is a highly aggressive neoplasm with a very rapid doubling time that includes 3 clinical variants: endemic (>90% EBV-associated), sporadic (15–20% EBV associated), and immunodeficiency-related 30–40% EBV-associated, see topic "Diagnosis of Burkitt Lymphoma and Related High-Grade B-cell Lymphomas" by Sohani and Hasserjian elsewhere in this issue. Importantly, although these clinical variants differ in their association with EBV, their pathologic features are overall similar. The clinical variants of BL also share a specific gene expression profile, supporting their inclusion within a single pathologic entity.[28,29]

Microscopic Features and Ancillary Studies

BL is composed of monotonous medium-sized B cells with finely dispersed chromatin, multiple nucleoli, and a scant amount of basophilic cytoplasm with a well-delineated cytoplasmic border (**Fig. 4**). As BL exhibits a very high rate of both mitosis and apoptosis, frequent phagocytic histiocytes impart a characteristic (but nonspecific) "starry-sky" appearance. By immunohistochemistry, BL is positive for B-cell markers and surface immunoglobulin M (sIgM), and strongly expresses CD10 and BCL-6, but is negative for BCL-2, an immunophenotype similar to that of germinal center B cells. Accordingly, BL cells also carry hypermutations in their immunoglobulin (*IG*) genes, indicating a germinal center cell origin. Ki67 reveals a proliferation fraction of near 100% (at least 95%). Irrespective of the EBV status, all cases of BL exhibit constitutive activation of the *MYC* gene at the 8q24 locus by translocation, most frequently to the *IGH* region (14q32), or less commonly to the *IGL* (22q11), *IGK* (2p12), or another, nonimmunoglobulin locus. *MYC* activation is a key factor in the oncogenesis of all clinical variants of BL.[6] Although not essential to the pathogenesis of BL, EBV supports tumor development. Most EBV-positive cases express only EBNA-1 and EBER (latency type I). The oncogenic potential of EBNA-1 is debated, but it plays a role in the maintenance and replication of the viral genome, and may promote genetic instability. Conversely,

Fig. 4. Burkitt lymphoma in an HIV-positive patient. (*A*) There is a diffuse lymphoid proliferation with a starry-sky pattern (H&E, ×200). (*B*) The neoplastic cells are medium-sized with round nuclei and multiple nucleoli (H&E, ×400). (*C*) On cytologic preparations, the cells have deeply basophilic and vacuolated cytoplasm (May-Grünwald Giemsa, ×10,200).

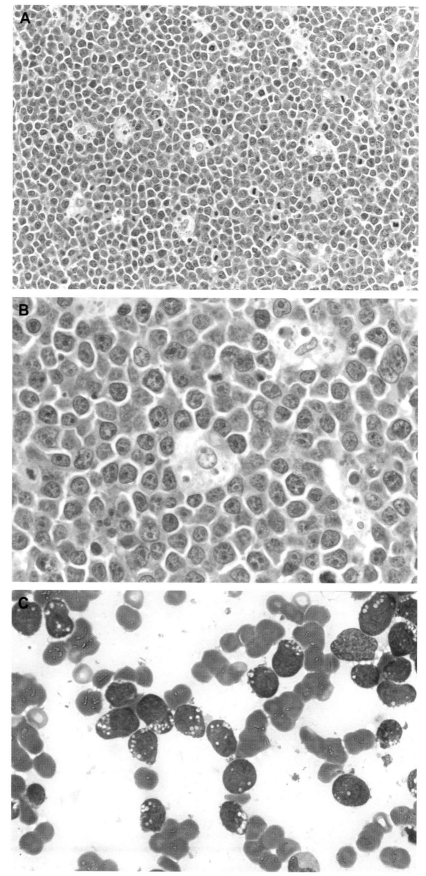

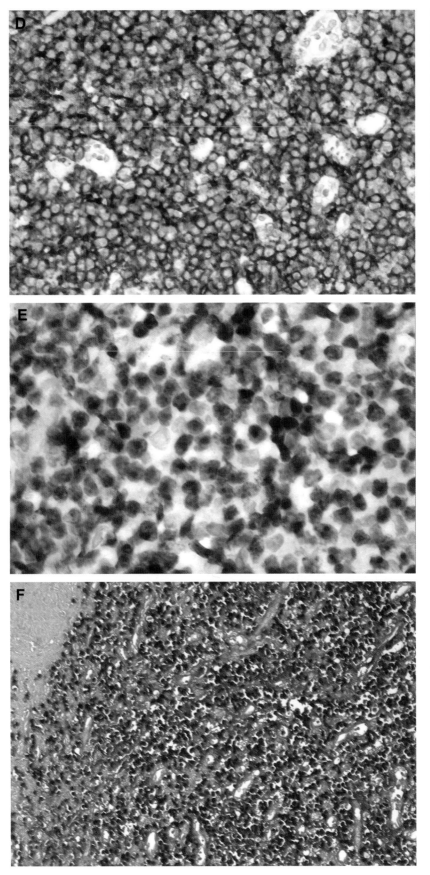

Fig. 4. Burkitt lymphoma in an HIV-positive patient. (*D*) By immunohistochemistry, the cells are strongly positive for CD20 (immunoperoxidase, ×200). The neoplastic cells display a nearly 100% proliferation fraction by Ki67 immunostaining (*E*) (immunoperoxidase, ×400) and are strongly positive for EBV by EBER in situ hybridization (*F*) (×200).

EBER seems to play a more important role by (1) counteracting the pro-apoptotic effects of c-MYC, (2) inducing the expression of IL-10, which might stimulate the growth of infected B cells, and (3) mediating resistance to interferon-alpha.[2,30,31] More recent data have shown that EBV encodes viral micro-inhibitory RNAs, which may interfere with the physiologic regulation exerted by cellular micro-inhibitory RNAs.[32]

Differential Diagnosis

The differential diagnosis of BL is discussed in detail in the article elsewhere in this publication by Sohani and Hasserjian, "Diagnosis of Burkitt Lymphoma and Related High-Grade B-cell Lymphomas."

Prognosis

BL is highly aggressive but potentially curable. With intensive chemotherapy, the cure rate is up to 90% in low-stage disease and 60% to 80% in patients with advanced-stage disease.[33] Because the EBV status does not influence the prognosis or response to therapy in BL, assessment of EBV status in BL samples in diagnostic practice is of little clinical relevance.

HODGKIN LYMPHOMA

Hodgkin lymphoma (HL) is characterized by scarce clonal neoplastic cells (Reed-Sternberg cells and variants [HRS cells]) dispersed among a reactive background. HL comprises classical and nonclassical types based on different morphologic, phenotypic, and molecular features.[34] Nodular lymphocyte-predominant HL (NLPHL) represents the nonclassical entity, whereas classical HL (cHL) includes the nodular-sclerosis, mixed-cellularity, lymphocyte-rich, and lymphocyte-depleted subtypes.

Clinical Features

EBV is found in the HRS cells in about 40% of cHL cases in the Western world, whereas NLPHL is with few exceptions not associated with EBV.[35–37] The rate of detection of EBV is higher in the mixed-cellularity and lymphocyte-depleted than in the lymphocyte-rich and nodular-sclerosis subtypes of cHL. Sex and ethnicity also influence the epidemiology of EBV in cHL cases: EBV is more frequent in cHL occurring in males than in females and is more frequent in Asian and Hispanic individuals than in whites and blacks. An increased incidence of EBV-positive cHL cases is also observed in underdeveloped nations as compared with Western countries. A bimodal age distribution is recognized for EBV-positive patients, with cHL in children and older age groups being more likely to be EBV-associated than cHL in young adults. This finding may be related to a reduced immune surveillance in children and older adults. Accordingly, EBV positivity is almost constant in HIV-associated cHL.[38]

Microscopic Features and Ancillary Studies

HRS cells in cHL are characterized by massive loss of the B-cell phenotype (absent or weak expression of CD20, negativity for CD79a, weak positivity for PAX-5, absent or weak expression of BOB.1 and/or OCT-2 transcription factors), strongly express CD30, and are positive for CD15 in most cases (**Fig. 5**).[39] They are probably derived from germinal center B cells that have acquired disadvantageous *IG* variable chain gene mutations (nonsense or crippling mutations)[40] and normally would have undergone apoptosis in the absence of a rescuing event. Accordingly, a central mechanism in cHL pathogenesis is the constitutive activation of the NF-kappaB and JAK/STAT signaling pathways that play a key role for promoting HRS cell survival and proliferation.[36,41] Conversely, the neoplastic cells in NLPHL phenotypically retain a complete B-cell immunophenotype, express BCL-6, and appear to derive from antigen-selected germinal center B cells.[36]

EBV-positive HRS cells exhibit a type II latency program, which includes expression of LMP-1, LMP-2, EBNA-1, and EBER.[2] Importantly, LMP-1 mimics an active CD40 receptor, thereby inducing NF-kappaB activation, and LMP-2A mimics the B-cell receptor. Thus, EBV provides two signals that are essential for the survival of germinal center B cells. The specific role of EBV in the pathogenesis of cHL is substantiated by the facts that EBV can rescue crippled germinal center B cells from apoptosis, and that all cases of cHL containing crippling *IG* mutations are EBV positive.[36,41]

Differential Diagnosis

Detection of EBV in the diagnostic workup of suspected HL is useful in at least two settings: (1) for the distinction between NLPHL and cHL, as the former is with few exceptions an EBV-negative neoplasm; (2) as an adjunct to other ancillary techniques in cases occurring in immunocompetent patients, where a differential diagnosis with non-Hodgkin lymphoma is entertained. For example, in the evaluation of difficult mediastinal lesions questionable for HL versus primary mediastinal large B-cell lymphoma,

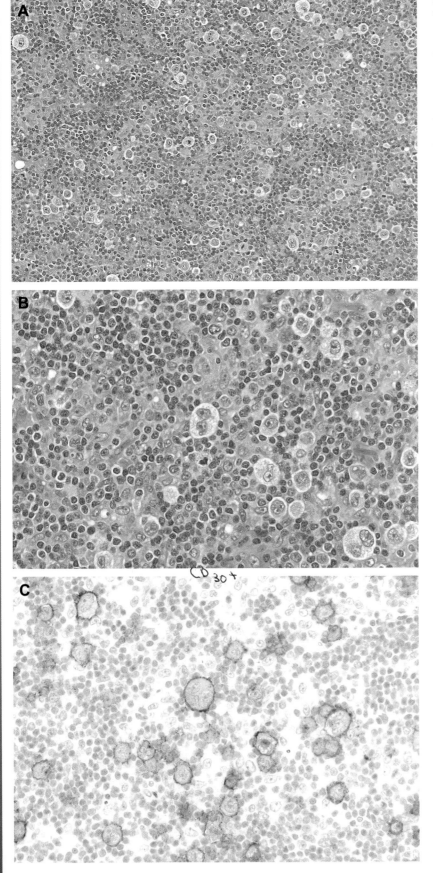

Fig. 5. EBV-positive mixed-cellularity classical Hodgkin lymphoma. (*A*) There is diffuse infiltrate with no dissecting fibrosis, comprising a histiocyte-rich background and numerous large atypical cells (H&E, ×200). (*B*) The atypical cells show cytologic features of Reed-Sternberg cells and variants (H&E, ×400). By immunohistochemistry, the Reed-Sternberg cells are positive for CD30 (*C*) (immunoperoxidase, ×400).

Fig. 5. EBV-positive mixed cellularity classical Hodgkin lymphoma. The Reed-Sternberg cells are partially positive for CD15 (*D*), show strong nuclear positivity for MUM1/IRF4 (*E*), and are positive for EBER by in situ hybridization (*F*) (*D–F*, ×400).

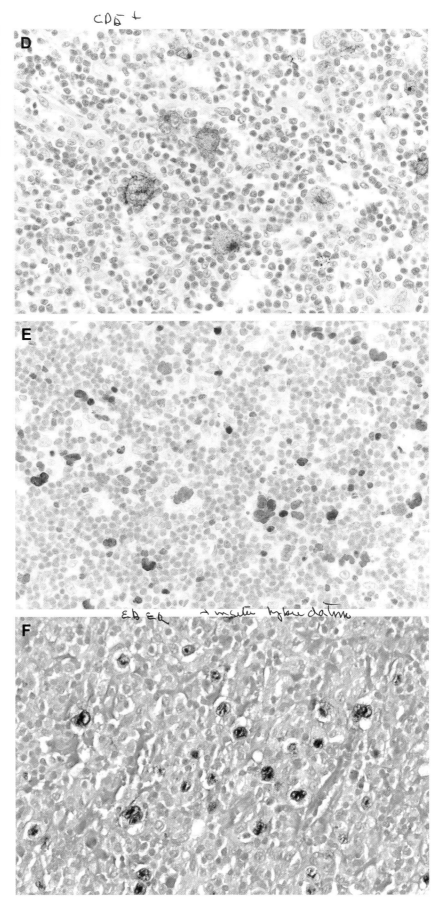

detection of EBV would strongly argue in favor of HL.[42] In immunocompromised individuals, EBV-positive cHL must be distinguished from other forms of EBV-positive B-cell lymphoid proliferations with Reed-Sternberg-like cells, such as EBV+ diffuse large B-cell lymphoma of the elderly.

Prognosis

Currently, cHL is curable in more than 85% of cases, usually with a combination of radiation and chemotherapy. Histologic subtyping influences the prognosis, with nodular sclerosis being more favorable than other subtypes.[39] The impact of EBV infection on clinical outcomes has been difficult to measure, because EBV association varies according to other variables, including age. For adult patients with cHL, EBV positivity has been found to correlate with an adverse clinical outcome in several studies.[43–45]

IMMUNODEFICIENCY-ASSOCIATED LYMPHOPROLIFERATIVE DISORDERS

EBV-positive lymphoid proliferations can often occur in the setting of immunodeficiency states that may be congenital, acquired, or iatrogenic. These include lymphoproliferative diseases associated with primary (ie, congenital) immune disorders, posttransplant lymphoproliferative disorders, lymphomas associated with HIV infection, and iatrogenic immunodeficiency-associated lymphoproliferative disorders.

Clinical Features

Patients with primary immune disorders (PIDs) carry an increased risk of developing lymphoproliferative disorders (LPDs), of which most are associated with EBV.[46] The PIDs most frequently associated with LPD are common variable immunodeficiency, severe combined immunodeficiency, ataxia telangiectasia, Wiskott-Aldrich syndrome, X-linked lymphoproliferative disorder, hyper-IgM syndrome, and autoimmune lymphoproliferative syndrome (ALPS). The types of lymphoid proliferation that occur in PID are variable (see later in this article) and the clinical context is the defining feature for the diagnosis of this category of lymphoid proliferations. EBV detection in this context may have therapeutic implications, as some of these disorders may be treated with antiviral agents.

Patients with HIV infection have a 60- to 200-fold increased risk of developing various lymphomas, predominantly aggressive B-cell neoplasms. Since the introduction of HAART (highly active antiretroviral therapy), the risk has,

however, been considerably reduced, and survival and outcomes have improved. HIV-associated lymphomas show an overall association with EBV in roughly 40% to 50% of the cases. Some specific HIV-associated histotypes are characterized by HHV-8 or dual HHV-8/EBV infection (discussed later in this article).[38,47]

Posttransplant lymphoproliferative disorders (PTLDs) occur in solid organ or bone marrow transplant recipients with an incidence related to the duration and intensity of the immune suppression. Iatrogenic immunodeficiency-associated LPDs encompass lymphoid proliferations arising in patients treated with immunosuppressive drugs for autoimmune disorders or conditions other than the posttransplant setting.[48] Immunosuppressive drugs reported in association with LPDs include methotrexate, antagonists of tumor necrosis factor (TNF)-alpha, and other immunomodulator agents.

Microscopic Features and Ancillary Studies

EBV-associated B-cell LPDs in PID include fatal IM (discussed previously in the Infectious Mononucleosis section), various B-cell lymphomas (diffuse large B-cell lymphoma, lymphomatoid granulomatosis, Burkitt lymphoma) and Hodgkin or Hodgkin-like lesions (**Fig. 6**). Their relative prevalence varies according to the type of underlying immune deficiency.

Table 5 summarizes the categories of HIV-associated lymphomas according to the World Health Organization (WHO) classification,[47] their association with lymphotropic viruses, and the correlation with the severity of immunodeficiency. BL and DLBCL each account for about 30% to 35% of HIV-associated lymphomas. HIV-associated lymphomas have a propensity to involve extranodal locations, especially the gastrointestinal tract and the central nervous system, but since the HAART era, nodal involvement has been observed to occur more often. Subtypes of lymphomas occurring more specifically in HIV-positive individuals will be described later in sections dealing with EBV-positive DLBCL and HHV-8-associated lymphomas.

Most PTLDs are of B-cell origin, and carry an association with EBV infection in most cases (60% to 80%). According to the WHO classification, B-cell PTLDs can be classified into 4 main categories[49]:

1. Early lesions, represented by polyclonal EBV-positive plasmacytic hyperplasia and IM-like lesions.
2. Polymorphic PTLDs, usually EBV-positive and monoclonal.

Fig. 6. EBV-positive lymphoid proliferation in primary immunodeficiency (autoimmune lymphoproliferative syndrome). (*A*) The palatal ulcer comprises a proliferation of large atypical lymphoid cells with foci of necrosis (H&E, ×200). (*B*) Some of the cells have Reed-Sternberg-like features (H&E, ×400).

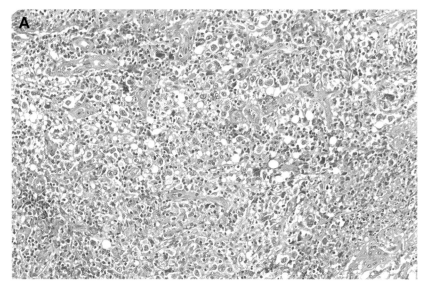

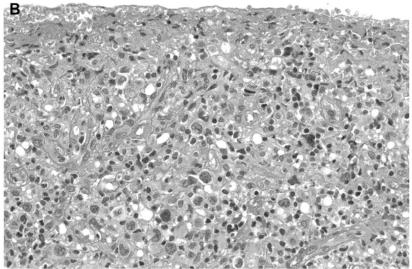

3. Monomorphic PTLDs represented by monoclonal B-cell lymphomas similar to those encountered in nonimmunosuppressed patients (usually DLBCL or BL), including a proportion of EBV-negative cases.
4. cHL, usually EBV-positive.

In PTLDs, the characteristic expression of the full spectrum of latent EBV genes (type III latency) indicates an important role for EBV in driving the proliferation of B cells. More aggressive clonal lymphoid proliferations may be associated with additional genetic alterations and a more restricted pattern of EBV latent gene expression.[2] Testing for EBV is essential in the workup of any LPD occurring in transplant recipient patients. Indeed early EBV-driven polyclonal lesions will often regress after withdrawal or reduction of the

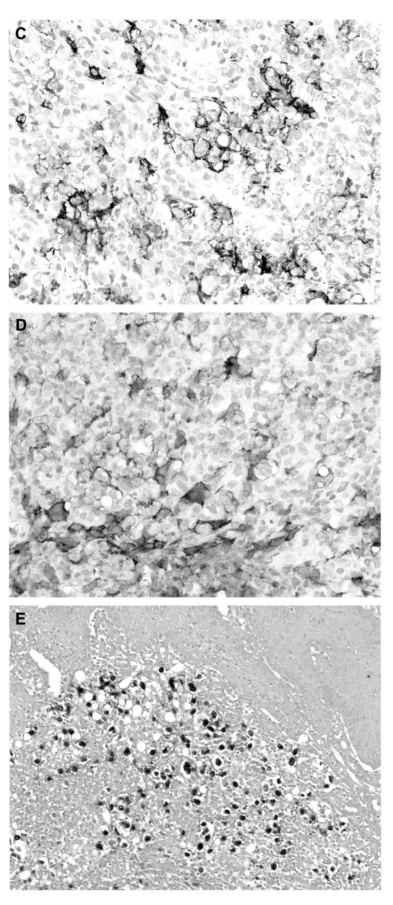

Fig. 6. EBV-positive lymphoid proliferation in primary immunodeficiency (autoimmune lymphoproliferative syndrome). By immunohistochemistry, the atypical cells show weak and partial expression of CD20 (*C*), with coexpression of CD30 (*D*) and positivity for EBER by in situ hybridization (*E*). A monoclonal IGH gene rearrangement was demonstrated by PCR (*C–E*, ×400).

Table 5
Lymphomas associated with HIV infection

	EBV	HHV-8	AIDS stage
LYMPHOMAS ALSO OCCURRING IN IMMUNOCOMPETENT PATIENTS			
Burkitt lymphoma	30–40%	No	Usually early
Diffuse large B-cell lymphoma subtypes			
• Centroblastic	>90%	No	Any time
• Immunoblastic (central nervous system or systemic)	30%	No	Late
Hodgkin lymphoma	>90%	No	Early
Others[a]			
LYMPHOMAS OCCURRING MORE SPECIFICALLY IN AIDS PATIENTS			
Plasmablastic lymphoma	80%	No	Late
Primary effusion lymphoma	80%	>90%	Late
Large B-cell lymphoma in HHV-8+ MCD	No	100%	Late
LYMPHOMAS OCCURRING IN OTHER IMMUNODEFICIENCY STATES			
Polymorphic B-cell lymphoid proliferations (PTLD-like)	>90%	No	Early

Abbreviations: EBV, Epstein-Barr virus; HHV, human herpesviruses; MCD, multicentric Castleman disease; PTLD, posttransplant lymphoproliferative disorder.

[a] Includes marginal zone lymphomas of MALT type and peripheral T/NK cell lymphomas.

immunosuppression and/or administration of EBV-specific T cells. From a diagnostic standpoint, as PTLDs frequently involve the transplanted organ, EBV testing can also be helpful for the assessment of dense lymphoid infiltrates raising the differential diagnosis between PTLD and severe rejection.

The histologic subtypes of iatrogenic immunodeficiency-associated LPDs are heterogeneous: most are of B-cell derivation and an association with EBV is found in fewer than half of the cases (**Fig. 7**).[50]

Differential Diagnosis

The diagnosis and resolution of the differential diagnosis in immunodeficiency-associated lymphoproliferative disorders rest on eliciting the appropriate history of congenital, acquired, or iatrogenic immunosuppression. These lymphomas and lymphoid proliferations share many features with comparable lesions that occur in nonimmunosuppressed patients.

Prognosis

The prognosis of EBV-associated B-cell PTLDs is variable. Early lesions tend to regress with reduction of the immune suppression, whereas a proportion of the polymorphic and many monomorphic lesions require chemotherapy. Cellular immunotherapy to restore EBV-specific cytotoxic T-cell immunity is another therapeutic strategy. The prognosis is overall better for patients who develop PTLD following solid organ allografts than bone marrow allografts. In HIV-positive patients, the mortality associated with B-cell lymphomas tends to be higher than for immunocompetent patients. However, since the introduction of HAART, more aggressive treatment protocols have been introduced and the overall survival has improved.[30,47] EBV infection in HIV-associated DLBCL does not appear to affect the outcome.[51] In iatrogenic immunodeficiency-associated EBV-positive LPDs, a variable proportion of cases regress at least partially after discontinuation of the drug, whereas others require chemotherapy.

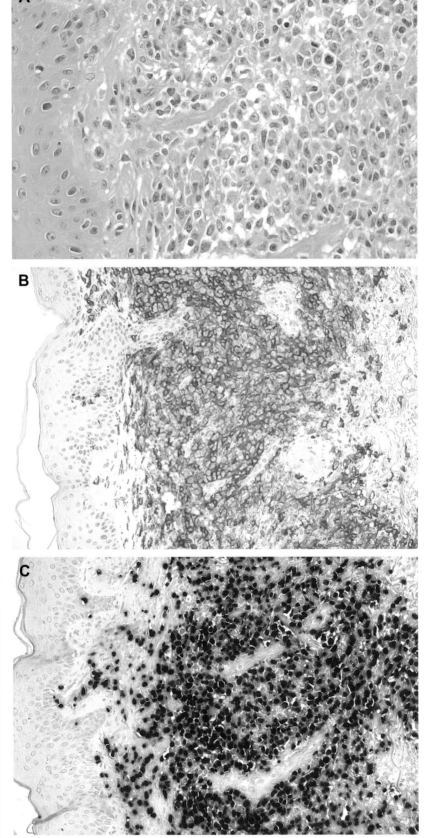

Fig. 7. Methotrexate-associated EBV-positive lymphoid proliferation (diffuse large B-cell lymphoma). (*A*) This cutaneous lesion comprises a diffuse proliferation of large lymphoid cells with centroblastic and immunoblastic features (H&E, ×400). (*B*) By immunohistochemistry, the large cells are CD20 positive (immunohistochemistry, alkaline phosphatase, ×200). (*C*) The large B cells are positive for EBV by EBER in situ hybridization (×200).

EBV-POSITIVE DIFFUSE LARGE B-CELL LYMPHOMAS

As described in the previous section, many EBV-associated lymphoid proliferations in immunocompromised individuals manifest histologically as proliferations of EBV-positive large B cells categorized as DLBCL, otherwise similar to the common form of EBV-negative DLBCL encountered in immunocompetent patients. Moreover, among the various subtypes or entities of DLBCL delineated because of peculiar clinicopathological features, several are defined at least in part by their association with EBV or with dual EBV/HHV-8 coinfection. The former are plasmablastic lymphoma, DLBCL associated with chronic inflammation, lymphomatoid granulomatosis, and EBV-positive DLBCL of the elderly and

the latter include primary effusion lymphoma and germinotropic lymphoproliferative disorder. The differential diagnosis and distinguishing features of these EBV-positive DLBCLs is provided in **Table 6**.

PLASMABLASTIC LYMPHOMA

Clinical Features

Plasmablastic lymphoma (PBL) was initially reported as a rare DLBCL variant occurring in the oral cavity in HIV-infected patients.[52] These tumors are locally invasive, disseminate to extraoral sites, and have a highly aggressive clinical behavior. Since the original description, the spectrum of PBL has been expanding: several reports have documented the occurrence of lymphomas with similar morphologic and phenotypic features

---

Table 6
EBV-positive large B-cell lymphomas

Type of Lymphoma	Clinical Setting	Presentation
EBV+ DLBCL (excluding EBV+ DLBCL of the elderly)	Primary immune disorders (congenital immunodeficiency syndromes) HIV infection Posttransplant Iatrogenic immunodeficiency-associated lymphoid proliferation (methotrexate, TNFα antagonists) With no known predisposing conditions and age <50 years old (rare)	Nodal or extranodal
Plasmablastic lymphoma	HIV infection (most cases)	Extranodal (oral cavity or other), less commonly nodal
DLBCL associated with chronic inflammation	Chronic pyothorax or chronic suppuration	Pleural-based mass, bone or joint tumor
Lymphomatoid granulomatosis	Congenital immunodeficiency syndromes, HIV infection Posttransplant	Lung, brain, skin; angiocentric multifocal involvement
EBV+ DLBCL of the elderly	Age >50 years old (immune senescence)	Extranodal (skin, tonsil) or nodal
Primary effusion lymphoma[a]	HIV infection Less often: posttransplant or elderly Mediterranean individuals	Body cavity effusion Solid extracavitary
Germinotropic lymphoproliferative disorder[a]	Immunocompetent individuals	Lymph nodes

Abbreviations: EBV, Epstein-Barr virus; HHV, human herpesviruses; DLBCL, diffuse large B-cell lymphoma.
[a] These disorders are characterized by coinfection by EBV and HHV-8.

in immunocompetent patients and in other anatomic locations in HIV-infected individuals, including nonoral extranodal sites (anorectal region, nasopharynx, and intestine) and lymph nodes.[53–58]

Microscopic Features and Ancillary Studies

PBL is characterized by a morphologic appearance suggestive of high-grade lymphoma and an immunophenotypic profile of plasma cells (**Fig. 8**).[34] It presents as a diffuse proliferation of medium to large immunoblastic cells harboring a central nucleolus and displaying a more or less cohesive appearance.[52,58] These tumors exhibit a high proliferation rate. A significant proportion of cases show frequent apoptotic cells and a starry-sky pattern may be seen.[58] A subset of tumors shows cytologic features suggestive of plasmacytic differentiation (perinuclear Hof, binucleation, "clockface" chromatin, eccentrically located nuclei) and contains a range of cells showing a morphologic continuum that includes mature plasma cells.[56,58]

Plasmablastic lymphoma is characterized by absent or weak expression of CD45 and B-cell-associated antigens (CD20–, PAX-5–, and CD79a±) and strong expression of plasma cell-associated antigens (MUM1+, CD138+, CD38+, and VS38c+). Monotypic expression of cytoplasmic immunoglobulins (usually IgG or IgA) is detected in a 50% to 70% of the cases. Expression of BCL-6 is usually lacking and expression of BCL-2 is heterogeneous. CD56 is usually negative, but may be seen in cases showing plasmacytic differentiation. In most cases the tumor cells carry EBV and show a type I latency of infection (expression of EBER and lack of EBNA-2 and LMP-1).[30,52,59,60] Although some investigators have suggested a role of HHV-8 infection in the pathogenesis of PBL,[61,62] most studies have found that PBL does not contain HHV-8, and the rare cases of HHV-8-positive large cell lymphomas reported in the oral cavity of AIDS patients likely represent examples of extracavitary primary effusion lymphomas (see below).[52,56,58,63,64]

At the molecular genetic level, PBL is heterogeneous: a subset of cases bear *IG* hypermutations with a pattern suggestive of antigen selection in some cases and thus conceivably derive from postgerminal center B cells, whereas another subset carry unmutated *IG* genes and appear to originate from naive B cells that have undergone differentiation outside the germinal center.[65] Genetic alterations associated with PBL are poorly characterized, but recent reports suggest that deregulation of *MYC* by translocation may be a recurrent aberration in PBL, which may correlate with a clinical presentation overlapping with plasma cell myeloma and appears to portend an aggressive clinical course.[66,67]

Differential Diagnosis

Because of its cohesive appearance and frequent occurrence in extranodal locations, PBL may be mistaken as nonhematolymphoid tumors (eg, carcinoma or melanoma). Moreover, because most of these tumors are negative for CD20 and fail to express CD45, a first-pass immunohistochemistry screen might suggest something other than lymphoma. Careful attention to morphologic detail should disclose characteristic plasmablastic morphologic features and lead to the appropriate staining panel (kappa and lambda light chains, CD138, EBER) confirming the plasmablastic nature of the proliferation. Once a plasmablastic phenotype is established, the differential diagnosis includes several entities in addition to PBL; their distinction from PBL is summarized in the Differential Diagnosis table of Lymphomas with Plasmablastic Features on page 1015. This differential diagnosis includes extramedullary plasma cell neoplasms (plasmacytoma and extramedullary dissemination of multiple myeloma), other high-grade B-cell neoplasms with plasmacytoid differentiation (immunoblastic lymphoma, BL), ALK-positive large B-cell lymphoma, and HHV-8-associated B-cell malignancies (large B-cell lymphoma arising in HHV-8-associated multicentric Castleman disease, primary effusion lymphoma and its extracavitary variant, and germinotropic lymphoproliferative disorder, which are discussed in the next sections).[56,58,63,68]

Extramedullary plasmacytoma has presenting features overlapping with those of PBL, as it also typically occurs in the upper respiratory tract. Extramedullary plasmacytomas may develop in patients with a history of myeloma and, conversely, PBL may present with osseous dissemination as multiple skeletal lesions and may even be associated with an M-component.[58] PBL and plasmablastic plasma cell neoplasms have a nearly identical immunophenotypic profile and aberrant expression of CD4, CD10, and CD56 expression may be seen in both.[63] Expression of cyclinD1 would favor a plasma cell neoplasm. In contrast to PBL, however, plasmablastic plasmacytomas are EBV negative. The distinction between PBL and DLBCL with immunoblastic features displaying plasmacytoid differentiation may be somewhat arbitrary and mostly relies on the expression of B-cell antigens (CD20 and PAX-5) in DLBCL that should be

Fig. 8. Plasmablastic lymphoma. (*A*) At low-power magnification, the tumor is densely cellular with a starry-sky appearance (H&E, ×100). (*B*) The large neoplastic cells have immunoblastic and plasmablastic features, showing a range of maturation up to plasma cells, as well as some cells showing frank anaplasia (H&E, ×400).

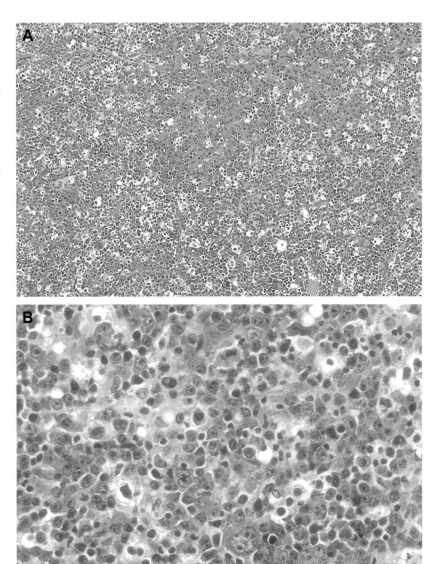

markedly downregulated in PBL. In HIV-infected patients, BL may show striking plasmacytoid features and morphologically resemble PBL. Moreover, *MYC* rearrangements are not specific for BL and may be found in PBL. However, BL is characterized by multiple nucleoli, a higher mitotic rate, and a starry-sky pattern, and is typically positive for CD20 and BCL-6, which are negative in PBL. The lack of B-cell antigens and monotonous large cells with prominent nucleoli in PBL may simulate ALK-positive large B-cell lymphoma.[69,70] However, PBL does not have the sinusoidal and nodular proliferation patterns associated with ALK+ B-cell lymphoma and expression of ALK has never been reported in PBL.

Prognosis

Plasmablastic lymphoma is a very aggressive disease, with most patients surviving less than

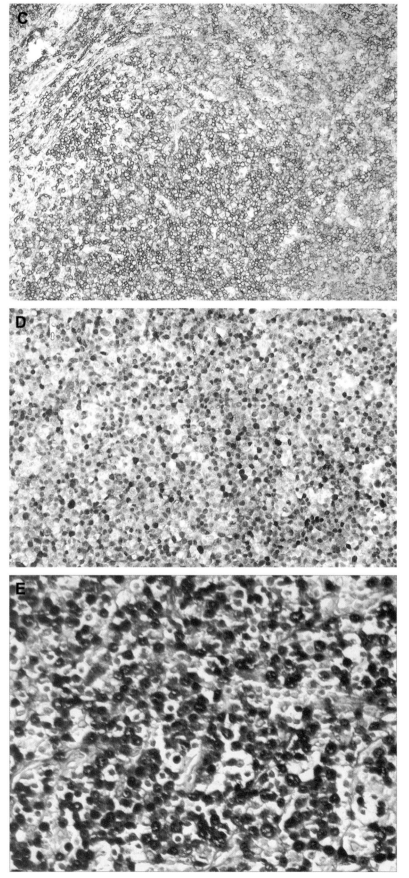

Fig. 8. Plasmablastic lymphoma. By immunohistochemistry, the lymphoma cells show strong CD138 positivity (*C*, immunoperoxidase ×100) as well as nuclear MUM1/IRF4 expression (*D*, immunoperoxidase ×200), indicating plasmacytic differentiation. The tumor cells are positive for EBV by in situ hybridization (*E*, ×400).

△△ *Differential Diagnosis*
OF LYMPHOMAS WITH PLASMABLASTIC FEATURES

Lymphoma Type	Morphology	Phenotype	EBV	HHV-8	Location	Clinical Course
Plasmablastic lymphoma	Immunoblasts, plasmablasts ± plasma cells	CD45− CD20− CD79a−/+ PAX-5− BCL-6− cIg± CD138+	+	−	Extranodal, rarely lymph nodes or bone marrow	Aggressive
Plasma cell neoplasms (myeloma, plasmacytoma)	Plasma cells ± plasmablasts	CD45− CD20− PAX-5− BCL-6− cIg+ CD138+, cyclinD1±	−	−	Bone marrow, extramedullary	Relatively indolent
Immunoblastic lymphoma	Immunoblasts ± plasmacytoid cells	CD45+ CD20+ PAX-5+ BCL-6− cIg± CD138±	+/−	−	Lymph nodes, extranodal, central nervous system	Aggressive
Burkitt lymphoma	Small noncleaved ± plasmacytoid cells	CD45+ CD20+ PAX-5+ BCL-6+ cIg− CD138−	+/−	−	Lymph nodes, extranodal	Aggressive
ALK+ DLBCL	Sinusoidal, nodular immunoblasts	CD45− CD20− BCL-6± ALK+ CD138+	−	−	Lymph nodes	Variable
Large B-cell lymphoma arising in HHV-8-associated MCD	Immunoblasts/ plasmablasts in mantle zones	CD45+ CD20± PAX-5− BCL-6− cIgM+ CD138−	−	+	Lymph nodes, spleen	Aggressive
Primary effusion lymphoma	Pleomorphic immunoblasts	CD45+ CD20− BCL-6− cIg− CD138+ CD30+	+	+	Body cavities	Aggressive
Extracavitary primary effusion lymphoma	Pleomorphic immunoblasts	CD45+ CD20− BCL-6− cIg± CD138±	+	+	Extranodal, lymph nodes	Variable
Germinotropic lympho-proliferative disorder	Intrafollicular, immunoblasts and plasmablasts	CD20− CD79a− BCL-6− cIg+ CD138−	+	+	Lymph nodes	Relatively indolent

Abbreviations: ALK, anaplastic lymphoma kinase; cIg, cytoplasmic immunoglobulin; DLBCL, diffuse large B-cell lymphoma; MCD, multicentric Castleman disease.

1 year, even with the use of HAART and chemotherapy.[30]

DIFFUSE LARGE B-CELL LYMPHOMA ASSOCIATED WITH CHRONIC INFLAMMATION

Clinical Features

Pyothorax-associated lymphoma (PAL) is the prototypic form of a DLBCL occurring in the context of chronic inflammation and showing association with EBV. PAL is a rare disease that develops in the pleural cavity of patients with a history of longstanding pyothorax. Most cases have been reported in Japan,[71–74] with only a few reported cases in Western countries.[75] PAL affects elderly patients with a strong male predominance. The patients typically have a 30- to 40-year history of pyothorax or chronic pleuritis resulting from artificial pneumothorax for treatment of pulmonary tuberculosis or, less often, tuberculous pleuritis. The most common presenting symptoms are chest and/or back pain, fever, and weight loss. Imaging studies demonstrate a pleural-based tumor mass that often shows direct invasion to adjacent structures such as the chest wall and lung.

Occasional cases of EBV-positive lymphomas complicating long-standing chronic suppuration have been described in other extranodal sites, such as bone or joint lymphomas in the setting of chronic osteomyelitis or in association with metallic implants, and skin lymphomas in patients with chronic venous ulcers. These cases have clinical and pathologic features similar to those of PAL and may be part of the same disease spectrum.[76,77]

Microscopic Features and Ancillary Studies

Histologically, PAL is similar to DLBCL of the immunoblastic type and often appears plasmacytoid or anaplastic. Angiocentric or angioinvasive features with areas of necrosis are often observed.[75,78] The tumor cells are CD45+, variably express CD20, and are usually positive for CD79a. They are negative for CD10 and BCL-6, while they uniformly express MUM1 and variably express CD138. Most cases are positive for BCL-2. CD30 can be expressed. Aberrant coexpression of T-cell-associated antigens (CD2, CD3, and/or CD4) has been reported in several cases. Some cases lack expression of lineage-specific antigens or express T-cell-associated antigens only.

Most cases are associated with EBV and display a type III latency phenotype.[79] Molecular genetic studies usually demonstrate monoclonal *IGH* rearrangement and polyclonal T-cell receptor gene rearrangement, even in cases with a dual B-cell and T-cell phenotype. PALs carry a high rate of somatic hypermutations without ongoing mutations of their *IG* genes, and in many cases the *IG* gene rearrangements appear to be nonproductive,[80,81] indicating derivation from post germinal center or "crippled" post germinal center B cells, similar to the neoplastic HRS cells of cHL.[81] The strong association with EBV and the viral gene expression pattern detected in most cases are features similar to those seen in posttransplant lymphoproliferative disorders, suggesting that a possibly localized immune defect may contribute to development of PAL. Chronic inflammation may create a micro-environment that is less accessible to T-cell immune surveillance, allowing the uncontrolled transformation of EBV-infected cells; indeed, the density of tumor-infiltrating T-cells has been found to be significantly lower in PAL as compared with other nodal or extranodal DLBCL.[82] Chronic inflammation may also contribute to the development of PAL by providing local production of cytokines such as IL-6, which acts as a growth factor on PAL cell lines.[83] Conversely, the immunosuppressive cytokine IL-10 produced in vitro by PAL cell lines may contribute to local immunosuppression.[84]

Differential Diagnosis

PAL may be confused with peripheral T-cell lymphomas, as the tumor cells may display an aberrant T-cell immunophenotype, but extensive phenotyping and genotypic studies will be the clue to the correct diagnosis. Primary or secondary involvement of the chest wall or pleura by DLBCL, not otherwise specified, must be distinguished from PAL, which is EBV-positive and occurs in the particular clinical setting as described previously. PAL forms solid tumor masses, in distinction from primary effusion lymphoma (PEL), which usually does not include a solid tumor component. Moreover, HHV-8 coinfection typical of PEL has not been detected in most cases of PAL.[85,86]

Prognosis

The estimated 5-year survival rate of PAL ranges between 20% and 35%.[73,74] Some patients may achieve durable remission with chemotherapy regimens.

LARGE B-CELL LYMPHOMA, LYMPHOMATOID GRANULOMATOSIS TYPE (LYG)

Clinical Features

Lymphomatoid granulomatosis (LYG), first reported as a rare and unique angiocentric and angiodestructive lymphoproliferative process in the lungs,[87] represents an EBV-positive B-cell proliferation associated with an exuberant T-cell reaction[88–91] and is currently listed as a rare DLBCL entity.[92] LYG affects patients of all ages, often between the fourth and sixth decades, with a slight male predominance.[93] Patients typically present with lung involvement and respiratory symptoms, with multiple bilateral nodular opacities predominating in the lower lobes on radiographic studies.[94] The central nervous system, kidneys, skin, and subcutaneous tissue are also commonly involved.[95] Lymphoid organs are usually spared. Immunosuppression is a predisposing factor. The lesions may occur in the setting of congenital immunodeficiencies, HIV, and posttransplantation, and in patients receiving iatrogenic immunosuppression with steroids and/or methotrexate for other disorders.[96]

Microscopic Features and Ancillary Studies

Lymphomatoid granulomatosis consists of a polymorphous cellular infiltrate including lymphocytes, histiocytes, plasma cells, and varying numbers of large atypical lymphoid cells, exhibiting an angiocentric and angioinvasive pattern with or without associated infarct-type necrosis (**Fig. 9**).[87] The large atypical cells may resemble immunoblasts or have a more pleomorphic appearance resembling Reed-Sternberg cells. LYG encompasses a spectrum of histologic grades (grades 1 to 3) related to the proportion of large, neoplastic, EBV-positive B cells.[97]

The neoplastic cells are EBV-positive B cells with a type III latency program, similar to that of PTLD. They are CD45+, CD20± and may weakly express CD30.[88,91] The small lymphocytes consist mostly of CD4+ T cells. EBER stains are useful for histologic grading:

- Grade 1 lesions, fewer than 5 EBER-positive cells/high power field (hpf).
- Grade 2 lesions, 5 to 20 EBER-positive cells/hpf.
- Grade 3 lesions, usually at least 50 EBER-positive cells/hpf.

The ability to demonstrate monoclonal *IGH* gene rearrangement by PCR correlates closely with the proportion of EBV-positive cells; *IGH* PCR is usually negative in grade 1 lesions. Analysis for *TCR* gene rearrangements is usually negative.[88,95] A peculiar feature of LYG is the abundant associated reactive T-cell-rich background in LYG, likely recruited from the circulation.[98] The chemokines interferon-gamma-inducible protein-10 (IP-10) and monokine induced by interferon-gamma (Mig), which are induced by EBV, are overexpressed by reactive cells in LYG lesions and have been implicated in mediating tissue necrosis and vascular damage in pulmonary LYG. These agents inhibit angiogenesis, promote T-cell adhesion to endothelial cells, and directly damage the endothelium. IP-10 is also increased in the serum of patients with LYG, suggesting that it could contribute to systemic constitutional symptoms.[99]

Differential Diagnosis

Grade 1 lesions contain few EBV-infected B cells and may be confused with non-neoplastic inflammatory processes. Clinical and pathologic features of LYG are frequently encountered in immunodeficiency-associated lymphoproliferative disorders and thus there is an overlap between LYG and other entities such as primary immunodeficiency-associated LPDs and PTLDs. Moreover, angiocentric features may be seen in other EBV-positive lymphoid proliferations, such as EBV-positive DLBCL of the elderly. Thus, the clinical distribution of disease (predominantly bilateral lung involvement with the presence of pulmonary nodules, with or without involvement of other extranodal sites and without lymphadenopathy) is critical in differentiating LYG from other EBV-positive entities.

Prognosis

Some patients experience a waxing and waning clinical course, but most cases are aggressive. Response to therapy and outcome correlate with the histologic grade.

EBV-POSITIVE DIFFUSE LARGE B-CELL LYMPHOMA OF THE ELDERLY

Clinical Features

EBV-positive DLBCL occurring in elderly patients (by definition older than 50 years, with a median age in the eighth decade) without any known immune deficiency syndrome has been incorporated as a new DLBCL subtype in the 2008 WHO classification.[26] Other EBV-positive DLBCL entities (see **Table 6**) and IM should be excluded. This neoplasm is believed to occur in the setting of altered immune function caused by immune senescence, and accordingly the proportion of EBV-positive tumors among large B-cell proliferations in individuals older than 50 years progressively increases with age.[100] The disease often involves extranodal sites (skin, tonsil, lung, or stomach), with or without lymph node involvement; B symptoms are common.

Microscopic Features and Ancillary Studies

The architecture of the involved tissues is effaced. The lymphoid proliferation consists of either a monomorphous large-cell lymphoma (in about two-thirds of the cases) or a polymorphous large cell infiltrate with a variable inflammatory background (in about one-third of the cases) (**Fig. 10**). Some cases may resemble T-cell/histiocyte-rich large B-cell lymphoma. Distinction between the monomorphous and polymorphous variants is not mandatory, as it appears to bear no clinical relevance.[25] Angiocentricity and extensive necrosis are frequent. In the polymorphous variant, Reed-Sternberg-like cells may be numerous, raising the differential diagnosis with classical Hodgkin lymphoma.

According to the disease definition, the EBV-positive tumor cells are positive for B-cell markers such as CD20, CD79a, and PAX-5, with light chain restriction that may be difficult to demonstrate in tissue sections. The tumor cells show a type III latency program: EBER and LMP-1 are detected in most cases, whereas the detection of EBNA-2

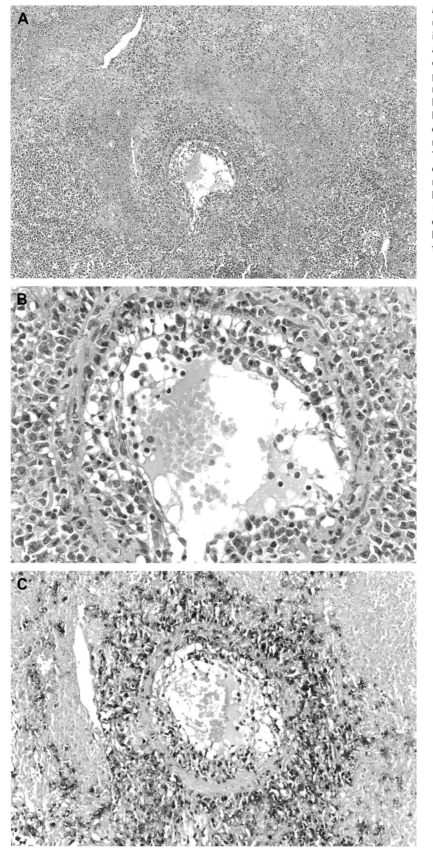

Fig. 9. Lymphomatoid granulomatosis, grade III, involving the lung in a patient with a history of bone marrow transplantation. (*A*) The lung nodule is characterized by an angiocentric lymphoid proliferation associated with areas of necrosis (H&E, ×100). (*B*) The neoplastic lymphoid cells are large and pleomorphic and invade blood vessel walls (H&E, ×400). (*C*) The tumor cells are positive for EBV by in situ hybridization for EBER (×200).

Fig. 10. Histology of EBV-positive diffuse large B cell lymphoma of the elderly. (*A*) These lymphomas often show large areas of geographic necrosis (H&E, ×100). (*B*) There are numerous large lymphoid cells in a histiocytic background (H&E, ×400). (*C*) In some areas, Reed-Sternberg-like cells are associated with an eosinophilic infiltrate, mimicking classical Hodgkin lymphoma (H&E, ×400).

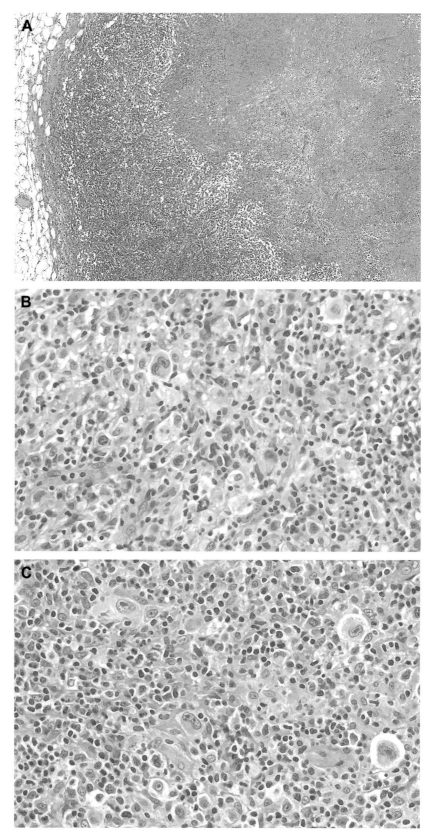

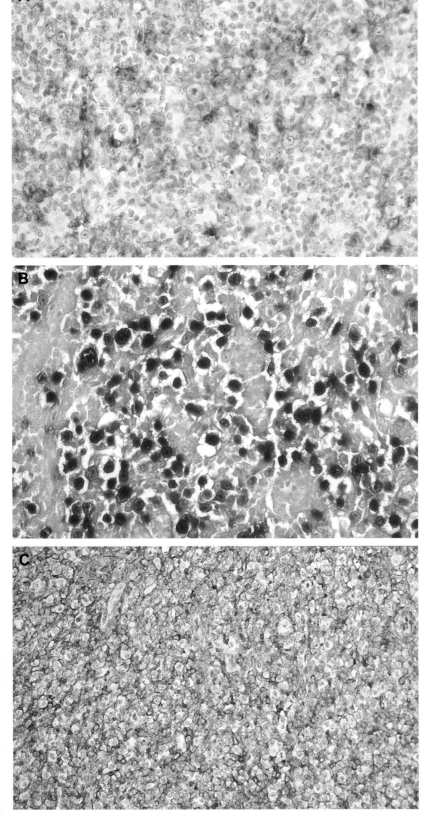

Fig. 11. Immunohistochemistry of EBV-positive diffuse large B-cell lymphoma of the elderly. Although many of the Reed-Sternberg like-cells are positive for CD30 (*A*) (immunoperoxidase, ×400) and show positivity for EBER by in situ hybridization (*B*) (×400), unlike classical Hodgkin lymphoma the cells are strongly positive for CD45 (*C*) (immunoperoxidase, ×200) and CD20 (*D*, see next page) (immunoperoxidase, ×200).

Fig. 11. Immunohistochemistry of EBV-positive diffuse large B-cell lymphoma of the elderly. There is also co-expression of both BOB-1 (*E*) (immunoperoxidase, ×400) and OCT-2 (*F*) (immunoperoxidase, ×400), which would be unusual for classical Hodgkin lymphoma.

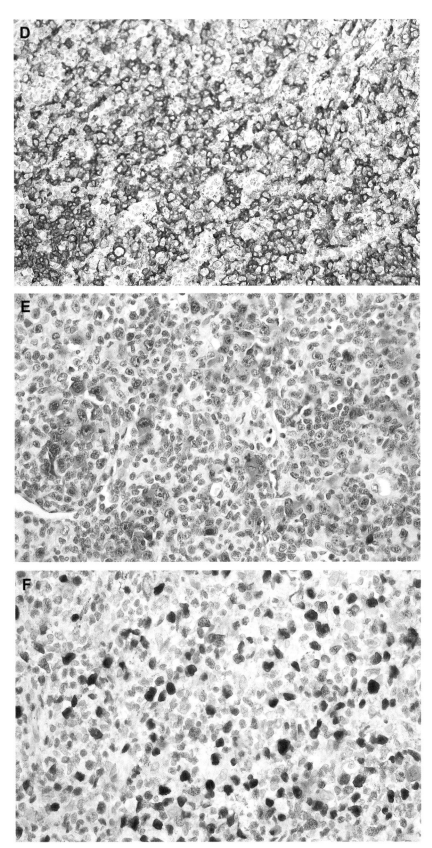

is more variable. The tumor cells variably express CD30, but are negative for CD15 (**Fig. 11**).[25,100–102] Monoclonal *IGH* gene rearrangement can usually be demonstrated by PCR.

Differential Diagnosis

The differential diagnosis of EBV-positive DLBCL of the elderly versus other EBV-positive DLBCLs is summarized in **Table 6**. By definition, other DLBCL subtypes must be excluded. In particular, because EBV-positive DLBCL of the elderly shares morphologic features with immunodeficiency-related LPDs, knowledge of the patient's clinical history and immune state is crucial to a proper diagnostic categorization. The polymorphous variant of EBV-positive DLBCL of the elderly may mimic EBV-positive cHL.[100] This differential diagnosis is commonly entertained and may be difficult to solve. In EBV-positive DLBCL of the elderly, the tumor cell population may consist mostly of HRS-like cells, which are often CD30+ but, in contrast to cHL, are negative for CD15. A key distinction is the recognition of the degree of expression of B-cell markers on the tumor cells. In cHL, usually only a minority of neoplastic cells express CD20 and B-cell associated transcription factors are negative or weakly expressed. Conversely in EBV-positive DLBCL of the elderly, despite variable EBV-associated downregulation of the B-cell program, at least 50% of the tumor cells should express B-cell markers. Geographic necrosis, commonly seen in EBV-positive DLBCL of the elderly, is uncommon in cHL.[100] Clonality studies are not helpful, as monoclonal *IGH* gene rearrangements typically found in DLBCL can also be detected in cHL. Clonality studies are however helpful to distinguish EBV-positive DLBCL from IM and reactivation of EBV-positive infection in elderly patients. The latter lesions, usually involving lymph nodes, are characterized by interfollicular expansion by large lymphoid cells and plasma cells, and the presence of EBV-positive cells in germinal centers and interfollicular areas.[100] EBV-positive mucocutaneous ulcers in elderly patients appear to represent a localized and more indolent form of EBV-positive DLBCL of the elderly.[27] These lesions, typically occurring in the oropharyngeal mucosa, comprise a proliferation of EBV-positive large B cells in a polymorphous background. These cases exhibit Hodgkin-like features, including the presence of HRS-like cells with frequent CD15 expression.

Prognosis

The prognosis is inferior to that of patients with EBV-negative DLBCLs or EBV-positive cHL[100];

the presence of B symptoms and age older than 70 are adverse prognostic factors.[25,103]

HHV-8-POSITIVE MULTICENTRIC CASTLEMAN DISEASE (MCD) AND ASSOCIATED LARGE B-CELL LYMPHOMAS

Clinical Features

HHV-8-positive MCD occurs in HIV-positive patients with profound immunodeficiency and in HIV-negative patients in areas where HHV-8 infection is endemic (Africa and Mediterranean countries). The disease manifests as disseminated lymphadenopathy and splenomegaly, associated with systemic symptoms as fever, night sweats, and weight loss. Kaposi's sarcoma is frequently present in patients with HHV-8-positive MCD and both lesions frequently coexist in affected lymph nodes (**Fig. 12**).[104]

Microscopic Features and Ancillary Studies

Histologically, HHV-8-positive MCD corresponds to the plasma cell variant of CD and is distinguished by the presence of HHV-8-positive plasmablasts distributed mostly within prominent follicular mantle zones (see **Fig. 12**).[105,106] The HHV-8-positive cells are negative for EBV and have morphologic features of plasmablasts (large cells with round nuclei and moderately abundant amphophilic cytoplasm). They weakly express B-cell antigens (CD20–/+, CD79a–, PAX-5–, OCT2+), are usually MUM1+ and CD138–, and are weakly positive for CD30.[107] Characteristically, they express high levels of cytoplasmic IgM lambda immunoglobulin, but are not monoclonal.[106] In contrast to the phenotypic features that suggest a postgerminal center B-cell derivation, genotypic studies indicate that HHV-8-positive plasmablasts arise from naïve, unmutated, pregerminal center B cells.[108] HHV-8-positive plasmablasts in MCD may expand and evolve toward HHV-8-positive large B-cell lymphoma. Clusters or aggregates of IgM lambda-positive, HHV-8-positive plasmablasts in mantle zones and interfollicular areas are called "microlymphomas" and can be polyclonal or monoclonal.[106] These foci of microlymphoma may have a smoldering evolution or progress toward an aggressive HHV-8-positive DLBCL with massive nodal or splenic involvement and/or a leukemic phase.

Differential Diagnosis

HHV-8-positive MCD may be underrecognized and misclassified as nonspecific lymphoid hyperplasia. Lymphadenopathy and/or splenomegaly

Fig. 12. HHV-8-associated multicentric Castleman disease in an HIV-positive patient. (*A*) Low-power view of the lymph node shows numerous small follicular structures, markedly increased vascularity, and a subcapsular focus of a solid spindle cell proliferation representing Kaposi's sarcoma (*upper right corner*) (H&E, ×50). (*B*) The follicles show markedly increased vascularity of the germinal centers and thickened mantle zones (H&E, ×200). (*C*) The interfollicular areas contain numerous plasma cells (H&E, ×400).

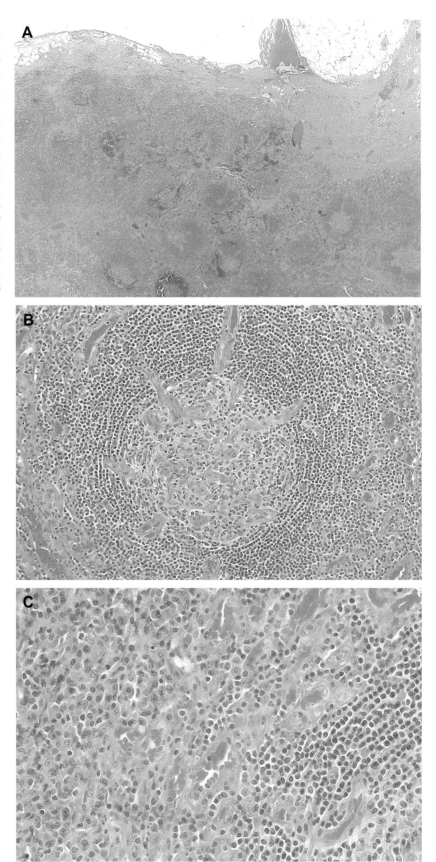

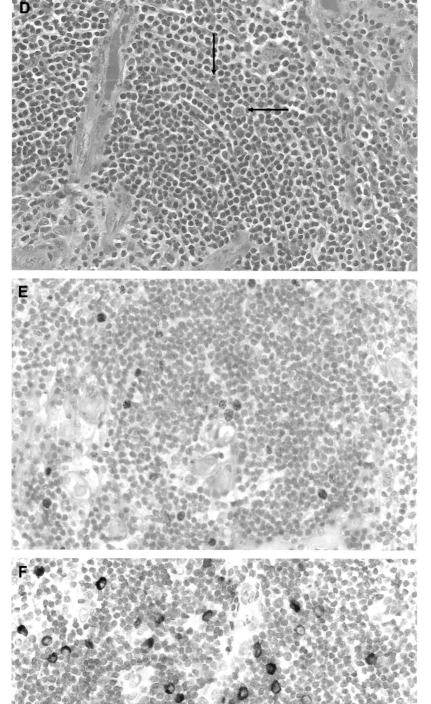

Fig. 12. HHV-8-associated multicentric Castleman disease in an HIV-positive patient. (*D*) The mantle zone contains scattered large plasmablastic cells (*arrows*) (H&E, ×400). By immunohistochemistry, the large plasmablastic cells are positive for HHV-8/LANA-1 (*E*) (immunoperoxidase, ×400) and show cytoplasmic expression of IgM heavy chain (*F*) (immunoperoxidase, ×400); the plasmablasts were lambda light chain-restricted (not shown).

in an HIV-positive patient should be a hint to look for a specific cause of the lymphoid expansion. The characteristic histopathologic features of MCD, including numerous follicles showing expanded mantles and perforating arterioles into the germinal centers as well as interfollicular plasmacytosis, are clues to help identify the disease. Immunohistochemistry to demonstrate HHV-8 is key to highlighting the infected plasmablasts. The relative paucity of HHV-8-positive plasmablasts defines the disorder as HHV-8-positive MCD versus large B-cell "microlymphomas" and lymphomas. HHV-8-positive lymphomas arising from MCD may be difficult to identify when the background of MCD is completely overrun by the large cell proliferation, and these lymphomas should enter into the differential diagnosis of any large B-cell lymphoma with plasmablastic features; in that setting, characterization of the viral associations (HHV-8 and EBV) are important features to guide the diagnosis and appropriate classification (see Differential Diagnosis table of Lymphomas with Plasmablastic Features, page 1015).

Prognosis

HHV-8-positive MCD has a very aggressive behavior, with most patients dying within 1 year.[106] A subset progress to develop large B-cell lymphomas arising from HHV-8-positive

MCD (formerly designated as "plasmablastic lymphomas" or "plasmablastic microlymphomas"), whereas others can develop a body cavity-based primary effusion lymphoma (PEL) or extracavitary PEL (see the following section). These progressed HHV-8-positive lymphomas herald a very short survival.[109]

PRIMARY EFFUSION LYMPHOMA AND OTHER HHV-8-POSITIVE LYMPHOMAS

Clinical Features

Primary effusion lymphoma (PEL), originally identified in AIDS patients and described as "body cavity-based lymphoma," is a rare B-cell neoplasm usually presenting as effusions in serous cavities (pleural, pericardial or peritoneal), generally with no formation of tumor masses. Most PELs occur exclusively as malignant effusions, but there are cases with concomitant or subsequent solid tissue involvement that are part of the same clinicopathologic spectrum. The disease occurs mainly in HIV-infected individuals, but has also been reported in solid organ transplant recipients and in elderly patients from areas where HHV-8 infection is endemic. HHV-8- and EBV-associated germinotropic lymphoproliferative disorder presents as localized lymphadenopathy in HIV-negative individuals.

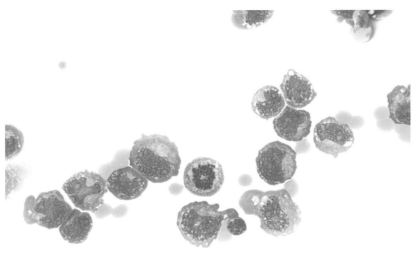

Fig. 13. Primary effusion lymphoma. On a Giemsa-stained cytologic preparation, the neoplastic cells appear large and pleomorphic, with irregularly shaped nuclei, multiple nucleoli, abundant cytoplasm, and frequently a clear paranuclear zone (May-Grünwald Giemsa, ×1000).

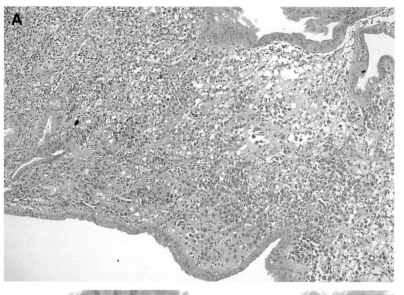

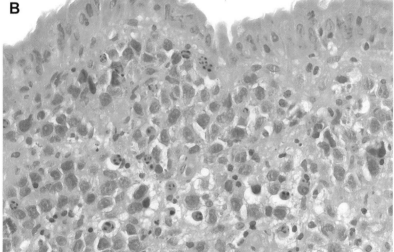

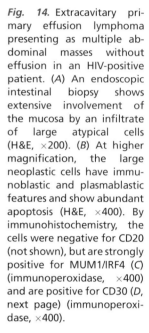

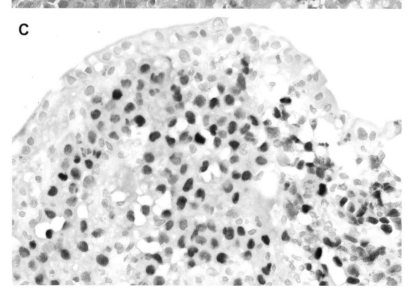

Fig. 14. Extracavitary primary effusion lymphoma presenting as multiple abdominal masses without effusion in an HIV-positive patient. (*A*) An endoscopic intestinal biopsy shows extensive involvement of the mucosa by an infiltrate of large atypical cells (H&E, ×200). (*B*) At higher magnification, the large neoplastic cells have immunoblastic and plasmablastic features and show abundant apoptosis (H&E, ×400). By immunohistochemistry, the cells were negative for CD20 (not shown), but are strongly positive for MUM1/IRF4 (*C*) (immunoperoxidase, ×400) and are positive for CD30 (*D*, next page) (immunoperoxidase, ×400).

Fig. 14. Extracavitary primary effusion lymphoma presenting as multiple abdominal masses without effusion in an HIV positive patient. The tumor cells are positive for EBER in situ hybridization (*E*) (×400) and are also positive for HHV-8/LANA-1 (*F*) (immunoperoxidase, ×400), indicating coinfection with both EBV and HHV-8.

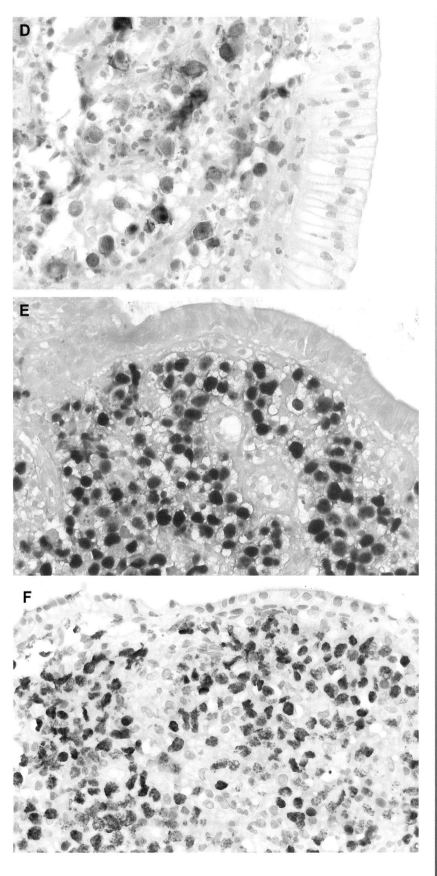

Microscopic Features and Ancillary Studies

Primary effusion lymphoma is composed of large pleomorphic cells with morphologic features bridging those of immunoblastic and anaplastic lymphoma (**Fig. 13**). Most PELs exhibit a distinctive immunophenotype: they express CD45 but lack expression of B-cell antigens (CD19, CD20, CD79a, PAX-5) and surface immunoglobulin and are positive for MUM1 and CD138 as well as for CD30, CD38, HLA-DR, and epithelial membrane antigen (EMA).[110,111] Detecting HHV-8 within the neoplastic cells is essential for the diagnosis of PEL. Most cases are coinfected with EBV with a latency type I pattern of gene expression.[112–114] Although most PEL cases are coinfected by both HHV-8 and EBV, studies on PEL pathogenesis suggest that HHV-8 plays a key role.[11,115–117] LANA-1 is the only HHV-8 gene that is consistently highly expressed. It plays a pivotal role in HHV-8 episomal persistence and interacts with and influences the expression of several cellular genes. LANA-1 thereby contributes to the growth of PEL cells, which also depends on cytokines and other host factors. In HIV-infected patients, in addition to systemic immunodeficiency a direct contribution to disease pathogenesis is exerted by the HIV protein Tat, which induces the expression of cellular and HHV-8 genes that are pro-proliferative and proinflammatory. Cases not associated with HIV infection are more likely to be EBV-negative. PEL harbors clonally rearranged and mutated *IG* whose sequences show evidence of antigen selection, but clonally rearranged *IGH* genes are detectable by PCR in only about half of the cases, likely because of false negativity secondary to the extensive somatic hypermutation.[118,119] Gene expression profile studies have documented that PELs are closely related to neoplastic plasma cells and EBV-positive immunoblasts, suggesting a plasmablastic derivation.[120,121]

HHV-8- and EBV-associated germinotropic lymphoproliferative disorder is a rare but distinctive lymphoproliferative disorder characterized by oligoclonal or polyclonal plasmablasts that involve the germinal centers of lymphoid follicles, forming confluent aggregates. These plasmablasts are negative for both CD20 and CD138, express CD30, are positive for both EBV and HHV-8, and express viral interleukin-6 (vIL-6). Recently, Seliem and colleagues[14] reported the occurrence of an HHV-8-positive, EBV-positive lymphoid proliferation manifesting as multicentric "microlymphomas" in an HIV-positive man, with pathologic features overlapping between a germinotropic lymphoproliferative disorder and MCD-associated DLBCL, and an aggressive clinical course.

Differential Diagnosis

Primary effusion lymphoma must be distinguished from other lymphomas primarily presenting as effusions without identifiable contiguous tumor masses as well as lymphomatous effusions secondary to systemic lymphomas or cavity-based solid lymphomas.[11] Other lymphomas primarily involving serous body cavities include some cases of BL (especially in AIDS patients), or, less commonly, extranodal DLBCLs. The correct recognition of PEL and its distinction from other lymphomatous effusions relies on the detection of HHV-8 as well as the pattern of phenotypic and genotypic markers associated with other lymphoma entities: for example, *MYC* rearrangements have not been reported in PEL. Secondary lymphomatous effusions closely mimic the features of the corresponding tissue-based lymphoma and consistently lack HHV-8.

After the original description of PEL, there have been reports of HHV-8-positive solid lymphomas presenting as extranodal masses involving the gastrointestinal tract, skin, lung, central nervous system, or, less commonly, lymph nodes, with no associated effusions. Most cases occurred in HIV-positive individuals. These lymphomas, termed *extracavitary primary effusion lymphomas*, are composed of large immunoblastic-like cells with pleomorphism and anaplastic features resembling PEL (**Fig. 14**). Their immunophenotypic and genotypic features are similar to those of PELs except for a slightly more frequent expression of B-cell antigens and surface immunoglobulin (both positive in 25% of the cases). Thus, these HHV-8-positive extracavitary tumors are thought to belong to the spectrum of PEL.[68,122,123]

Prognosis

Primary effusion lymphoma carries an adverse prognosis, with a median survival of 6 months.[124] In contrast, HHV-8- and EBV-associated germinotropic lymphoproliferative disorder shows a favorable response to chemotherapy or radiotherapy.[13]

REFERENCES

1. Norberg P. Divergence and genotyping of human alpha-herpesviruses: an overview. Infect Genet Evol 2010;10(1):14–25.

2. Kuppers R. B cells under influence: transformation of B cells by Epstein-Barr virus. Nat Rev Immunol 2003;3(10):801–12.

3. Wen KW, Damania B. Kaposi sarcoma-associated herpesvirus (KSHV): molecular biology and oncogenesis. Cancer Lett 2010;289(2):140–50.

4. Epstein M, Achong B, Barr Y. Virus particles in cultured lymphoblasts from Burkitt's lymphoma. Lancet 1964;1:702–3.

5. Henle G, Henle W, Diehl V. Relation of Burkitt's tumor-associated herpes-type virus to infectious mononucleosis. Proc Natl Acad Sci U S A 1968;59(1):94–101.

6. Young LS, Rickinson AB. Epstein-Barr virus: 40 years on. Nat Rev Cancer 2004;4(10):757–68.

7. Williams H, Crawford DH. Epstein-Barr virus: the impact of scientific advances on clinical practice. Blood 2006;107(3):862–9.

8. Delecluse HJ, Feederle R, O'Sullivan B, et al. Epstein Barr virus-associated tumours: an update for the attention of the working pathologist. J Clin Pathol 2007;60(12):1358–64.

9. Carbone A, Gloghini A, Dotti G. EBV-associated lymphoproliferative disorders: classification and treatment. Oncologist 2008;13(5):577–85.

10. Chang Y, Cesarman E, Pessin MS, et al. Identification of herpesvirus-like DNA sequences in AIDS-associated Kaposi's sarcoma. Science 1994;266(5192):1865–9.

11. Carbone A, Gloghini A. KSHV/HHV8-associated lymphomas. Br J Haematol 2008;140(1):13–24.

12. Du MQ, Bacon CM, Isaacson PG. Kaposi sarcoma-associated herpesvirus/human herpesvirus 8 and lymphoproliferative disorders. J Clin Pathol 2007;60(12):1350–7.

13. Du MQ, Diss TC, Liu H, et al. KSHV- and EBV-associated germinotropic lymphoproliferative disorder. Blood 2002;100(9):3415–8.

14. Seliem RM, Griffith RC, Harris NL, et al. HHV8+, EBV+ multicentric plasmablastic microlymphoma in an HIV+ man: the spectrum of HHV8+ lymphoproliferative disorders expands. Am J Surg Pathol 2007;31(9):1439–45.

15. Ferry JA, Sohani AR, Longtine JA, et al. HHV8-positive, EBV-positive Hodgkin lymphoma-like large B-cell lymphoma and HHV8-positive intravascular large B-cell lymphoma. Mod Pathol 2009;22(5):618–26.

16. Edelman DC. Human herpesvirus 8—a novel human pathogen. Virol J 2005;2:78.

17. Laurent C, Meggetto F, Brousset P. Human herpesvirus 8 infections in patients with immunodeficiencies. Hum Pathol 2008;39(7):983–93.

18. Dupin N, Fisher C, Kellam P, et al. Distribution of human herpesvirus-8 latently infected cells in Kaposi's sarcoma, multicentric Castleman's disease, and primary effusion lymphoma. Proc Natl Acad Sci U S A 1999;96(8):4546–51.

19. Yamamoto M, Kimura H, Hironaka T, et al. Detection and quantification of virus DNA in plasma of patients with Epstein-Barr virus-associated diseases. J Clin Microbiol 1995;33(7):1765–8.

20. Abbondanzo SL, Sato N, Straus SE, et al. Acute infectious mononucleosis. CD30 (Ki-1) antigen expression and histologic correlations. Am J Clin Pathol 1990;93(5):698–702.

21. Louissant A, Ganguly A, Hassserjian RP, et al. Infectious mononucleosis: morphology and immunophenotype in cervical lymph nodes and Waldeyer's ring. Mod Pathol 2008;21:236A.

22. Plumbley JA, Fan H, Eagan PA, et al. Lymphoid tissues from patients with infectious mononucleosis lack monoclonal B and T cells. J Mol Diagn 2002;4(1):37–43.

23. Wick MJ, Woronzoff-Dashkoff KP, McGlennen RC. The molecular characterization of fatal infectious mononucleosis. Am J Clin Pathol 2002;117(4):582–8.

24. Childs CC, Parham DM, Berard CW. Infectious mononucleosis. The spectrum of morphologic changes simulating lymphoma in lymph nodes and tonsils. Am J Surg Pathol 1987;11(2):122–32.

25. Oyama T, Yamamoto K, Asano N, et al. Age-related EBV-associated B-cell lymphoproliferative disorders constitute a distinct clinicopathologic group: a study of 96 patients. Clin Cancer Res 2007;13(17):5124–32.

26. Nakamura S, Jaffe E, Swerdlow S. EBV positive diffuse large B-cell lymphoma of the elderly. In: Swerdlow S, Campo E, Harris N, et al, editors. WHO classification of tumours of haematopoietic and lymphoid tissues. Lyon (France): IARC; 2008. p. 243–4.

27. Dojcinov SD, Venkataraman G, Raffeld M, et al. EBV positive mucocutaneous ulcer—a study of 26 cases associated with various sources of immunosuppression. Am J Surg Pathol 2010;34(3):405–17.

28. Dave SS, Fu K, Wright GW, et al. Molecular diagnosis of Burkitt's lymphoma. N Engl J Med 2006;354(23):2431–42.

29. Hummel M, Bentink S, Berger H, et al. A biologic definition of Burkitt's lymphoma from transcriptional and genomic profiling. N Engl J Med 2006;354(23):2419–30.

30. Carbone A, Cesarman E, Spina M, et al. HIV-associated lymphomas and gamma-herpesviruses. Blood 2009;113(6):1213–24.

31. Allday MJ. How does Epstein-Barr virus (EBV) complement the activation of Myc in the pathogenesis of Burkitt's lymphoma? Semin Cancer Biol 2009;19(6):366–76.

32. De Falco G, Antonicelli G, Onnis A, et al. Role of EBV in microRNA dysregulation in Burkitt lymphoma. Semin Cancer Biol 2009;19(6):401–6.

33. Leoncini L, Raphael M, Stein H, et al. Burkitt lymphoma. In: Swerdlow S, Campo E, Harris N, et al, editors. WHO classification of tumours of

haematopoietic and lymphoid tissues. Lyon (France): International Agency for Research on Cancer; 2008. p. 262–4.

34. Swerdlow S, Campo E, Harris N, et al. WHO classification of tumours of haematopoietic and lymphoid tissues. Lyon (France): IARC Press; 2008.

35. Kapatai G, Murray P. Contribution of the Epstein Barr virus to the molecular pathogenesis of Hodgkin lymphoma. J Clin Pathol 2007;60(12):1342–9.

36. Kuppers R. The biology of Hodgkin's lymphoma. Nat Rev Cancer 2009;9(1):15–27.

37. Quintanilla-Martinez L, de Jong D, de Mascarel A, et al. Gray zones around diffuse large B cell lymphoma. Conclusions based on the workshop of the XIV meeting of the European Association for Hematopathology and the Society of Hematopathology in Bordeaux, France. J Hematop 2009; 2(4):211–36.

38. Grogg KL, Miller RF, Dogan A. HIV infection and lymphoma. J Clin Pathol 2007;60(12):1365–72.

39. Stein H, Delsol G, Pileri S, et al. Classical Hodgkin lymphoma, introduction. In: Swerdlow S, Campo E, Harris N, et al, editors. WHO classification of tumours of haematopoietic and lymphoid tissues. Lyon (France): IARC; 2008. p. 326–9.

40. Kanzler H, Kuppers R, Hansmann ML, Rajewsky K. Hodgkin and Reed-Sternberg cells in Hodgkin's disease represent the outgrowth of a dominant tumor clone derived from (crippled) germinal center B cells. J Exp Med 1996;184(4):1495–505.

41. Kuppers R. Molecular biology of Hodgkin lymphoma. Hematology Am Soc Hematol Educ Program 2009;491–6.

42. Hasserjian RP, Ott G, Elenitoba-Johnson KS, et al. Commentary on the WHO classification of tumors of lymphoid tissues (2008): "Gray zone" lymphomas overlapping with Burkitt lymphoma or classical Hodgkin lymphoma. J Hematop 2009; 2(2):89–95.

43. Keegan TH, Glaser SL, Clarke CA, et al. Epstein-Barr virus as a marker of survival after Hodgkin's lymphoma: a population-based study. J Clin Oncol 2005;23(30):7604–13.

44. Jarrett RF, Stark GL, White J, et al. Impact of tumor Epstein-Barr virus status on presenting features and outcome in age-defined subgroups of patients with classic Hodgkin lymphoma: a population-based study. Blood 2005;106(7):2444–51.

45. Diepstra A, van Imhoff GW, Schaapveld M, et al. Latent Epstein-Barr virus infection of tumor cells in classical Hodgkin's lymphoma predicts adverse outcome in older adult patients. J Clin Oncol 2009;27(23):3815–21.

46. Van Krieken J, Onciu M, Elenitoba-Johnson K, et al. Lymphoproliferative diseases associated with primary immune disorders. In: Swerdlow S, Campo E, Harris N, et al, editors. WHO

classification of tumours of the haematopoietic and lymphoid tissues. Lyon (France): IARC; 2008. p. 336–9.

47. Raphael M, Said J, Borisch B, et al. Lymphomas associated with HIV infection. In: Swerdlow S, Campo E, Harris N, et al, editors. WHO classification of tumours of haematopoietic and lymphoid neoplasms. Lyon (France): IARC; 2008. p. 340–2.

48. Gaulard P, Swerdlow S, Harris N, et al. Other iatrogenic immunodeficiency-associated lymphoproliferative disorders. In: Swerdlow S, Campo E, Harris N, et al, editors. WHO classification of tumours of haematopoietic and lymphoid tissues. Lyon (France): IARC; 2008. p. 350–1.

49. Swerdlow S, Webber S, Chadburn A, et al. Post-transplant lymphoproliferative disorders. In: Swerdlow S, Campo E, Harris N, et al, editors. WHO classification of tumours of haematopoietic and lymphoid tissues. Lyon (France): IARC; 2008. p. 343–9.

50. Hasserjian RP, Chen S, Perkins SL, et al. Immunomodulator agent-related lymphoproliferative disorders. Mod Pathol 2009;22(12):1532–40.

51. Chadburn A, Chiu A, Lee JY, et al. Immunophenotypic analysis of AIDS-related diffuse large B-cell lymphoma and clinical implications in patients from AIDS Malignancies Consortium clinical trials 010 and 034. J Clin Oncol 2009;27(30):5039–48.

52. Delecluse HJ, Anagnostopoulos I, Dallenbach F, et al. Plasmablastic lymphomas of the oral cavity: a new entity associated with the human immunodeficiency virus infection. Blood 1997;89(4):1413–20.

53. Chetty R, Hlatswayo N, Muc R, et al. Plasmablastic lymphoma in HIV+ patients: an expanding spectrum. Histopathology 2003;42(6):605–9.

54. Lin Y, Rodrigues GD, Turner JF, et al. Plasmablastic lymphoma of the lung: report of a unique case and review of the literature. Arch Pathol Lab Med 2001; 125(2):282–5.

55. Hausermann P, Khanna N, Buess M, et al. Cutaneous plasmablastic lymphoma in an HIV-positive male: an unrecognized cutaneous manifestation. Dermatology 2004;208(3):287–90.

56. Colomo L, Loong F, Rives S, et al. Diffuse large B-cell lymphomas with plasmablastic differentiation represent a heterogeneous group of disease entities. Am J Surg Pathol 2004;28(6):736–47.

57. Schichman SA, McClure R, Schaefer RF, et al. HIV and plasmablastic lymphoma manifesting in sinus, testicles, and bones: a further expansion of the disease spectrum. Am J Hematol 2004;77(3):291–5.

58. Dong HY, Scadden DT, de Leval L, et al. Plasmablastic lymphoma in HIV-positive patients: an aggressive Epstein-Barr virus-associated extramedullary plasmacytic neoplasm. Am J Surg Pathol 2005;29(12):1633–41.

59. Teruya-Feldstein J, Chiao E, Filippa DA, et al. CD20-negative large-cell lymphoma with plasmablastic

features: a clinically heterogeneous spectrum in both HIV-positive and -negative patients. Ann Oncol 2004;15(11):1673–9.

60. Carbone A, Gloghini A, Larocca LM, et al. Expression profile of MUM1/IRF4, BCL-6, and CD138/syndecan-1 defines novel histogenetic subsets of human immunodeficiency virus-related lymphomas. Blood 2001;97(3):744–51.

61. Cioc AM, Allen C, Kalmar JR, et al. Oral plasmablastic lymphomas in AIDS patients are associated with human herpesvirus 8. Am J Surg Pathol 2004; 28(1):41–6.

62. Zanetto U, Martin CA, Sapia S, et al. Re: Cioc AM, Allen C, Kalmar J, et al. Oral plasmablastic lymphomas in AIDS patients are associated with human herpesvirus 8. Am J Surg Pathol 2004; 25:41–46. Am J Surg Pathol 2004;28(11):1537–8 [author reply: 1538].

63. Vega F, Chang CC, Medeiros LJ, et al. Plasmablastic lymphomas and plasmablastic plasma cell myelomas have nearly identical immunophenotypic profiles. Mod Pathol 2005;18(6):806–15.

64. Goedhals J, Beukes CA, Hardie D. HHV8 in plasmablastic lymphoma. Am J Surg Pathol 2008; 32(1):172.

65. Gaidano G, Cerri M, Capello D, et al. Molecular histogenesis of plasmablastic lymphoma of the oral cavity. Br J Haematol 2002;119(3):622–8.

66. Bogusz AM, Seegmiller AC, Garcia R, et al. Plasmablastic lymphomas with MYC/IgH rearrangement: report of three cases and review of the literature. Am J Clin Pathol 2009;132(4): 597–605.

67. Taddesse-Heath L, Meloni-Ehrig A, Scheerle J, et al. Plasmablastic lymphoma with MYC translocation: evidence for a common pathway in the generation of plasmablastic features. Mod Pathol 2010; 23(7):991–9.

68. Chadburn A, Hyjek E, Mathew S, et al. KSHV-positive solid lymphomas represent an extra-cavitary variant of primary effusion lymphoma. Am J Surg Pathol 2004;28(11):1401–16.

69. Delsol G, Lamant L, Mariame B, et al. A new subtype of large B-cell lymphoma expressing the ALK kinase and lacking the 2;5 translocation. Blood 1997;89(5):1483–90.

70. Gascoyne RD, Lamant L, Martin-Subero JI, et al. ALK-positive diffuse large B-cell lymphoma is associated with Clathrin-ALK rearrangements: report of 6 cases. Blood 2003;102(7):2568–73.

71. Iuchi K, Ichimiya A, Akashi A, et al. Non-Hodgkin's lymphoma of the pleural cavity developing from long-standing pyothorax. Cancer 1987;60(8): 1771–5.

72. Iuchi K, Aozasa K, Yamamoto S, et al. Non-Hodgkin's lymphoma of the pleural cavity developing from long-standing pyothorax. Summary of clinical

and pathological findings in thirty-seven cases. Jpn J Clin Oncol 1989;19(3):249–57.

73. Nakatsuka S, Yao M, Hoshida Y, et al. Pyothorax-associated lymphoma: a review of 106 cases. J Clin Oncol 2002;20(20):4255–60.

74. Narimatsu H, Ota Y, Kami M, et al. Clinicopathological features of pyothorax-associated lymphoma: a retrospective survey involving 98 patients. Ann Oncol 2007;18(1):122–8.

75. Petitjean B, Jardin F, Joly B, et al. Pyothorax-associated lymphoma: a peculiar clinicopathologic entity derived from B cells at late stage of differentiation and with occasional aberrant dual B- and T-cell phenotype. Am J Surg Pathol 2002;26(6): 724–32.

76. Copie-Bergman C, Niedobitek G, Mangham DC, et al. Epstein-Barr virus in B-cell lymphomas associated with chronic suppurative inflammation. J Pathol 1997;183(3):287–92.

77. Cheuk W, Chan AC, Chan JK, et al. Metallic implant-associated lymphoma: a distinct subgroup of large B-cell lymphoma related to pyothorax-associated lymphoma? Am J Surg Pathol 2005; 29(6):832–6.

78. Androulaki A, Drakos E, Hatzianastassiou D, et al. Pyothorax-associated lymphoma (PAL): a western case with marked angiocentricity and review of the literature. Histopathology 2004;44(1):69–76.

79. Fukayama M, Ibuka T, Hayashi Y, et al. Epstein-Barr virus in pyothorax-associated pleural lymphoma. Am J Pathol 1993;143(4):1044–9.

80. Miwa H, Takakuwa T, Nakatsuka S, et al. DNA sequences of the immunoglobulin heavy chain variable region gene in pyothorax-associated lymphoma. Oncology 2002;62(3):241–50.

81. Takakuwa T, Tresnasari K, Rahadiani N, et al. Cell origin of pyothorax-associated lymphoma: a lymphoma strongly associated with Epstein-Barr virus infection. Leukemia 2008;22(3):620–7.

82. Yamato H, Ohshima K, Suzumiya J, et al. Evidence for local immunosuppression and demonstration of c-myc amplification in pyothorax-associated lymphoma. Histopathology 2001;39(2):163–71.

83. Kanno H, Aozasa K. Mechanism for the development of pyothorax-associated lymphoma. Pathol Int 1998;48(9):653–64.

84. Kanno H, Naka N, Yasunaga Y, et al. Role of an immunosuppressive cytokine, interleukin-10, in the development of pyothorax-associated lymphoma. Leukemia 1997;11(Suppl 3):525–6.

85. Ascani S, Piccioli M, Poggi S, et al. Pyothorax-associated lymphoma: description of the first two cases detected in Italy. Ann Oncol 1997;8(11):1133–8.

86. O'Donovan M, Silva I, Uhlmann V, et al. Expression profile of human herpesvirus 8 (HHV8) in pyothorax associated lymphoma and in effusion lymphoma. Mol Pathol 2001;54(2):80–5.

87. Liebow AA, Carrington CR, Friedman PJ. Lymphomatoid granulomatosis. Hum Pathol 1972;3(4):457–558.

88. Guinee D Jr, Jaffe E, Kingma D, et al. Pulmonary lymphomatoid granulomatosis. Evidence for a proliferation of Epstein-Barr virus infected B-lymphocytes with a prominent T-cell component and vasculitis. Am J Surg Pathol 1994;18(8):753–64.

89. Haque AK, Myers JL, Hudnall SD, et al. Pulmonary lymphomatoid granulomatosis in acquired immunodeficiency syndrome: lesions with Epstein-Barr virus infection. Mod Pathol 1998;11(4):347–56.

90. Katzenstein AL, Peiper SC. Detection of Epstein-Barr virus genomes in lymphomatoid granulomatosis: analysis of 29 cases by the polymerase chain reaction technique. Mod Pathol 1990;3(4):435–41.

91. Myers JL, Kurtin PJ, Katzenstein AL, et al. Lymphomatoid granulomatosis. Evidence of immunophenotypic diversity and relationship to Epstein-Barr virus infection. Am J Surg Pathol 1995;19(11):1300–12.

92. Pittaluga S, Wilson W, Jaffe E. Lymphomatoid granulomatosis. In: Swerdlow S, Campo E, Harris N, et al, editors. WHO classification of tumours of haemaopoietic and lymphoid tissues. Lyon (France): IARC; 2008. p. 247–9.

93. Katzenstein A, Carrington C, Liebow A. Lymphomatoid granulomatosis: a clinicopathologic study of 152 cases. Cancer 1979;43:360–73.

94. Cadranel J, Wislez M, Antoine M. Primary pulmonary lymphoma. Eur Respir J 2002;20(3):750–62.

95. Beaty MW, Toro J, Sorbara L, et al. Cutaneous lymphomatoid granulomatosis: correlation of clinical and biologic features. Am J Surg Pathol 2001;25(9):1111–20.

96. Saxena A, Dyker KM, Angel S, et al. Posttransplant diffuse large B-cell lymphoma of "lymphomatoid granulomatosis" type. Virchows Arch 2002;441(6):622–8.

97. Lipford E, Margolich J, Longo D, et al. Angiocentric immunoproliferative lesions: a clinicopathologic spectrum of post-thymic T cell proliferations. Blood 1988;5:1674–81.

98. Guinee DG Jr, Perkins SL, Travis WD, et al. Proliferation and cellular phenotype in lymphomatoid granulomatosis: implications of a higher proliferation index in B cells. Am J Surg Pathol 1998;22(9):1093–100.

99. Teruya-Feldstein J, Jaffe ES, Burd PR, et al. The role of Mig, the monokine induced by interferon-gamma, and IP-10, the interferon-gamma-inducible protein-10, in tissue necrosis and vascular damage associated with Epstein-Barr virus-positive lymphoproliferative disease. Blood 1997;90(10):4099–105.

100. Shimoyama Y, Asano N, Kojima M, et al. Age-related EBV-associated B-cell lymphoproliferative disorders: diagnostic approach to a newly recognized clinicopathological entity. Pathol Int 2009;59(12):835–43.

101. Oyama T, Ichimura K, Suzuki R, et al. Senile EBV+ B-cell lymphoproliferative disorders: a clinicopathologic study of 22 patients. Am J Surg Pathol 2003;27(1):16–26.

102. Shimoyama Y, Oyama T, Asano N, et al. Senile Epstein-Barr virus-associated B-cell lymphoproliferative disorders: a mini review. J Clin Exp Hematop 2006;46(1):1–4.

103. Park S, Lee J, Ko YH, et al. The impact of Epstein-Barr virus status on clinical outcome in diffuse large B-cell lymphoma. Blood 2007;110(3):972–8.

104. Naresh KN, Rice AJ, Bower M. Lymph nodes involved by multicentric Castleman disease among HIV-positive individuals are often involved by Kaposi sarcoma. Am J Surg Pathol 2008;32(7):1006–12.

105. Soulier J, Grollet L, Oksenhandler E, et al. Kaposi's sarcoma-like herpesvirus-like DNA sequences in multicentric Castleman's disease. Blood 1995;84:1276–80.

106. Dupin N, Diss TL, Kellam P, et al. HHV8 is associated with a plasmablastic variant of Castleman disease that is linked to HHV8-positive plasmablastic lymphoma. Blood 2000;95(4):1406–12.

107. Chadburn A, Hyjek EM, Tam W, et al. Immunophenotypic analysis of the Kaposi sarcoma herpesvirus (KSHV; HHV8)-infected B cells in HIV+ multicentric Castleman disease (MCD). Histopathology 2008;53(5):513–24.

108. Du MQ, Liu H, Diss TC, et al. Kaposi sarcoma-associated herpesvirus infects monotypic (IgM lambda) but polyclonal naive B cells in Castleman disease and associated lymphoproliferative disorders. Blood 2001;97(7):2130–6.

109. Oksenhendler E, Boulanger E, Galicier L, et al. High incidence of Kaposi sarcoma-associated herpesvirus-related non-Hodgkin lymphoma in patients with HIV infection and multicentric Castleman disease. Blood 2002;99(7):2331–6.

110. Carbone A, Cilia AM, Gloghini A, et al. Establishment and characterization of EBV-positive and EBV-negative primary effusion lymphoma cell lines harbouring human herpesvirus type-8. Br J Haematol 1998;102(4):1081–9.

111. Gaidano G, Gloghini A, Gattei V, et al. Association of Kaposi's sarcoma-associated herpesvirus-positive primary effusion lymphoma with expression of the CD138/syndecan-1 antigen. Blood 1997;90(12):4894–900.

112. Cesarman E, Chang Y, Moore PS, et al. Kaposi's sarcoma-associated herpesvirus-like DNA sequences in AIDS-related body-cavity-based lymphomas. N Engl J Med 1995;332(18):1186–91.

113. Horenstein MG, Nador RG, Chadburn A, et al. Epstein-Barr virus latent gene expression in primary effusion lymphomas containing Kaposi's sarcoma-associated herpesvirus/human herpesvirus-8. Blood 1997;90(3):1186–91.

114. Cesarman E, Nador RG, Aozasa K, et al. Kaposi's sarcoma-associated herpesvirus in non-AIDS related lymphomas occurring in body cavities. Am J Pathol 1996;149(1):53–7.

115. Cesarman E, Knowles DM. The role of Kaposi's sarcoma-associated herpesvirus (KSHV/HHV8) in lymphoproliferative diseases. Semin Cancer Biol 1999;9(3):165–74.

116. Ascoli V, Lo-Coco F. Body cavity lymphoma. Curr Opin Pulm Med 2002;8(4):317–22.

117. Fan W, Bubman D, Chadburn A, et al. Distinct subsets of primary effusion lymphoma can be identified based on their cellular gene expression profile and viral association. J Virol 2005;79(2):1244–51.

118. Matolcsy A, Nador RG, Cesarman E, et al. Immunoglobulin VH gene mutational analysis suggests that primary effusion lymphomas derive from different stages of B cell maturation. Am J Pathol 1998; 153(5):1609–14.

119. Fais F, Gaidano G, Capello D, et al. Immunoglobulin V region gene use and structure suggest antigen selection in AIDS-related primary effusion lymphomas. Leukemia 1999;13(7):1093–9.

120. Klein U, Gloghini A, Gaidano G, et al. Gene expression profile analysis of AIDS-related primary effusion lymphoma (PEL) suggests a plasmablastic derivation and identifies PEL-specific transcripts. Blood 2003;101(10):4115–21.

121. Jenner RG, Maillard K, Cattini N, et al. Kaposi's sarcoma-associated herpesvirus-infected primary effusion lymphoma has a plasma cell gene expression profile. Proc Natl Acad Sci U S A 2003; 100(18):10399–404.

122. Carbone A, Gloghini A, Vaccher E, et al. Kaposi's sarcoma-associated herpesvirus/human herpesvirus type 8-positive solid lymphomas: a tissue-based variant of primary effusion lymphoma. J Mol Diagn 2005;7(1):17–27.

123. Deloose ST, Smit LA, Pals FT, et al. High incidence of Kaposi sarcoma-associated herpesvirus infection in HIV-related solid immunoblastic/plasmablastic diffuse large B-cell lymphoma. Leukemia 2005; 19(5):851–5.

124. Boulanger E, Gerard L, Gabarre J, et al. Prognostic factors and outcome of human herpesvirus 8-associated primary effusion lymphoma in patients with AIDS. J Clin Oncol 2005;23(19):4372–80.

DIAGNOSIS OF BURKITT LYMPHOMA AND RELATED HIGH-GRADE B-CELL NEOPLASMS

Aliyah R. Sohani, MD*, Robert Paul Hasserjian, MD

KEYWORDS

- Burkitt lymphoma • MYC • Epstein-Barr virus • High-grade B-cell lymphoma unclassifiable
- Diffuse large B-cell lymphoma • Acute lymphoblastic lymphoma

ABSTRACT

Burkitt lymphoma (BL) is an aggressive B-cell neoplasm with an extremely short doubling time that mainly affects children and young adults. Despite having several characteristic features, none is entirely specific for BL and the differential diagnosis may include diffuse large B-cell lymphoma (DLBCL), B lymphoblastic leukemia/lymphoma, and B-cell lymphoma unclassifiable with features intermediate between DLBCL and BL. We outline a practical approach to establish a diagnosis of BL and distinguish it from other high-grade B-cell malignancies. We pay particular attention to B-cell lymphomas with features intermediate between DLBCL and BL, a new diagnostic category in the 2008 World Health Organization classification system that provides a framework for categorizing challenging cases not meeting diagnostic criteria for either "classic" BL or DLBCL.

BURKITT LYMPHOMA

OVERVIEW

The pathogenesis of BL appears to be multifactorial, as evidenced by its occurrence in different populations and clinical settings and its varying association with Epstein-Barr virus (EBV) infection; the 3 clinical variants of BL are described in **Table 1**. The vast majority of cases of endemic BL are EBV

Pathologic Key Features
OF BURKITT LYMPHOMA

1. Morphology is characterized by a diffuse proliferation of small to medium-sized monomorphous cells with round nuclei, finely clumped chromatin, multiple small paracentric nucleoli, and scant deeply basophilic cytoplasm. Numerous mitoses and apoptotic histiocytes give the tumor a characteristic "starry-sky" pattern on low magnification.

2. Slight nuclear pleomorphism, nuclear membrane irregularities, or nucleolar prominence is acceptable, particularly in immunodeficiency-associated cases, provided other key immunophenotypic and genetic criteria are met.

3. The immunophenotype of BL is CD10 strongly positive, BCL6-positive, BCL2-negative (or occasionally weakly positive), and a Ki-67 proliferation index greater than 95%.

4. The main genetic feature of BL is the presence of a *MYC* translocation, present in 95% of cases. This is most often an *IGH-MYC* translocation, or less commonly, *IGK-MYC* or *IGL-MYC* translocation.

positive and their geographic distribution closely parallels that of holoendemic malaria. Evidence suggests that endemic BL may result from polyclonal B-cell activation and reactivation of latently

Department of Pathology, Massachusetts General Hospital, and Harvard Medical School, 55 Fruit Street, Boston, MA 02114, USA
* Corresponding author. Massachusetts General Hospital, 55 Fruit Street, WRN 219, Boston, MA 02114.
E-mail address: arsohani@partners.org

Surgical Pathology 3 (2010) 1035–1059
doi:10.1016/j.path.2010.09.010

Table 1
Clinical variants of Burkitt lymphoma

Clinical Variant	Age of Onset and Incidence	Male:Female Ratio	Geographic Distribution	Sites of Disease	EBV Association
Endemic BL	Mainly children, peak incidence 4–7 years. Most common childhood malignancy in equatorial Africa	2:1	Equatorial Africa and Papua New Guinea	Commonly extranodal: jaws, orbit or other facial bones (50% of cases); also ileocecal region, omentum, gonads, kidneys, long bones, thyroid, salivary glands and breasts	>90% of cases
Sporadic BL	Children and young adults (median age of adult patients 30 years). 1%–2% of all lymphomas in Western Europe and North America and 30%–50% of childhood lymphomas	2–3:1 in adults, higher in children	Worldwide	Commonly extranodal: ileocecal region (most frequent site); also ovaries, kidneys, breasts. Nodal presentation more common in adults. Jaw tumors, Waldeyer ring and mediastinal disease rare	15%–30% of cases
Immunodeficiency-associated BL	HIV+ adults and patients with congenital or iatrogenic immunodeficiency	Males more commonly affected	Worldwide	Nodal and bone marrow involvement more common than Endemic or Sporadic BL	25%–40% of cases

Abbreviations: EBV, Epstein-Barr virus; HIV, human immunodeficiency virus.
Data from Refs.[2,8,11,12]

infected memory B cells. In addition to the presumed effect of *Plasmodium falciparum* on T-cell immunity and EBV-specific T-cell responses, other factors, including arboviruses and tumor promoters derived from plants, are hypothesized to play a role in the high incidence of BL in endemic regions.[1-6] Potentially oncogenic, mosquito-borne arboviruses appear to be associated with case clusters of endemic BL, and symptoms of arboviral infection have been noted in patients immediately before the onset of lymphoma. Extracts of a plant commonly used in endemic regions for medicinal purposes, *Euphorbia tirucalli*, have been shown to induce the t(8;14) in EBV-infected cell lines, activate latent EBV in infected cells and enhance EBV-mediated cell transformation; the distribution of *E tirucalli* closely parallels that of the lymphoma belt in sub-Saharan Africa, suggesting a potential pathogenetic role.[1-6] In cases of sporadic BL, low socioeconomic status and young age of EBV infection correlate with EBV-positive cases, whereas immunodeficiency-associated cases of BL are intriguing in that most cases lack EBV expression.[7,8] BL is more common in HIV than in other forms of immunosuppression and tends to occur early in the course of disease, when the CD4-positive T-cell count is still relatively preserved, suggesting that factors other than immunosuppression might explain the increased incidence of BL in this group of patients.[9] Roles for HIV in promoting polyclonal B-cell activation or in direct oncogenic activation have been postulated.[10]

CLINICAL FEATURES

BL has the highest doubling time of any tumor. For this reason, patients often present acutely, with bulky disease, a high tumor burden, and symptoms often lasting only several days to a few weeks. The 3 clinical variants differ in epidemiology, geographic distribution, clinical presentation, and pathogenesis (see **Table 1**), but extranodal sites of involvement are common in all subtypes and all show a striking predilection for central nervous system (CNS) involvement. BL may involve the bone marrow and peripheral blood in advanced, disseminated disease. Despite its designation in prior classification systems as the "L3" type of acute lymphoblastic leukemia (ALL), involvement limited to bone marrow and peripheral blood with a purely leukemic presentation is rare in immunocompetent patients. In the current 2008 World Health Organization (WHO) classification, leukemic BL is not considered to represent a variant of ALL, but is regarded as a mature B-cell lymphoma.[2,8,11,12]

DIAGNOSIS: MICROSCOPIC FEATURES

BL has a diffuse growth pattern and is classically composed of medium-sized lymphocytes with nuclei similar in size or slightly smaller than a histiocyte nucleus. The tumor cells are monomorphous with round nuclei, absent to minimal nuclear irregularities, finely clumped chromatin with multiple small paracentric nucleoli, and scant, deeply basophilic cytoplasm (**Fig. 1**A). In tissue sections, the cells may have a cohesive appearance with angulated cell borders. In air-dried touch imprints or smears, lipid-filled cytoplasmic vacuoles are usually visible (see **Fig. 1**B, C). Because of its high proliferation fraction, BL contains numerous mitotic figures and apoptotic bodies, making interspersed phagocytic histiocytes readily visible; the resulting "starry-sky" appearance on low magnification is a characteristic, but nonspecific, finding (**Fig. 2**A).[2] Some cases may contain patchy or extensive areas of geographic necrosis.

In the 2008 WHO classification, no formal morphologic variants of BL are recognized. Some cases, particularly those associated with immunodeficiency, may exhibit single central nucleoli and plasmacytoid features with eccentric scant basophilic cytoplasm. Some cases of BL (including most cases arising in adults) may have more variable morphology, such as mild nuclear irregularities, slight nuclear pleomorphism with minor variability in nuclear size, or more prominent, single nucleoli as compared with "classic" BL (see **Fig. 2**B). In the past, such cases were referred to as "atypical BL." However, recent gene expression profiling studies show that such cases with variable morphology have a similar molecular signature to classic BL, supporting the concept that the morphologic spectrum of BL is wider than previously thought. Thus, cases with slight morphologic variations, but that otherwise fulfill all immunophenotypic and genetic criteria for BL should be classified as such and are no longer considered to comprise a discrete BL variant.[2,13,14]

DIAGNOSIS: ANCILLARY STUDIES

BL is positive for pan-B-cell markers (CD19, CD20, CD22, CD79a, Pax5) and demonstrates moderate to strong expression of surface IgM and either kappa or lambda light chain. The classic immunophenotype, present in nearly all cases, is strong positivity for CD10, expression of BCL6, and negativity for BCL2 (**Fig. 3**).[2,15] If BCL2 expression is present (seen in only a minority of cases), its level of expression is weak. The tumor cells are also positive for CD38, CD43, and TCL1, and are

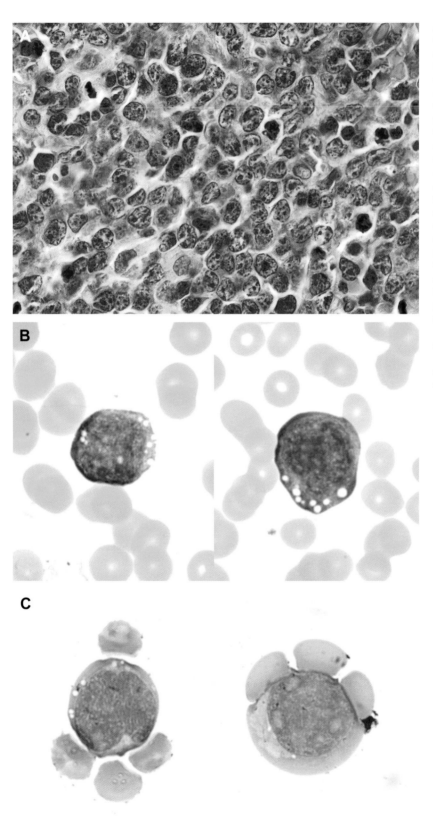

Fig. 1. Examples of typical cases of BL. (*A*) BL in a pediatric patient, with classic high-power morphology characterized by monomorphous, medium-sized cells with round to slightly angulated nuclei, finely clumped chromatin, and multiple, small paracentrally located nucleoli. Mitotic figures and apoptotic cells are conspicuous (H&E, ×1000). (*B*) BL cells in the peripheral blood of a leukemic case, with multiple small nucleoli and basophilic, vacuolated cytoplasm; BL cells may appear more irregular in smear preparations than in tissue sections (Wright-Giemsa, ×1000). (*C*) BL cells in the cerebrospinal fluid specimen of an adult patient exhibiting similar features (Wright-Giemsa, ×1000).

Fig. 2. Morphologic features of BL. (*A*) Characteristic low-power "starry-sky" appearance of BL with scattered phagocytic histiocytes (H&E, ×200). (*B*) HIV-associated BL occurring in an adult patient with more variable nuclear morphology (H&E, ×1000). Overall, the cells are medium-sized (compare with size of histiocyte nucleus in lower left); however, some cells are slightly larger with more prominent central nucleoli (*arrow*) and a greater degree of nuclear irregularity as compared with **Fig. 1A**.

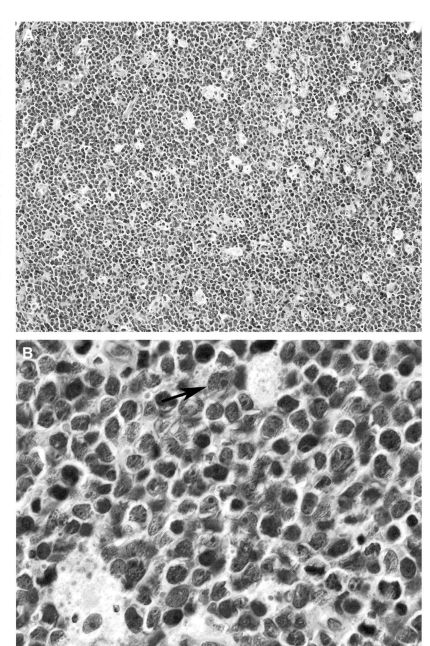

negative for CD5, CD23, CD44, CD138, and precursor cell markers (CD34, CD99, and TdT). Positivity for MUM1/IRF4 is seen in relatively few cases.[16,17] Nearly 100% of the cells are positive for the proliferation marker Ki-67 (MIB1). Staining for pan-T-cell markers (CD2, CD3, CD5, CD7) reveals only rare admixed non-neoplastic small T cells, fewer than typically seen in most cases of diffuse large B-cell lymphoma (DLBCL). EBV expression may be detected by in situ hybridization for EBV-encoded RNA (EBER) and the frequency of positivity differs among clinical variants (see **Table 1**).[2,8,11,12,16–19] EBV-LMP1 immunohistochemistry is usually negative owing to the latency phase of EBV that characterizes BL.

Nearly all cases of BL have a demonstrable translocation involving the *MYC* gene at 8q24, most commonly partnered with the immunoglobulin heavy chain gene (*IGH*) at 14q32. Less frequently, the partner is another *IG* gene, either lambda light chain (*IGL*) at 22q11 or kappa light chain (*IGK*) at 2p12.[12] A *MYC* rearrangement may be demonstrated either by conventional cytogenetics or interphase fluorescent in situ

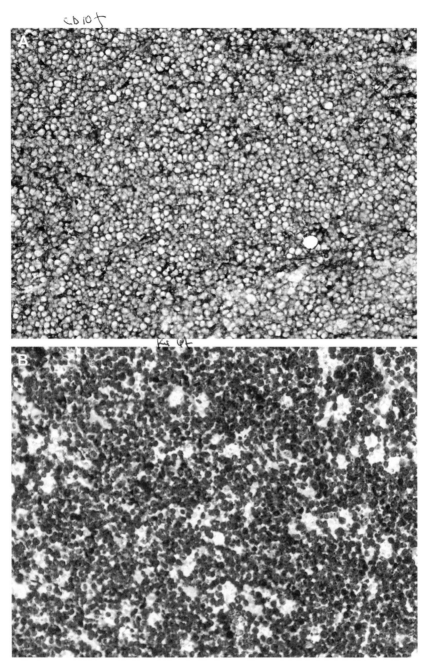

Fig. 3. Classic immunophenotype of BL. (*A*) By immunohistochemistry, the tumor cells show strong positivity for CD10 (×200). (*B*) Nearly all tumor cells show nuclear staining for Ki-67 (MIB1); the negatively stained cells correspond to phagocytic histiocytes (×200).

hybridization (FISH) analysis (**Fig. 4**). If the former is performed, a relatively simple background karyotype is usually seen, with few additional rearrangements or aneuploidies (see **Fig. 4**A).[14,20] In many instances, however, fresh tissue is not sent at the time of biopsy for cytogenetic analysis, either because of insufficient tissue or lack of recognition of the importance of such analysis to a particular case at the time of surgery. In such circumstances, FISH with a dual-color break-apart probe performed on unstained smear preparations or paraffin-embedded tumor tissue may be used

to detect the presence of a *MYC* rearrangement at 8q24 (see **Fig. 4**B).

Because a *MYC* rearrangement is not specific for BL and may be seen in up to 15% of cases of DLBCL, one should be cautious in interpreting a positive *MYC* rearrangement by FISH as definitive evidence for BL.[14,20–22] Correlation with morphologic and immunophenotypic findings is required: if a high degree of morphologic or immunophenotypic variability exists, classification as DLBCL or B-cell lymphoma unclassifiable with features intermediate between DLBCL and BL (U-DLBCL/BL)

Fig. 4. Genetic features of BL. (*A*) Conventional cytogenetics demonstrates a t(8;14)(q24;q32) indicative of an *IGH-MYC* rearrangement (*black arrows*). Although this case also contains one other abnormality in the form of additional unknown genetic material within the long arm of chromosome 1 (*red arrow*), the karyotype is relatively simple. (*B*) Interphase FISH analysis of the same case with a dual-color break-apart probe for the *MYC* locus. Each cell contains a single fused red/green signal that represents the non-rearranged copy of *MYC*, as well as separated red and green signals indicative of a *MYC* rearrangement.

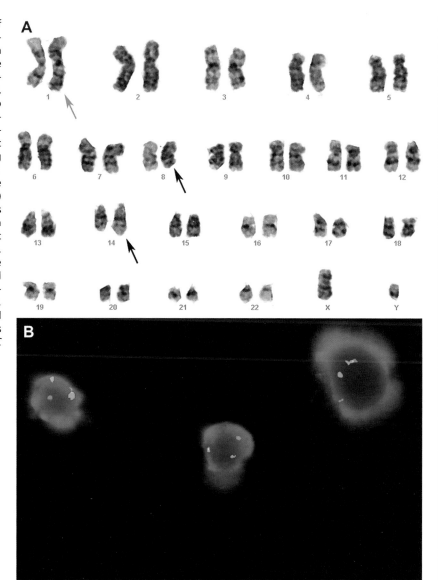

may be appropriate (see next section). In such cases, additional FISH studies to identify the partner gene using probes for *IG* loci may be informative: in BL, *MYC* is juxtaposed to an *IG* gene, most commonly *IGH*. However, these probes are not available in most cytogenetics laboratories. Finally, additional FISH analysis to exclude both *BCL2* and *BCL6* translocations should be considered, as the presence of either of these rearrangements effectively excludes the diagnosis of BL.[15,23] Because of the wide range of *IGH* breakpoints in BL and the occurrence of other translocation partners such as *IGL* and *IGK*, polymerase chain reaction (PCR) is relatively insensitive to detect a *MYC* rearrangement.[4,11,24]

Rare cases that are otherwise characteristic of BL lack a *MYC* translocation; the percentage of these cases is variable in published studies, likely reflecting differing pathologic inclusion criteria.[25] These cases contain a molecular signature similar to other BL cases that have detectable *MYC* rearrangement, thereby validating their classification as BL.[13,14]

DIFFERENTIAL DIAGNOSIS

Florid Reactive Follicular Hyperplasia

The differential diagnosis between BL and florid reactive follicular hyperplasia (RFH) may be a consideration in small biopsy or fine-needle aspiration (FNA) specimens, in which the amount of tissue biopsied is small, precluding adequate assessment for the presence of diffuse architectural effacement (**Fig. 5**A, B). In our experience,

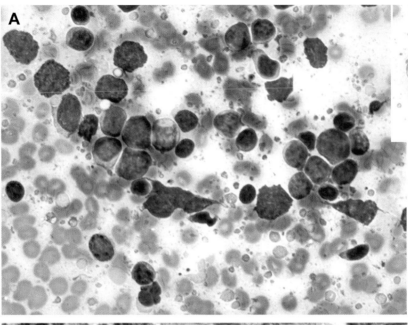

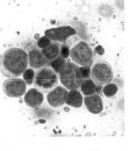

Fig. 5. The differential diagnosis of BL versus reactive follicular hyperplasia. (A) Fine needle aspiration specimen from a cervical lymph node, with numerous centroblasts mimicking the neoplastic cells of BL; mitotic figures were also evident (*inset*) (Giemsa, ×1000). (B) Subsequent excisional biopsy revealed florid reactive follicular hyperplasia. A high-power view of a reactive germinal center illustrates its resemblance to the starry-sky pattern of BL (H&E, ×1000).

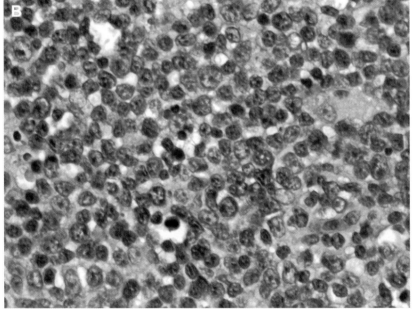

extensively fragmented excisional biopsy specimens of sites that would be unusual for BL involvement, such as tonsil, can make the distinction of BL from RFH challenging (see **Fig. 5**C—E).[26] In addition, BL may invade adjacent reactive lymphoid tissue and such cases of partial nodal involvement may be particularly difficult to diagnose.[2]

In small or fragmented tissue samples, reactive follicles can appear cytologically and immunophenotypically identical to BL: they contain numerous medium-sized centroblasts with multiple small peripheral nucleoli and scant basophilic cytoplasm; they exhibit a "starry-sky" growth pattern with numerous tingible-body macrophages; they express a germinal center phenotype (CD10+, BCL6+) with absent expression for BCL2; and have a very high proliferation index. In the absence of obvious follicle structures, immunohistochemical stains for CD21, CD23, or CD35 may help to identify follicular dendritic cell aggregates in RFH, which should be absent in BL. For a definitive

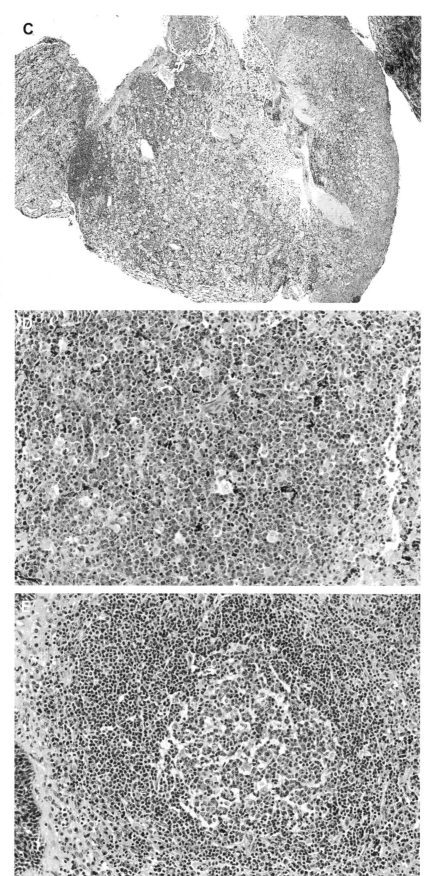

Fig. 5. The differential diagnosis of BL versus reactive follicular hyperplasia. (*C*) A fragmented, focally crushed tonsil biopsy specimen partially involved by BL (note the low-power starry-sky pattern) that could be mistaken for enlarged germinal centers (H&E, ×100). The sheetlike proliferation in the areas of BL (*D*) contrasts with the defined germinal centers in the residual reactive follicles (*E*). Ultimately, frozen section immunohistochemistry (not shown) helped to confirm B-cell clonality and the diagnosis of lymphoma.

diagnosis of lymphoma, demonstration of B-cell clonality by flow cytometry or frozen section immunohistochemistry is required and identification of a *MYC* rearrangement by karyotype or interphase FISH may be used to support the diagnosis of BL. In most circumstances, the turnaround time for *IGH* gene rearrangement by PCR to confirm clonality may be unacceptably long if BL is strongly suspected clinically. In cases with insufficient tissue for these confirmatory ancillary studies, open rebiopsy should be undertaken for a definitive diagnosis.

Diffuse Large B-cell Lymphoma, Not Otherwise Specified (DLBCL, NOS)

Diffuse large B-cell lymphoma (DLBCL) is a neoplasm with a diffuse growth pattern composed of large B lymphocytes, defined as having a nuclear size equal to or exceeding that of a histiocyte nucleus. Cases of DLBCL may exhibit diverse morphologies, including cases composed predominantly of centroblasts (cells with oval to round nuclei, vesicular chromatin, and small, peripherally located nucleoli), immunoblasts (large cells with prominent central nucleoli and moderately abundant basophilic cytoplasm), or an admixture of these two cell types.[27] Some cases demonstrate anaplastic features with large cells containing bizarre, pleomorphic nuclei, some of which may resemble Reed-Sternberg cells. The proliferation fraction may vary from moderate to high, but exceeds 95% in only rare cases. In most cases of DLBCL, therefore, the distinction from BL is relatively straightforward because of the large cell size, polymorphous nature of the infiltrate with a relatively high degree of nuclear irregularity, and the absence of a "starry-sky" pattern (**Fig. 6A**). However, cases of DLBCL with cytologic monomorphism, a predominance of medium-sized cells, and a high proliferation index with conspicuous mitoses and apoptotic bodies may raise the differential diagnosis of BL. In such cases, a panel of immunohistochemical stains that includes CD10, BCL2, MUM1/IRF4, and Ki-67 may help to distinguish DLBCL from BL (see **Fig. 6B**). BL should be strongly positive for CD10 and negative for BCL2; therefore, cases with weak or absent expression of CD10 or strong positivity for BCL2 are unlikely to be BL.[2,16] In addition, positivity for MUM1/IRF4 has been reported in only a few cases of BL.[16,17] Finally, most cases of DLBCL, including those with a high proliferation index, typically show absent staining in a visible subset of neoplastic cells with Ki-67 antibody, whereas virtually all tumor cells appear positive for Ki-67 in BL (**Table 2**).

If tissue is available for cytogenetic analysis, karyotypic findings in DLBCL may help to distinguish it from BL. Aberrations involving the *BCL6* locus at 3p27 are most common, and may be seen in up to 30% of cases, whereas an *IGH-BCL2* translocation or t(14;18) occurs in 20% to 30% of cases and often points to derivation from an underlying follicular lymphoma; the presence of either of these abnormalities would exclude a diagnosis of BL.[22] As mentioned previously, a *MYC* translocation, although characteristic of BL, may be seen in 5% to 15% of DLBCL.[14,20–22] In cases of DLBCL harboring a *MYC* rearrangement, karyotypic features that help to support a diagnosis of DLBCL over BL include the presence of additional structural or numerical abnormalities (at least 3 abnormalities in addition to the *MYC* translocation), *MYC* rearranged with a non-*IG* partner (often manifesting as additional unknown genetic material at 8q24 on the karyotype), and/or the presence of a *BCL6* or *BCL2* rearrangement in addition to the *MYC* rearrangement. If a karyotype is unavailable, FISH for *BCL6*, *BCL2,* and *MYC* rearrangements may be considered in morphologically and immunophenotypically ambiguous cases. If FISH shows evidence of a *BCL6* or *BCL2* rearrangement, the diagnosis of BL can be excluded regardless of *MYC* status (see **Table 2**). Cases with morphologic, immunophenotypic, or genetic features that appear to fall in a spectrum between BL and DLBCL may be more appropriately placed in the U-DLBCL/BL category (see later in this article).

B-lymphoblastic Leukemia/Lymphoma

B-lymphoblastic leukemia/lymphoma (B-LBL) is a neoplasm derived from precursor B cells (B lymphoblasts) and is typically composed of small to medium-sized cells with round, irregular, or convoluted nuclei, scant cytoplasm, dispersed chromatin, and absent or small, inconspicuous nucleoli. Occasional cases contain more abundant cytoplasm that may appear vacuolated or contain coarse azurophilic granules. Most patients present with bone marrow and blood involvement; however, occasionally primary presentation in lymph nodes or in extranodal sites may occur. In most circumstances, the morphologic characteristics of B-LBL (finely dispersed chromatin, nuclear convolutions and irregularities, inconspicuous to absent nucleoli) and clinical characteristics (usually primary leukemic presentation) are sufficient to distinguish it from BL (**Fig. 7A**). In some

Fig. 6. A case of DLBCL, NOS harboring concurrent *IGH-BCL2* and *MYC* rearrangements. (*A*) Some cells are medium in size, but most are larger with vesicular chromatin and conspicuous nuclear irregularities, including occasional multilobated forms (H&E, ×1000). (*B*) By immunohistochemistry, many nuclei show absent staining for Ki-67 (MIB1), with an overall proliferation index of about 60% (×400).

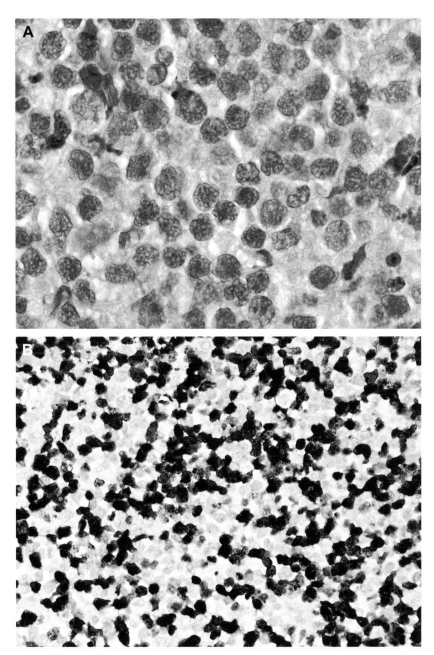

cases with overlapping morphologic and/or clinical features, immunohistochemistry or flow cytometry for markers of immaturity (CD34 and TdT) should be sufficient to exclude BL with certainty, as BL is a mature B-cell neoplasm that lacks expression of these precursor cell antigens (see **Fig. 7**B).[28] Finally, many cases of B-LBL exhibit characteristic cytogenetic abnormalities, such as hyperdiploid or hypodiploid karyotype, t(9;22), t(12;21), or *MLL* rearrangements, that are distinct from rearrangements involving *MYC* at 8q24.[29] Rare cases of B-LBL with *MYC* and *IGH-BCL2* gene rearrangements have been reported; the classification of such cases is controversial,

Table 2
Clinical and pathologic features distinguishing Burkitt lymphoma from other high-grade B-cell lymphomas

Characteristic	BL	U-DLBCL/BL	DLBCL, NOS
Clinical features	Child or young adult; male predominance Malaria exposure in endemic cases History of immunosuppression in some patients Often extranodal, including BM and CNS involvement	Middle-aged or older adult Prior history of FL in some cases Most cases not associated with immunosuppression Widespread extranodal disease common, including BM and CNS involvement	Variable age of presentation, but usually middle-aged or older adult Prior history of FL in some cases History of immunosuppression in some patients Nodal or extranodal disease, localized or advanced
Serum LDH Level	Usually elevated, but typically ≤3 times upper limit of normal	Very high (>3 times upper limit of normal)	Normal or elevated
Morphology	Starry-sky growth pattern with abundant mitoses and apoptotic figures Monomorphous small or medium-sized cells with round, regular nuclei and multiple small, paracentral nucleoli Cases with mild nuclear pleomorphism acceptable if all other immunophenotypic and genetic criteria met (see below)	Starry-sky growth pattern with abundant mitoses and apoptotic figures Monomorphous small or medium-sized cells with greater variation in nuclear size, nuclear contour or nucleolar prominence than seen in "classic" BL May have blastoid cytology Morphology may also resemble BL if immunophenotypic or genetic features exclude a diagnosis of BL	Uniformly large cells or mixture of small and large cells More polymorphous appearance, with variability of nuclear shape and chromatin quality
Proliferation Index (Ki-67 immunostaining)	>95% and homogeneous[a]	Usually <95% and heterogeneous[a]	Usually <95% and heterogeneous Rarely >95%[b]
Immunophenotype	Germinal center phenotype (strongly CD10+ and BCL6+) BCL2 negative or weakly expressed in rare cases[a] Rare to few cases are MUM1/IRF4+ Strong expression of sIg	Germinal center phenotype in most cases (CD10+, BCL6+) BCL2 strongly expressed in most cases, especially those with *IGH-BCL2* rearrangement Subset of cases are MUM1/IRF4+ sIg expression may be weak or absent	Subset of cases are CD10+ and/or BCL6+ Some cases are BCL2+ Subset of cases are MUM1/IRF4+ sIg expression may be weak or absent

	Most sporadic and immunodeficiency-associated cases are EBV− Most endemic cases are EBV+	No reported association with EBV infection	Certain cases are EBV+ (immunodeficiency-associated DLBCL and DLBCL of the elderly)
EBV association	Most sporadic and immunodeficiency-associated cases are EBV− Most endemic cases are EBV+	No reported association with EBV infection	Certain cases are EBV+ (immunodeficiency-associated DLBCL and DLBCL of the elderly)
Genetic features	MYC rearrangement detectable by FISH in 95% of cases No IGH-BCL2 or BCL6 rearrangement[a] MYC rearranged with an IG partner, typically IGH (14q32) Background karyotype simple with no or few (<3) additional cytogenetic abnormalities	MYC rearrangement common; if present, more likely to have non-IGH partner (either IGK, IGL, or unknown) Often concurrent MYC and IGH-BCL2 rearrangements or (less commonly) MYC and BCL6 rearrangements May rarely have IGH-BCL2 or BCL6 rearrangements without MYC rearrangement Background karyotype complex with >3 cytogenetic abnormalities	BCL6 translocation (30%) or IGH-BCL2 translocation (20%–30% of cases) common MYC translocation in 5%–15% of cases; may have non-IG partner[b] Complex karyotype with >3 cytogenetic abnormalities

Abbreviations: BL, Burkitt lymphoma; BM, bone marrow; CNS, central nervous system; DLBCL, NOS, diffuse large B-cell lymphoma, not otherwise specified; EBV, Epstein-Barr virus; FL, follicular lymphoma; LDH, lactate dehydrogenase; sIg, surface immunoglobulin; U-DLBCL/BL, B-cell lymphoma unclassifiable with features intermediate between DLBCL and BL.

[a] Strong BCL2 expression by immunohistochemistry, presence of IGH-BCL2 or BCL6 rearrangement, or Ki-67 <95% (under conditions of optimal immunohistochemical staining) are absolute contraindications to the diagnosis of BL.

[b] Cases of morphologically typical DLBCL with a MYC translocation or with a very high proliferation index by Ki-67 staining should be diagnosed as DLBCL, NOS and should not be included in the U-DLBCL/BL category.

Data from Refs.[17,23,47,65]

DIFFERENTIAL DIAGNOSIS OF BURKITT LYMPHOMA

CONSIDER A DIAGNOSIS OF U-DLBCL/BL IF

- Morphologic overlap with BL, but greater nuclear size variation, nuclear irregularity or nucleolar prominence than considered acceptable for classic BL[a]
- Blastoid cytologic features (small cells with dispersed chromatin and absent nucleoli)[a]
- BCL2-positive, MUM1/IRF4-positive, or Ki-67 less than 95%[a]
- Presence of *BCL2* and/or *BCL6* rearrangement in addition to *MYC* by karyotype or FISH
- If a karyotype is available, the presence of 3 or more structural or numeric aberrations in addition to *MYC* rearrangement or a non-IG *MYC* translocation partner

CONSIDER DIAGNOSIS OF DLBCL, NOS IF

- Uniformly large cells resembling typical centroblasts or immunoblasts
- High degree of nuclear size variability
- Nuclear irregularity or nucleolar prominence
- Presence of pleomorphic, bizarre-appearing cells

CONSIDER DIAGNOSIS OF B-LBL IF

- Blast-like cytologic features (small to medium-sized cells with dispersed chromatin, absent nucleoli, and round or lobulated nuclear contours)
- Immature precursor B-cell immunophenotype: CD191, but CD20-negative or weakly positive
- Surface light-chain-negative
- Presence of markers of immaturity (TdT and/or CD34)

CONSIDER DIAGNOSIS OF FLORID REACTIVE HYPERPLASIA AND SUGGEST RE-BIOPSY IF

- Limited or fragmented FNA or biopsy specimen containing starry-sky pattern which could represent floridly reactive germinal centers
- No clonal B-cell population demonstrated by flow cytometry or frozen section
- Immunohistochemistry
- No *MYC* rearrangement demonstrated by FISH

[a] Consider performing FISH for *MYC* and *BCL2* in these circumstances.

---

but some may be best categorized in the U-DLBCL/BL category (see next section).[17,23,30] However, if TdT or CD34 is expressed, the diagnosis of B-LBL may still be appropriate.[17,23]

B-cell Lymphoma, Unclassifiable, with Features Intermediate between Diffuse Large B-cell Lymphoma and Burkitt Lymphoma

The differential diagnosis between this group of recently defined cases and BL will be discussed in the next section.

PROGNOSIS

BL is a highly aggressive but potentially curable lymphoma. Importantly, it is not effectively treated by moderate intensity regimens typically used in DLBCL, such as CHOP-R (rituximab, cyclophosphamide, doxorubicin, vincristine, and prednisone) or CHOP-like regimens.[31] However, both adult and pediatric patients with BL can be cured by highly intensive chemotherapy containing high-dose methotrexate, ifosfamide, etoposide, and cytarabine, and more recently, rituximab, given in alternating

Fig. 7. A case of B lymphoblastic leukemia/lymphoma with concurrent rearrangements of *MYC* and *IGH-BCL2*. (*A*) The bone marrow aspirate contains numerous medium-sized blasts with finely dispersed chromatin, small nucleoli, and occasional cytoplasmic vacuoles (Wright-Giemsa, ×1000). (*B*) Flow cytometric analysis of peripheral blood leukemic cells shows CD19+, CD10+, TdT+ B lymphoblasts (*green population*). The cells were also CD45dim+ and negative for CD20 and surface light chain (not shown).

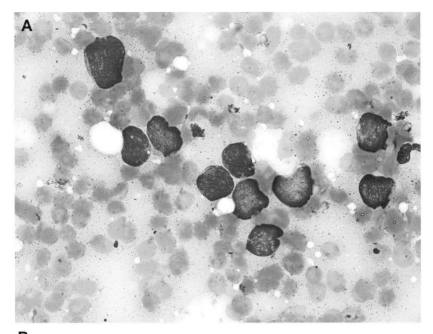

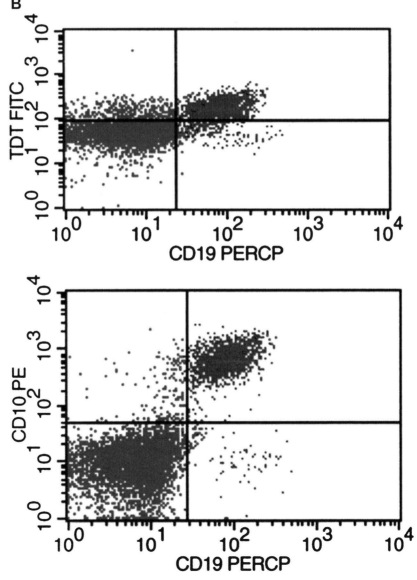

cycles with a CHOP-like regimen (CODOX/M-IVAC).[32–39] BL also requires the administration of intrathecal chemotherapy, as it carries a high risk of CNS relapse. Most patients with BL present with disseminated high-stage disease. The bone marrow is involved in 10% to 30% of cases of sporadic and immunodeficiency-associated BL.[12,40] BL has a superior prognosis when it is limited-stage and when it occurs in children rather than adults. In adults, risk factors include bone marrow and/or CNS involvement, elevated serum lactate dehydrogenase (LDH), older age, and unresected tumor size exceeding 10 cm.[2,41] In patients with a single site of disease and in children, the 5-year overall survival rate is 90% or more, but even in advanced stages and in patients with a leukemic presentation, the 5-year survival rate is at least 50% and may be as high as 80% with high-intensity treatment.[37,41–45] Recent studies suggest that the addition of rituximab (anti-CD20 monoclonal antibody therapy) to standard high-intensity regimens may lead to further benefit.[35,36,38,39] Relapse, if it occurs, is usually seen within the first year after diagnosis.[37] Despite its potential curability, many patients worldwide continue to die of BL, because of the high burden of disease in developing countries and the continued high rates of prevalence of *Plasmodium falciparum* malaria in these regions.[2,46]

B-CELL LYMPHOMA, UNCLASSIFIABLE, WITH FEATURES INTERMEDIATE BETWEEN DIFFUSE LARGE B-CELL LYMPHOMA AND BURKITT LYMPHOMA

BACKGROUND

In the 2008 WHO classification, this group of neoplasms (U-DLBCL/BL) is defined as aggressive lymphomas that share morphologic, immunophenotypic, and genetic features with both DLBCL and BL, but that should not be included in either of these categories due to their particular biologic and/or clinical reasons. Some cases categorized as "atypical" BL or "Burkitt-like" lymphoma in previous classification schemes may currently fit best in this category. In addition, cases of high-grade B-cell lymphoma with morphologic features resembling lymphoblasts but lacking expression of markers of immaturity or cases of transformed follicular lymphoma may be best classified in this category. This category therefore represents a heterogeneous group of tumors rather than a single entity and the WHO classification authors recommend that it be used to classify rare cases not meeting diagnostic criteria for either BL or

DLBCL, so that such cases may be identified and further studied.[23] As we develop better understanding of cases falling between the defined borders of DLBCL and BL, it is possible that more clearly defined entities will emerge and will be recognized in future classification systems; this would restrict the use of the U-DLBCL/BL category to only select cases or even allow for its eventual elimination.

CLINICAL FEATURES

The clinical features of U-DLBCL/BL are not well characterized and most reported information is from the subset of "double-hit" lymphoma cases bearing both *MYC* and *BCL2* rearrangements. These patients are middle-aged to older adults who present with advanced-stage disease and commonly have involvement of extranodal sites, including bone marrow and CNS.[17,47,48] The median LDH at the time of presentation is usually high, and has been found to be significantly higher when compared with BL and International Prognostic Index (IPI)-matched DLBCL control patients.[17,48,49] Some patients have a prior history of low-grade follicular lymphoma.

DIAGNOSIS: MICROSCOPIC FEATURES AND ANCILLARY STUDIES

Because of the heterogeneity of this diagnostic category, it is not possible to assign strict morphologic, immunophenotypic, or genetic definitions. U-DLBCL/BL cases are typically composed of a diffuse proliferation of small, medium-sized, or slightly larger lymphoid cells. On low magnification, some cases may contain numerous mitoses or apoptotic bodies and at higher magnification, the cells may closely resemble BL cells because of their relative monomorphism and small to medium size. In contrast, other cases may demonstrate greater variability in cell size, nuclear shape, or nucleolar prominence than is typically seen in classic BL.[23] Ultimately, most cases within the U-DLBCL/BL category have additional clinical, immunophenotypic, and/or genetic features that exclude a diagnosis of BL or that make it highly unlikely. Clinical and pathologic features that should prompt consideration of placement of a case of high-grade B-cell lymphoma within the intermediate U-DLBCL/BL category are summarized in **Table 2**.

Cases harboring concurrent *MYC* and *IGH-BCL2* and/or *BCL6* translocations, so-called "double-hit lymphomas," have emerged as a putative subgroup within the U-DLBCL/BL category.[17] Despite their variable morphology and immunophenotype, they appear to share highly aggressive clinical features.[15,17,30,47−56] In addition, gene expression profiling and comparative genomic hybridization studies suggest a molecular signature intermediate between DLBCL and BL, with significant alterations from pediatric and adult BL and DLBCL.[14,57] In patients with a prior history of follicular lymphoma, the double-hit lymphoma is presumed to represent transformation of the underlying follicular lymphoma harboring a t (14;18) with acquisition of a MYC translocation.[47,49,52,55,56,58−64] Importantly, the poor prognosis of cases of double-hit lymphoma (see below) underscores the need for pathologists and clinicians to identify these patients as having an aggressive high-grade B-cell neoplasm distinct from either BL or DLBCL.

In a recent study that applied the 2008 WHO classification to cases of MYC and IGH-BCL2 rearranged double-hit lymphomas, 12 (60%) of 20 cases were classified in the U-DLBCL/BL category. Among the remaining 8 cases, 7 were classified as DLBCL-NOS (35%) and 1 case was classified as B-LBL because of the patient's leukemic presentation and expression of TdT by the neoplastic cells (see **Figs. 6** and **7**).[17] Detailed examination of the 12 cases classified in the U-DLBCL/BL category allowed division of these cases into 3 subgroups: one group closely resembled BL, with conspicuous mitoses and apoptotic bodies, starry-sky pattern, and a monomorphous small to medium-sized cell population (**Fig. 8**); another showed some morphologic overlap with BL, but cell size was variable and a proportion of cells contained more irregular nuclei and more prominent nucleoli than classic BL (**Fig. 9**); in the third group, the cells were small with dispersed chromatin resembling lymphoblasts (**Fig. 10**).

Various studies have also outlined certain immunophenotypic features that help to distinguish cases of double-hit lymphoma from BL, including weak or negative expression of CD10, positivity for BCL2 or MUM1/IRF4, and/or Ki-67 proliferation index less than 95%.[16,17,47] Double-hit lymphoma cases with karyotypic analysis generally demonstrate a complex karyotype, a finding only rarely seen in BL (**Fig. 11**).[13,14,17,47,56,65] Among double-hit lymphoma cases, the MYC partner is frequently one of the light chain loci or an unidentified non-IG partner, while in BL the MYC partner is usually IGH or, less commonly, one of the light chain loci.[12−14,17,47,56,65]

Differential Diagnosis: An Algorithmic Approach

Based on the previously mentioned studies that have documented the clincopathologic spectrum of U-DLBCL/BL, we recommend consideration of the diagnosis of U-DLBCL/BL in the following circumstances:

1. High-grade B-cell lymphoma patients who present with advanced stage disease with extranodal or CNS involvement or with a serum lactate dehydrogenase (LDH) level exceeding 3 times the upper limit of normal.
2. Immunocompetent adult patients whose tumors have morphologic resemblance to BL, such as medium-sized cells with nuclear monomorphism, high mitotic rate, and abundant apoptotic debris (starry-sky growth pattern).
3. Lymphomas resembling BL morphologically but with an atypical immunophenotype, including strong positivity for BCL2, Ki-67 less than 95%, and/or MUM1/IRF4 positivity.
4. Patients with a history of low-grade follicular lymphoma (FL) who relapse with a high-grade B-cell neoplasm with unusual features for DLBCL (such as intermediate cell size or blastoid cytologic features).
5. Tumors resembling low-grade FL with unusual features, such as an entirely diffuse growth pattern (absent staining for follicular dendritic cell antigens), blastoid cytologic features, very high proliferation index by Ki-67 staining, starry-sky pattern, and/or necrosis.
6. Lymphomas resembling BL morphologically but with atypical genetic features, such as an IGH-BCL2 rearrangement or a BCL6 rearrangement (designated by some investigators as "double-hit" lymphomas), a non-IG MYC partner, or a complex karyotype (3 or more structural or numerical abnormalities in addition to MYC).

In scenarios 1 to 5, consideration should be given to performing FISH analysis for MYC, BCL6, and BCL2 translocations to confirm or exclude the possibility of double-hit lymphoma if fresh tissue is not available for full karyotypic analysis. An algorithmic approach to the diagnosis of diagnosis of BL and related high-grade B-cell neoplasms is outlined in **Fig. 12**.

PROGNOSIS

Unlike cases of BL, lymphomas classified in the U-DLBCL/BL category tend to have an aggressive clinical course and a poor prognosis, even with the administration of highly aggressive chemotherapy typically used to treat BL.[17,48,49,52,56] Evidence for the inferior clinical outcome in such patients may be inferred from studies of patients with MYC/IGH-BCL2 rearranged double-hit lymphomas, as many such cases are classified in the U-DLBCL/BL

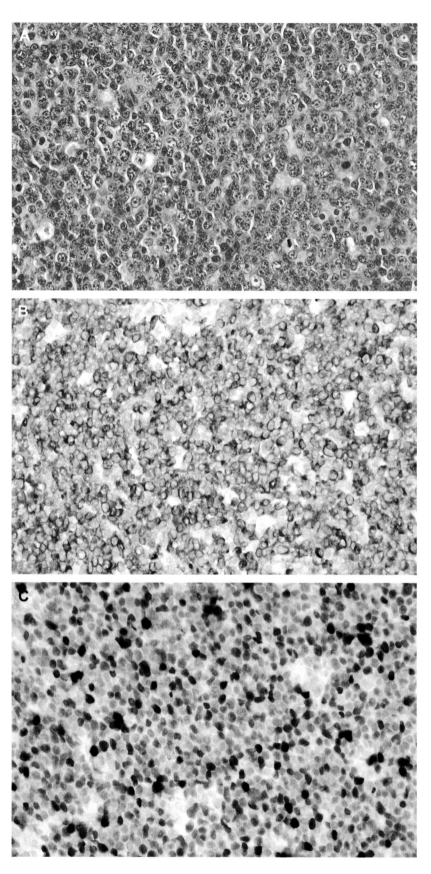

Fig. *8.* An example of U-DLBCL/BL with morphology resembling BL. (*A*) The morphologic features of this case are similar to BL, although some cells have single, relatively prominent nucleoli (H&E, ×400). (*B*) The diagnosis of BL is excluded on the basis of the immunohistochemical findings, as the tumor cells show strong staining for BCL2 (×400). (*C*) In addition, the neoplastic cells show positive staining for MUM1/IRF4, which would be unusual for BL (×400). Cytogenetic analysis revealed a complex karyotype with a t(14;18)(q32;q21) indicating a *IGH-BCL2* rearrangement in addition to a *MYC* rearrangement ("double-hit" lymphoma) (not shown).

Fig. 9. An example of U-DLBCL/BL with morphology intermediate between BL and DLBCL. (*A*) This subcutaneous mass shows some degree of morphologic overlap with BL; however, at high power (*B*), some cells exhibit a greater degree of nuclear irregularity and nucleolar prominence than typically seen in BL. The diagnosis of BL is excluded in this case on the basis of strong BCL2 expression by immunohistochemistry (*C*) and a complex karyotype containing a t(14;18) in addition to a t(8;22) (*IGL-MYC*) (not shown) (*A*: H&E, ×400; *B*: H&E, ×1000; *C*: ×400).

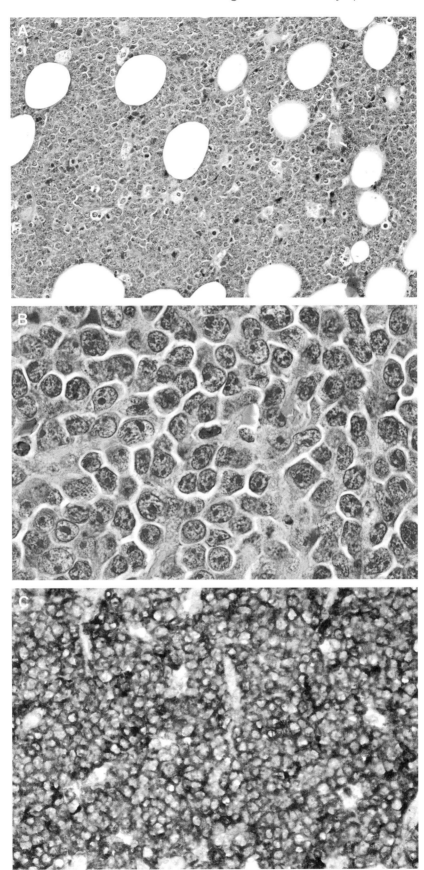

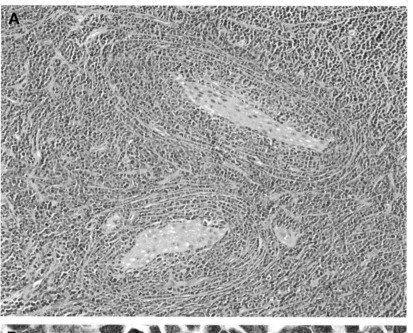

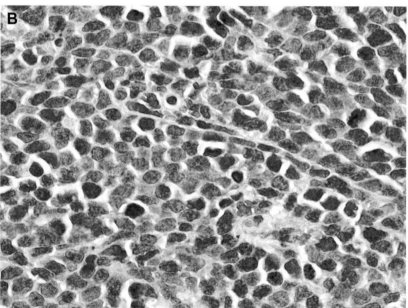

Fig. 10. Example of U-DLBCL/BL with blastoid morphology. (*A*) This patient presented with a testicular mass, with sheets of lymphoid cells infiltrating around the residual seminiferous tubules (H&E, ×200). (*B*) The cells are small to medium-sized with finely dispersed chromatin and absent nucleoli resembling lymphoblasts; the tumor cells were strongly positive for CD20, negative for TdT, expressed surface kappa light chain by flow cytometry, and had a *MYC* rearrangement as well as multiple copies of the *BCL2* gene demonstrated by FISH (not shown) (H&E, ×1000).

category.[17,56] In one prospective study, Mead and colleagues[54] demonstrated that 5 patients with double-hit lymphoma treated with a Burkitt-like regimen (CODOX/M-IVAC) had a median overall survival of less than 6 months, which was significantly inferior to that of BL patients treated with the same high-intensity regimen. In a retrospective study of 54 double-hit lymphoma patients, Johnson

and colleagues[56] showed that DLBCL morphology, low IPI score, absence of bone marrow involvement, a non-*IG MYC* translocation partner, and treatment with a rituximab-containing regimen were features associated with a significantly superior overall survival in univariate analyses. However, the overall survival was still poor, with nearly 60% of patients succumbing to disease within 6 months of

Fig. 11. Cytogenetic features of double-hit U-DBLCL/BL. (*A*) In contrast to the simple BL karyotype shown in **Fig. 4A**, this karyotype is highly complex with numerous structural and numeric aberrations (*arrows*), including a t(8;22)(q24;q11). (*B*) *MYC* rearrangement is confirmed by metaphase FISH, showing separation of the 5′ (*red*) and 3′ (*green*) *MYC* signals. (*C*) Metaphase FISH with a dual-color dual-fusion probe for *IGH-BCL2* demonstrates 2 red/green (*yellow*) fusion signals, indicative of a concurrent t(14;18) rearrangement.

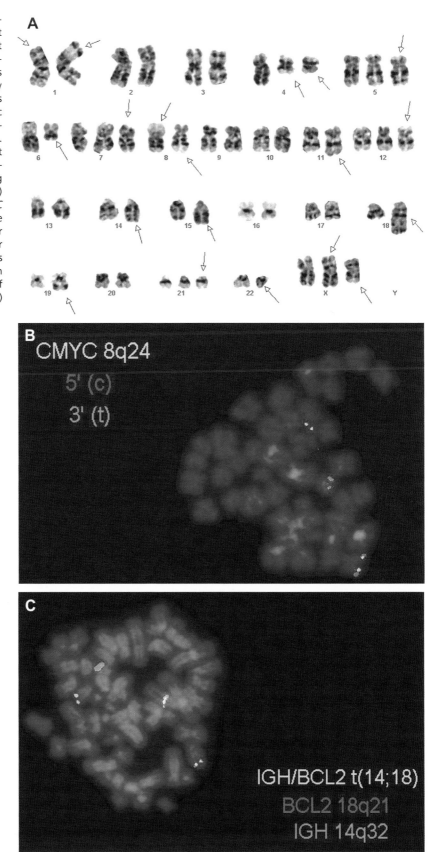

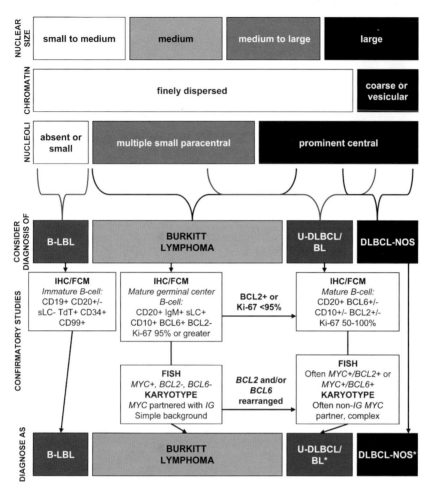

Fig. 12. An algorithmic approach to the diagnosis of BL and related high-grade B-cell neoplasms. *Abbreviations:* B-LBL, B lymphoblastic lymphoma; U-DLBCL/BL, B-cell lymphoma, unclassifiable, with features intermediate between diffuse large B-cell lymphoma and Burkitt lymphoma; DLBCL-NOS, diffuse large B-cell lymphoma, not otherwise specified; FCM, flow cytometry; IHC, immunohistochemistry; sLC, surface light chain. (*Data from* Refs.[21,22,67])

*Cases with concurrent *MYC* and *BCL2* and/or *BCL6* translocations are highly aggressive

diagnosis, irrespective of treatment regimen. In another retrospective study, Snuderl and colleagues[17] compared the clinical outcome of 20 cases of double-hit lymphoma to BL and IPI-matched DLBCL patients. Double-hit lymphoma patients had a significantly worse overall survival (median 4.5 months) in comparison with IPI-matched patients with DLBCL and BL, with 70% of patients dying within 8 months of diagnosis. DLBCL morphology was associated with superior overall survival in the double-hit lymphoma series of Johnson and colleagues.[56] Neither moderate-intensity regimens used to treat DLBCL nor high-intensity regimens used in BL have emerged as significantly associated with improved progression-free or overall survival in U-DLBCL/BL cases. The latter finding, in particular, highlights the challenges inherent in treating patients with U-

DLBCL/BL, as little prospective data for treatment of such patients exist and most of the retrospective data, as outlined previously, suggest that highly intensive chemotherapy successfully used in BL may not offer clear benefit in patients with U-DLBCL/BL.[17,54,66] Inclusion of CNS-directed therapy should be considered because of the high risk of CNS disease. In addition, inclusion of rituximab in multiagent chemotherapy regimens may offer some benefit.[17,56] Needless to say, additional prospective studies and the development of novel therapeutic approaches are required. Perhaps most importantly for the diagnostic pathologist, these findings underscore the need to distinguish double-hit lymphomas and U-DLBCL/BL cases from BL and DLBCL, as identification of such cases is a critical issue from both a prognostic and therapeutic standpoint (see **Fig. 12** and **Table 2**).[17,49,56]

PITFALLS IN BURKITT LYMPHOMA

BL should not be diagnosed if there is:

! Strong positivity for BCL2 by immunohistochemistry.

! Presence of *BCL2* or *BCL6* rearrangement in addition to *MYC*.

! Ki-67 proliferation index less than 95% under optimal staining conditions.

Question the diagnosis of BL and consider the possibility of U-DLBCL/BL or DLBCL, NOS in the following circumstances:

! Unusual clinical features, such as older age at diagnosis in absence of immunosuppression or a predominantly leukemic presentation.

! High degree of morphologic variability in terms of nuclear size, nuclear irregularity, or nucleolar prominence.

! Unusual immunohistochemical features, including weak positivity for BCL2, positivity for MUM1/IRF4, or negativity for BCL6 or CD10.

REFERENCES

1. Thorley-Lawson DA, Gross A. Persistence of the Epstein-Barr virus and the origins of associated lymphomas. N Engl J Med 2004;350:1328–37.

2. Leoncini L, Raphael M, Stein H, et al. Burkitt lymphoma. In: Swerdlow SH, Campo E, Harris NL, et al, editors. WHO classification of tumours of haematopoietic and lymphoid tissues. 4th edition. Lyon (France): IARC Press; 2008. p. 262–4.

3. Rochford R, Cannon MJ, Moormann AM. Endemic Burkitt's lymphoma: a polymicrobial disease? Nat Rev Microbiol 2005;3:182–7.

4. Bellan C, Lazzi S, Hummel M, et al. Immunoglobulin gene analysis reveals 2 distinct cells of origin for EBV-positive and EBV-negative Burkitt lymphomas. Blood 2005;106:1031–6.

5. Rainey JJ, Omenah D, Sumba PO, et al. Spatial clustering of endemic Burkitt's lymphoma in high-risk regions of Kenya. Int J Cancer 2007;120:121–7.

6. van den Bosch CA. Is endemic Burkitt's lymphoma an alliance between three infections and a tumour promoter? Lancet Oncol 2004;5:738–46.

7. Hamilton-Dutoit SJ, Raphael M, Audouin J, et al. In situ demonstration of Epstein-Barr virus small RNAs (EBER 1) in acquired immunodeficiency syndrome-related lymphomas: correlation with tumor morphology and primary site. Blood 1993;82: 619–24.

8. Raphael M, Gentilhomme O, Tulliez M, et al. Histopathologic features of high-grade non-Hodgkin's lymphomas in acquired immunodeficiency syndrome. The French Study Group of Pathology for Human Immunodeficiency Virus-Associated Tumors. Arch Pathol Lab Med 1991;115:15–20.

9. Lim ST, Karim R, Tulpule A, et al. Prognostic factors in HIV-related diffuse large-cell lymphoma: before versus after highly active antiretroviral therapy. J Clin Oncol 2005;23:8477–82.

10. Bellan C, De Falco G, Lazzi S, et al. Pathologic aspects of AIDS malignancies. Oncogene 2003;22: 6639–45.

11. Burmeister T, Schwartz S, Horst HA, et al. Molecular heterogeneity of sporadic adult Burkitt-type leukemia/lymphoma as revealed by PCR and cytogenetics: correlation with morphology, immunology and clinical features. Leukemia 2005;19:1391–8.

12. Hecht JL, Aster JC. Molecular biology of Burkitt's lymphoma. J Clin Oncol 2000;18:3707–21.

13. Dave SS, Fu K, Wright GW, et al. Molecular diagnosis of Burkitt's lymphoma. N Engl J Med 2006; 354:2431–42.

14. Hummel M, Bentink S, Berger H, et al. A biologic definition of Burkitt's lymphoma from transcriptional and genomic profiling. N Engl J Med 2006;354: 2419–30.

15. Cogliatti SB, Novak U, Henz S, et al. Diagnosis of Burkitt lymphoma in due time: a practical approach. Br J Haematol 2006;134:294–301.

16. Chuang SS, Ye H, Du MQ, et al. Histopathology and immunohistochemistry in distinguishing Burkitt lymphoma from diffuse large B-cell lymphoma with very high proliferation index and with or without a starry-sky pattern: a comparative study with EBER and FISH. Am J Clin Pathol 2007;128:558–64.

17. Snuderl M, Kolman OK, Chen YB, et al. B-cell lymphomas with concurrent IGH-BCL2 and MYC rearrangements are aggressive neoplasms with clinical and pathologic features distinct from Burkitt lymphoma and diffuse large B-cell lymphoma. Am J Surg Pathol 2010;34:327–40.

18. Rodig SJ, Vergilio JA, Shahsafaei A, et al. Characteristic expression patterns of TCL1, CD38, and CD44 identify aggressive lymphomas harboring a MYC translocation. Am J Surg Pathol 2008;32:113–22.

19. Dogan A, Bagdi E, Munson P, et al. CD10 and BCL-6 expression in paraffin sections of normal lymphoid tissue and B-cell lymphomas. Am J Surg Pathol 2000;24:846–52.

20. Boerma EG, Siebert R, Kluin PM, et al. Translocations involving 8q24 in Burkitt lymphoma and other malignant lymphomas: a historical review of cytogenetics in the light of today's knowledge. Leukemia 2009;23:225–34.

21. Kramer MH, Hermans J, Wijburg E, et al. Clinical relevance of BCL2, BCL6, and MYC rearrangements in diffuse large B-cell lymphoma. Blood 1998;92: 3152–62.

22. Abramson JS, Shipp MA. Advances in the biology and therapy of diffuse large B-cell lymphoma: moving toward a molecularly targeted approach. Blood 2005;106:1164–74.

23. Kluin PM, Harris NL, Stein H, et al. B-cell lymphoma, unclassifiable, with features intermediate between diffuse large B-cell lymphoma and Burkitt lymphoma. In: Swerdlow SH, Campo E, Harris NL, et al, editors. WHO classification of tumours of haematopoietic and lymphoid tissues. 4th edition. Lyon (France): IARC Press; 2008. p. 265–6.

24. Shiramizu B, Barriga F, Neequaye J, et al. Patterns of chromosomal breakpoint locations in Burkitt's lymphoma: relevance to geography and Epstein-Barr virus association. Blood 1991;77:1516–26.

25. Leucci E, Cocco M, Onnis A, et al. MYC translocation-negative classical Burkitt lymphoma cases: an alternative pathogenetic mechanism involving miRNA deregulation. J Pathol 2008;216: 440–50.

26. Ferry JA, Harris NL. Atlas of lymphoid hyperplasia and lymphoma. Philadelphia: W.B. Saunders Co; 1997.

27. Stein H, Warnke RA, Chan WC, et al. Diffuse large B-cell lymphoma, not otherwise specified. In: Swerdlow SH, Campo E, Harris NL, et al, editors. WHO classification of tumours of haematopoietic and lymphoid tissues. 4th edition. Lyon (France): IARC Press; 2008. p. 233–7.

28. Borowitz MJ, Chan JK. B lymphoblastic leukaemia/lymphoma, not otherwise specified. In: Swerdlow SH, Campo E, Harris NL, et al, editors. WHO classification of tumours of haematopoietic and lymphoid tissues. 4th edition. Lyon (France): IARC Press; 2008. p. 168–70.

29. Borowitz MJ, Chan JK. B lymphoblastic leukaemia/lymphoma with recurrent genetic abnormalities. In: Swerdlow SH, Campo E, Harris NL, et al, editors. WHO classification of tumours of haematopoietic and lymphoid tissues. 4th edition. Lyon (France): IARC Press; 2008. p. 171–5.

30. Stamatoullas A, Buchonnet G, Lepretre S, et al. De novo acute B cell leukemia/lymphoma with t(14;18). Leukemia 2000;14:1960–6.

31. Nomura Y, Karube K, Suzuki R, et al. High-grade mature B-cell lymphoma with Burkitt-like morphology: results of a clinicopathological study of 72 Japanese patients. Cancer Sci 2008;99: 246–52.

32. Magrath I, Adde M, Shad A, et al. Adults and children with small non-cleaved-cell lymphoma have a similar excellent outcome when treated with the same chemotherapy regimen. J Clin Oncol 1996; 14:925–34.

33. Mead GM, Sydes MR, Walewski J, et al. An international evaluation of CODOX-M and CODOX-M alternating with IVAC in adult Burkitt's lymphoma: results of United Kingdom Lymphoma Group LY06 study. Ann Oncol 2002;13:1264–74.

34. Lacasce A, Howard O, Lib S, et al. Modified Magrath regimens for adults with Burkitt and Burkitt-like lymphomas: preserved efficacy with decreased toxicity. Leuk Lymphoma 2004;45:761–7.

35. Barnes JA, Lacasce A, Feng Y, et al. Rituximab added to CODOX-M/IVAC has no clear benefit compared to CODOX-M/IVAC alone in adult patients with Burkitt lymphoma [abstract]. Blood 2009;114:665.

36. Li Y, Huang S, Wang X, et al. Rituximab combined with autologous peripheral blood stem cell transplantation improve therapeutic effects of chemotherapy in pediatric patients with Burkitt's lymphoma. J Trop Pediatr 2010;56:337–41.

37. Magrath IT, Janus C, Edwards BK, et al. An effective therapy for both undifferentiated (including Burkitt's) lymphomas and lymphoblastic lymphomas in children and young adults. Blood 1984;63:1102–11.

38. de Vries MJ, Veerman AJ, Zwaan CM. Rituximab in three children with relapsed/refractory B-cell acute lymphoblastic leukaemia/Burkitt non-Hodgkin's lymphoma. Br J Haematol 2004;125:414–5.

39. Thomas DA, Faderl S, O'Brien S, et al. Chemoimmunotherapy with hyper-CVAD plus rituximab for the treatment of adult Burkitt and Burkitt-type lymphoma or acute lymphoblastic leukemia. Cancer 2006;106: 1569–80.

40. Blum KA, Lozanski G, Byrd JC. Adult Burkitt leukemia and lymphoma. Blood 2004;104:3009–20.

41. Divine M, Casassus P, Koscielny S, et al. Burkitt lymphoma in adults: a prospective study of 72 patients treated with an adapted pediatric LMB protocol. Ann Oncol 2005;16:1928–35.

42. Cairo MS, Sposto R, Perkins SL, et al. Burkitt's and Burkitt-like lymphoma in children and adolescents: a review of the Children's Cancer Group experience. Br J Haematol 2003;120:660–70.

43. Patte C, Auperin A, Gerrard M, et al. Results of the randomized international FAB/LMB96 trial for intermediate risk B-cell non-Hodgkin lymphoma in children and adolescents: it is possible to reduce treatment for the early responding patients. Blood 2007;109:2773–80.

44. Soussain C, Patte C, Ostronoff M, et al. Small non-cleaved cell lymphoma and leukemia in adults. A retrospective study of 65 adults treated with the LMB pediatric protocols. Blood 1995;85:664–74.

45. Cairo MS, Gerrard M, Sposto R, et al. Results of a randomized international study of high-risk central nervous system B non-Hodgkin lymphoma and B

acute lymphoblastic leukemia in children and adolescents. Blood 2007;109:2736–43.

46. Harif M, Barsaoui S, Benchekroun S, et al. [Treatment of childhood cancer in Africa. Preliminary results of the French-African paediatric oncology group]. Arch Pediatr 2005;12:851–3 [in French].

47. Kanungo A, Medeiros LJ, Abruzzo LV, et al. Lymphoid neoplasms associated with concurrent t(14;18) and 8q24/c-MYC translocation generally have a poor prognosis. Mod Pathol 2006;19:25–33.

48. Niitsu N, Okamoto M, Miura I, et al. Clinical features and prognosis of de novo diffuse large B-cell lymphoma with t(14;18) and 8q24/c-MYC translocations. Leukemia 2009;23:777–83.

49. Le Gouill S, Talmant P, Touzeau C, et al. The clinical presentation and prognosis of diffuse large B-cell lymphoma with t(14;18) and 8q24/c-MYC rearrangement. Haematologica 2007;92:1335–42.

50. D'Achille P, Seymour JF, Campbell LJ. Translocation (14;18)(q32;q21) in acute lymphoblastic leukemia: a study of 12 cases and review of the literature. Cancer Genet Cytogenet 2006;171:52–6.

51. Haralambieva E, Boerma EJ, van Imhoff GW, et al. Clinical, immunophenotypic, and genetic analysis of adult lymphomas with morphologic features of Burkitt lymphoma. Am J Surg Pathol 2005;29:1086–94.

52. Macpherson N, Lesack D, Klasa R, et al. Small non-cleaved, non-Burkitt's (Burkitt-like) lymphoma: cytogenetics predict outcome and reflect clinical presentation. J Clin Oncol 1999;17:1558–67.

53. McClure RF, Remstein ED, Macon WR, et al. Adult B-cell lymphomas with Burkitt-like morphology are phenotypically and genotypically heterogeneous with aggressive clinical behavior. Am J Surg Pathol 2005;29:1652–60.

54. Mead GM, Barrans SL, Qian W, et al. A prospective clinicopathologic study of dose-modified CODOX-M/IVAC in patients with sporadic Burkitt lymphoma defined using cytogenetic and immunophenotypic criteria (MRC/NCRI LY10 trial). Blood 2008;112:2248–60.

55. Tomita N, Tokunaka M, Nakamura N, et al. Clinicopathological features of lymphoma/leukemia patients carrying both BCL2 and MYC translocations. Haematologica 2009;94:935–43.

56. Johnson NA, Savage KJ, Ludkovski O, et al. Lymphomas with concurrent BCL2 and MYC translocations: the critical factors associated with survival. Blood 2009;114:2273–9.

57. Salaverria I, Zettl A, Bea S, et al. Chromosomal alterations detected by comparative genomic hybridization in subgroups of gene expression-defined Burkitt's lymphoma. Haematologica 2008;93:1327–34.

58. De Jong D, Voetdijk BM, Beverstock GC, et al. Activation of the c-myc oncogene in a precursor-B-cell blast crisis of follicular lymphoma, presenting as composite lymphoma. N Engl J Med 1988;318:1373–8.

59. Gauwerky CE, Hoxie J, Nowell PC, et al. Pre-B-cell leukemia with a t(8;14) and a t(14;18) translocation is preceded by follicular lymphoma. Oncogene 1988;2:431–5.

60. Lee JT, Innes DJ Jr, Williams ME. Sequential bcl-2 and c-myc oncogene rearrangements associated with the clinical transformation of non-Hodgkin's lymphoma. J Clin Invest 1989;84:1454–9.

61. Thangavelu M, Olopade O, Beckman E, et al. Clinical, morphologic, and cytogenetic characteristics of patients with lymphoid malignancies characterized by both t(14;18)(q32;q21) and t(8;14)(q24;q32) or t(8;22)(q24;q11). Genes Chromosomes Cancer 1990;2:147–58.

62. Tomita N, Nakamura N, Kanamori H, et al. Atypical Burkitt lymphoma arising from follicular lymphoma: demonstration by polymerase chain reaction following laser capture microdissection and by fluorescence in situ hybridization on paraffin-embedded tissue sections. Am J Surg Pathol 2005;29:121–4.

63. Voorhees PM, Carder KA, Smith SV, et al. Follicular lymphoma with a Burkitt translocation—predictor of an aggressive clinical course: a case report and review of the literature. Arch Pathol Lab Med 2004;128:210–3.

64. Young KH, Xie Q, Zhou G, et al. Transformation of follicular lymphoma to precursor B-cell lymphoblastic lymphoma with c-myc gene rearrangement as a critical event. Am J Clin Pathol 2008;129:157–66.

65. Harris NL, Horning SJ. Burkitt's lymphoma—the message from microarrays. N Engl J Med 2006;354:2495–8.

66. Lin P, Medeiros LJ. High-grade B-cell lymphoma/leukemia associated with t(14;18) and 8q24/MYC rearrangement: a neoplasm of germinal center immunophenotype with poor prognosis. Haematologica 2007;92:1297–301.

67. Savage KJ, Johnson NA, Ben-Neriah S, et al. MYC gene rearrangements are associated with a poor prognosis in diffuse large B-cell lymphoma patients treated with R-CHOP chemotherapy. Blood 2009;114:3533–7.

UPDATE ON THE DIAGNOSIS AND CLASSIFICATION OF THE PLASMA CELL NEOPLASMS

Robert B. Lorsbach, MD, PhD

KEYWORDS

- Plasma cell • Myeloma • MGUS • Amyloidosis • M-protein • Plasmacytoma
- Plasma cell dyscrasia

ABSTRACT

The plasma cell neoplasms are malignancies of the most terminally differentiated cells in B-cell ontogeny and are usually associated with the production of a monoclonal immunoglobulin molecule or M protein. These malignancies include tumors whose clinical manifestations are directly attributable to the end-organ damage induced by the dysregulated proliferation of neoplastic plasma cells. In contrast, disorders, such as primary amyloidosis, have a paradoxically low burden of neoplastic plasma cells, rendered highly pathogenic by the end-organ damage induced by deposition of the secreted paraprotein. In this article, discussion focuses on plasma cell myeloma. The molecular pathogenesis of plasma cell myeloma is reviewed and the diagnosis of the plasma cell neoplasms discussed.

OVERVIEW

Plasma cell myeloma (PCM) is derived from a post-germinal B-cell, which has undergone productive immunoglobulin (Ig) heavy chain class switching and somatic hypermutation. In most if not all instances, PCM derives from a precursor state, so-called monoclonal gammopathy of undetermined significance (MGUS).[1,2] Extensive cytogenetic and molecular characterization has identified two major groups of PCM: those

containing primarily numerical chromosomal abnormalities, so-called hyperdiploid PCM, and those myelomas harboring chromosomal translocations targeting the Ig heavy chain locus located at chromosome 14q32 (**Table 1**).[3,4] These two groups are not absolutely mutually exclusive, however, because hyperdiploid PCM may contain Ig chromosomal translocations.

The classification and diagnostic criteria for the plasma cell (PC) neoplasms have been revised as part of the updated World Health Organization (WHO) classification of hematolymphoid malignancies (**Table 2**).[5] The major and minor criteria for the diagnosis of symptomatic PCM have been eliminated, and the criteria refined to require the presence of a clonal plasma cell population with no minimum level specified (**Table 3**). The rationale for this is that a significant minority of patients with unequivocal symptomatic myeloma, based on clinical and radiologic findings, have fewer than 30% PCs in random iliac crest bone marrow samples.

IMMUNOPHENOTYPIC EVALUATION OF NORMAL AND NEOPLASTIC PLASMA CELLS

Normal PCs retain the expression of some B-cell–associated markers, including CD19 and CD79a as well as CD45 (leukocyte common antigen).[6] The expression of most B-cell antigens, however, including that of CD20, CD22, CD24, and

Department of Pathology, University of Arkansas for Medical Sciences, 4301 West Markham Street, Mail Slot 517, Little Rock, AR 72205, USA
E-mail address: rlorsbach@uams.edu

Surgical Pathology 3 (2010) 1061–1089
doi:10.1016/j.path.2010.09.005

Table 1
Most frequent primary chromosomal translocations targeting chromosome 14q32 in plasma cell myeloma

Translocation	Frequency (%)	Target Gene
t(11;14)(q13;q32)	15	CCND1
t(6;14)(p21;q32)	3	CCND3
t(4;14)(p16;q32)	15	MMSET, FGFR3
t(14;16)(q32;q23)	5	C-MAF
t(14;20)(q23;q11)	2	MAFB

PAX5, is down-regulated on plasmacytic differentiation, with the commensurate up-regulation of several PC-associated antigens (**Fig. 1**).[7] Those most commonly used for immunophenotypic analysis include CD138, CD38, VS38c, MUM1/IRF4, and the Ig heavy and light chains.[8–11] CD38 and CD138 can be used to identify PCs by flow cytometry (FC), because they are expressed at significantly higher levels in PCs than in mature B cells.

Diagnostic immunohistochemistry (IHC) of PC neoplasms exploits the fact that malignant PCs retain many of the immunophenotypic characteristics of their normal counterparts. The most widely used plasmacytic marker is CD138, whose expression within the hematolymphoid system is normally restricted to PCs. CD138 is strongly expressed in virtually all PCMs.[12–14] In addition to supporting a PC lineage, CD138 IHC permits more accurate assessment of the extent of myelomatous involvement than can be obtained by morphologic evaluation alone.[15,16] CD138 is also expressed in other lymphoid malignancies with

Table 2
WHO classification of plasma cell neoplasms

Plasma cell myeloma	Symptomatic myeloma Asymptomatic myeloma Nonsecretory myeloma Plasma cell leukemia
Plasmacytoma	Solitary osseous plasmacytoma Extramedullary plasmacytoma
Immunoglobulin deposition diseases	Primary amyloidosis Systemic light and heavy chain deposition diseases
Osteosclerotic myeloma (POEMS syndrome)	

plasmacytic differentiation, however, including lymphoplasmacytic lymphoma, marginal zone lymphomas, and plasmablastic lymphoma as well as variants of diffuse large B-cell lymphoma (DLBCL) manifesting plasmacytic differentiation[12–14,17]; CD138 is also weakly expressed in some cases of classical Hodgkin lymphoma.[13,14] CD138 is expressed by most normal epithelia and by a high fraction of pulmonary, gastrointestinal, genitourinary, and breast carcinomas.[18,19] Thus, CD138 immunoreactivity of a tumor should be interpreted with caution when evaluating poorly differentiated plasmacytoid neoplasms at extramedullary sites.

The transcription factor, MUM1/IRF4, is highly expressed in nearly all PCMs, where it seems to play a critical pathogenetic role.[11,20] MUM1/IRF4 is normally expressed in PCs and a subset of germinal center B-cells. In contrast to CD138, MUM1/IRF4 is more broadly expressed in lymphoid neoplasia, being expressed at varying frequencies in several subtypes of B- and T-lineage lymphoma as well as in the Reed-Sternberg cells of classical Hodgkin lymphoma.[11,21] MUM1/IRF4 IHC has diagnostic usefulness where the differential diagnosis includes carcinoma and anaplastic myeloma, because MUM1/IRF4 is not expressed in epithelial malignancies, in contrast to CD138.[21] The antibody VS38c recognizes p63, which is strongly expressed by normal PCs as well as osteoblasts.[10,22,23] VS38c is strongly positive in essentially all PCMs, plasmacytomas, and lymphoplasmacytic lymphomas, and is either negative or only weakly positive in other B-cell lymphomas.[10] Although VS38c antigen expression in nonhematolymphoid malignancies has not been well characterized, more than 90% of melanomas are VS38c positive.[24]

Evaluation of Ig expression to establish clonality is critical in the pathologic evaluation of PC neoplasms. Assessment of light chain expression using IHC can often be problematic due to high background imparted by ambient serum Ig levels. The use of a chromogenic in situ hybridization (ISH) assay to assess Ig light chain expression largely circumvents these technical problems.[25] Cyclin D1 is overexpressed in approximately 20% of PCM. Cyclin D1 positivity can be particularly helpful in distinction of PCM from low-grade lymphomas with plasmacytic differentiation. This can sometimes be diagnostically challenging, especially with small lymphocyte-like PCM, which is often cyclin D1 positive due to the frequent presence of the t(11;14).

FC provides an alternative and often complementary approach to the immunophenotypic evaluation of PC neoplasia (**Fig. 2**). With improvements

Table 3
WHO diagnostic criteria for plasma cell myeloma

Monoclonal gammopathy of undetermined significance	Serum M protein present, <30 g/L Bone marrow: • Clonal plasma cells comprising <10% of nucleated cells in aspirate • Interstitial infiltration pattern present in biopsy No lytic bone lesions No myeloma-related end-organ injury or impairment[a] No evidence of other B-cell lymphoproliferative disorder
Plasma cell myeloma	*Symptomatic* • Serum or urine M protein present • Presence of either clonal plasma cells in bone marrow or plasmacytoma • Myeloma-related end organ injury or impairment[a] *Asymptomatic* • Serum M protein present, >30 g/L and/or • Presence of clonal plasma cells in bone marrow, >10% of nucleated cells • No myeloma-related end-organ injury or impairment[a]
Plasma cell leukemia[b]	• Presence of clonal plasma cells in peripheral blood, >2 × 10⁹/L or >20% of leukocytes

[a] End-organ damage due directly to either destructive activity of the neoplastic plasma cells (eg, lytic bone lesions, hypercalcemia, anemia) or indirectly secondary to deposition of or damage induced by the M protein (eg, hypercalcemia, renal insufficiency, or anemia).
[b] Plasma cell leukemia is considered primary if present at initial diagnosis; secondary plasma cell leukemia develops during subsequent disease evolution.

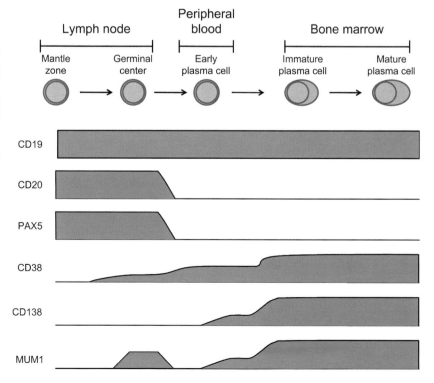

Fig. 1. Kinetics of cell surface antigen and transcription factor expression during B-cell development. With the onset of plasma cell differentiation, the expression of several transcription factors is induced commensurate with the down-regulation of several B-cell–associated transcription factors and cell surface markers.

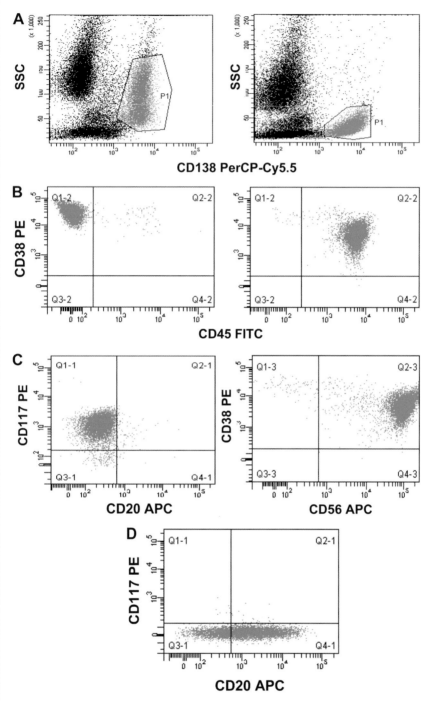

Fig. 2. FC analysis of PCM. (*A*) PC neoplasms often manifest heterogenous light scatter properties, due to variable quantities of cytoplasm and coexistence of cytoplasmic vacuoles and inclusions, which should be taken into account when setting analysis gates. (*B*) Most PCM cases are negative or only weakly positive for CD45 (*left panel*), but occasional cases show strong CD45 expression mimicking that seen in lymphomas (*right panel*). (*C*) Many PCM cases express CD117 and/or CD56. (*D*) A subset of PCM cases express CD20, which is typically weak or heterogenous in contrast to the uniformly bright expression characteristic of most B-cell lymphomas.

in instrumentation and reagents, six-color FC assays for PC neoplasms are currently used in many laboratories.[26,27] FC often underestimates the level of tumor involvement when compared with morphologic assessment, due to hemodilution or under-representation of PCs in the single cell suspensions required for FC analysis.[28,29] In addition, PCs seem to be more mechanically fragile than other hematopoietic cells and as a result may be preferentially lost during red cell lysis and other processing steps required for FC.

Using FC, several diagnostically useful immunophenotypic differences can be exploited to distinguish between neoplastic PCs and their benign counterparts. For example, in contrast to normal PCs, myeloma cells are CD19 negative in more than 95% of cases and are frequently either negative or express an aberrantly low level of CD45 (see **Fig. 2**B).[27,30,31] CD117 (c-KIT), which is expressed in hematopoietic progenitors and in many acute myeloid leukemias (AMLs), is also expressed in 30% to 40% of PCMs, whereas normal PCs are negative for this marker (see **Fig. 2**C).[30,32–34] CD56, or N-CAM, is aberrantly expressed in 60% to 88% of PCM, where its expression is typically bright and uniform (see **Fig. 2**C).[30,34–38] Given its normal role in mediating homotypic adhesion in neurons and other cell types, it is not surprising that PCMs with reduced expression of CD56 are associated with higher levels of peripherally circulating PCs.[39] The pan-B-cell marker CD20, whose expression is normally extinguished with commitment to plasmacytic differentiation, is expressed in 10% to 17% of myelomas.[30,38] The frequency of CD20 positivity is significantly higher in PCMs harboring the t(11;14).[40–42] The expression of CD20 in myeloma is typically heterogeneous or weak (see **Fig. 2**D), in contrast to the strong, uniform expression that characterizes most B-cell lymphomas; this variable weak expression of CD20 likely accounts for the modest antimyeloma effect of rituximab therapy.[43,44]

The aberrant over- or underexpression of a host of other cell surface markers in PCM has been described, including CD27, CD28, CD33, CD81, CD126, and CD221.[45] The aberrant expression of several myeloid markers (eg, CD13, CD33, and CD15) in a small subset of PCM is notable, because this could lead to an erroneous diagnosis of AML.[46,47] Although not expressed on normal PCs, the costimulatory receptor CD28 is expressed in approximately 30% of PCM, and the frequency of its expression increases with disease progression.[48,49]

In addition to confirming the plasmacytic differentiation and clonality in PC neoplasia, FC is diagnostically useful in distinguishing PC neoplasms from low-grade B-cell lymphomas with plasmacytic differentiation. The latter are characterized by the presence of a mature, surface light chain-restricted B-cell component, which may be difficult to identify using immunohistochemical approaches, particularly in cases with marked plasmacytic differentiation. In this setting, FC can readily permit characterization of both the PC and mature B-cell components. Furthermore, plasmacytic cells in low-grade B-cell lymphomas usually express CD19, whereas PCM is almost always negative for this marker.[50,51] In addition, myeloma tends to be negative for CD45 and expresses CD56 in a high fraction of cases, in contrast to lymphomas with plasmacytic differentiation, which are CD45+ and generally CD56−.[50]

GENERAL APPROACH TO THE DIAGNOSIS OF PLASMA CELL MYELOMA

The pathologic diagnosis of bone marrow involvement by a PC neoplasm is straightforward in most instances. Evaluation of the marrow should include an assessment of the extent of bone marrow involvement as well as confirmation of the clonality of the PC infiltrate. The pathologic reporting should also take into account the biologic peculiarities of PCM. Marrow involvement by PCM is notoriously heterogeneous and may be localized, similar to that of metastatic nonhematolymphoid malignancies. Thus, patients with PCM not infrequently have a negative random iliac crest bone marrow examination. Conversely, in involved marrows, the pathologist may have no access to clinical or radiologic data to determine whether or not there is disseminated involvement. In such cases, rendering a diagnosis of PC neoplasm is appropriate, with inclusion of a comment indicating that the bone marrow findings must be interpreted in the context of the clinical, laboratory, and radiologic data. Similarly, in directed bone biopsies of osseous lesions, it may be impossible on a pathologic basis alone to ascertain whether or not such a lesion represents a solitary plasmacytoma or a manifestation of systemic disease. Thus, the final, definitive classification of every PC neoplasm requires thorough clinical-pathologic correlation.

Several different myeloma grading schemes have been developed, most of which rely on assessment of the relative number of myeloma cells with plasmablastic or other high-grade cytologic features. Despite significant variations in the grading criteria of each of these schemes, most have shown a clear correlation between myeloma grade and clinical prognosis.[52–58] Nearly all of these grading systems, however, predate the advent of newer antimyeloma therapies (eg, thalidomide, bortezomib, and autologous stem cell transplantation); thus, their current relevance to clinical outcome is largely unknown. Using the criteria of Bartl,[52] in the author's experience, high-grade myelomas frequently yield complex karyotypes with genetic lesions associated with poor clinical prognosis, suggesting that grading may still have some clinical relevance.

MONOCLONAL GAMMOPATHY OF UNDETERMINED SIGNIFICANCE

CLINICAL FEATURES

Monoclonal gammopathy of undetermined significance (MGUS) is defined clinically by the presence of a serum monoclonal paraprotein and low-level bone marrow plasmacytosis (see **Table 3**). Nearly all cases of PCM are believed to evolve from an underlying MGUS.[1,2] The incidence of MGUS is 3% in individuals older than 50 years, and the incidence of both MGUS and PCM increases with advancing age.[59] The frequency of MGUS and myeloma is significantly influenced by ethnicity, with higher and lower rates of these disorders in individuals of African American and Asian ancestry, respectively, when compared with white patients.[60,61]

DIAGNOSIS: MICROSCOPIC FEATURES AND ANCILLARY STUDIES

Monoclonal gammopathy of undetermined significance (MGUS) is characterized by an interstitial infiltrate of PCs in the bone marrow without effacement of normal bone marrow architecture. By definition, PCs comprise fewer than 10% of nucleated cells in the marrow. In MGUS, PCs may be localized in a purely interstitial pattern or may show perivascular tropism, similar to normal PCs. Cytologically, the PCs usually have a mature morphology with clumped chromatin and ample basophilic cytoplasm, although scattered nucleolated forms may be present. The bone marrow PCs in MGUS usually demonstrate light chain restriction by either IHC, ISH, or FC.

DIFFERENTIAL DIAGNOSIS

MGUS should be distinguished from reactive plasmacytoses, which are frequently encountered and may be due to a wide array of etiologies (**Table 4**). Demonstration of light chain restriction distinguishes MGUS from reactive plasmacytoses. Distinction of MGUS from PCM is often not possible on the basis of the findings of a bone marrow

| **Table 4** |
| **Causes of reactive bone marrow plasmacytosis** |
| HIV/AIDS |
| Inflammatory disorders (eg, sarcoidosis) |
| Autoimmune disorders (eg, rheumatoid arthritis and systemic lupus erythematosus) |
| Hypersensitivity reactions (eg, drug induced) |
| Hemophagocytic syndrome |
| Castleman disease |
| Aplastic anemia |
| Postchemotherapy (plasmacytosis may be relative) |
| Non-plasma cell malignancy (eg, Hodgkin lymphoma, angioimmunoblastic T-cell lymphoma, carcinomas) |

examination alone. In some patients with so-called macrofocal PCM, the growth of neoplastic PCs is predominantly confined to focal lesions with very low-level involvement of the intervening marrow. In a nondirected bone marrow biopsy and aspirate sampling this intervening marrow, the findings may be indistinguishable from the low-level plasmacytosis seen in MGUS. Cytologically atypical PCs (ie, those with prominent nucleoli or with plasmablastic or anaplastic features) are infrequently seen in MGUS and are a helpful clue to the diagnosis of PCM in such cases.

In those occasional instances where there is a coexisting MGUS and marrow lymphocytosis, a concurrent low-grade B-cell lymphoma with plasmacytic differentiation (such as chronic lymphocytic leukemia with plasmacytic differentiation, lymphoplasmacytic lymphoma, or marginal zone lymphomas) must be considered; the diagnostic approach in this setting is discussed later.

PROGNOSIS

MGUS is considered a precursor condition to virtually all PCMs. The rate of progression of MGUS to PCM, however, is low (approximately 1% annually).[62]

PLASMA CELL MYELOMA, INCLUDING PLASMA CELL LEUKEMIA

CLINICAL FEATURES

Plasma cell myeloma (PCM) is one of the most common hematologic malignancies, with an estimated 20,000 newly diagnosed patients and approximately 10,000 deaths in 2009 in the United States.[63] PCM originates from antecedent MGUS

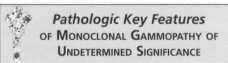

Pathologic Key Features
OF MONOCLONAL GAMMOPATHY OF UNDETERMINED SIGNIFICANCE

- Low-level, interstitial pattern of bone marrow involvement without effacement of marrow architecture
- Usually mature PC cytology

Pathologic Key Features
OF PLASMA CELL MYELOMA

- Neoplasm derived from a post-germinal center B cell

- Pattern of bone marrow involvement may be interstitial, focal, or obliterative

- Neoplastic cells manifest wide range of cytologic features, including mature, small lymphocyte-like, plasmablastic and anaplastic types

- Typical immunophenotype is CD138+, CD38+, CD56+/−, CD117−/+, CD19−

- Genetic features include hyperdiploidy with gains of odd-numbered chromosomes or translocations involving the *IGH* locus (see Table 1)

in virtually all cases. Plasma cell leukemia (PCL) is recognized as a variant form of PCM in the WHO classification (see **Table 3**). Primary PCL is uncommon, occurring in fewer than 5% of patients with PCM; secondary PCL most often develops during late stages of disease in patients with disseminated myeloma. PCL is more commonly associated with light chain only, IgD, or IgE paraprotein synthesis.

DIAGNOSIS: GROSS AND MICROSCOPIC FEATURES AND ANCILLARY STUDIES

The bony lesions of PCM often manifest grossly evident osseous destruction. Myelomatous involvement in the form of a gray, fleshy mass may be apparent on gross examination of affected bones.[64] With the advent of sophisticated radiologic imaging techniques, such as positron emission tomography, as well as more effective therapies, the gross pathology of myelomatous lesions is only rarely encountered by pathologists.

In the bone marrow biopsy, the degree of marrow involvement varies widely in PCM, ranging from a low-level interstitial infiltration to a diffuse obliterative effacement of the marrow with a commensurate reduction in normal hematopoiesis. The cytologic spectrum in PCM is comparably broad. Although most cases have cytologic features resembling normal mature PCs (so-called Marschalko morphology), small lymphocyte-like myelomas comprised of small PCs with scant cytoplasm are not infrequently encountered (**Fig. 3**). Higher-grade myelomas are characterized by blastic or anaplastic cytologic features (**Fig. 4**).

In such high-grade tumors, the neoplastic cells are often significantly larger than normal PCs, may be multinucleated or have multilobated nuclei, frequently have prominent nucleoli, and often manifest increased mitotic activity. Plasmablastic myeloma is characterized by large neoplastic cells with relatively scant cytoplasm and often prominent central nucleoli; in the aspirate, these may resemble other hematolymphoid neoplasms, such as AML or DLBCL (see **Fig. 4**). Necrosis is uncommon in PCM, even those with high-grade morphology.

Plasma cell leukemia can occur either as a primary disease manifestation or as a phase of progression in conventional PCM. Although such secondary PCLs usually do not pose a diagnostic dilemma, primary PCL can be diagnostically more challenging, particularly in the absence of other clinical information. Morphologically recognizable circulating myeloma cells are present in most cases; however, in some instances the neoplastic cells possess scant cytoplasm and thus may not be recognized as PCs. On occasion, circulating tumor cells may be dysplastic and can closely resemble large cell lymphoma cells or myeloblasts (**Fig. 5**). PCL shares many immunophenotypic similarities with PCM, although there are a few notable differences. In comparison with PCM, PCL is more likely to be negative for CD56 and CD117 and more frequently expresses CD20.[65] The latter finding is compatible with the observation that a high fraction of primary PCL harbors the t(11;14), which is also associated with CD20 expression.[66]

DIFFERENTIAL DIAGNOSIS

Because of its cytologic features as well as its frequent coexpression of CD20, small lymphocyte-like PCM may be confused with a B-cell lymphoma with plasmacytic differentiation, in particular, lymphoplasmacytic lymphoma (see **Fig. 3**). In contrast to B-cell lymphoma, the neoplastic cells in this myeloma subtype uniformly express CD138 and lack surface light chain expression. In addition, by virtue of the strong association with the t(11;14), small lymphocyte-like PCM is usually cyclin D1 positive, in contrast to other B-cell lymphomas with plasmacytic differentiation. Fortunately, mantle cell lymphoma and hairy cell leukemia, two B-cell lymphomas that express cyclin D1, do not show plasmacytic differentiation and thus do not usually enter into the differential diagnosis. Because PCM with the t(11;14) can rarely present in extramedullary sites, cyclin D1 IHC should be performed in unusual cases.

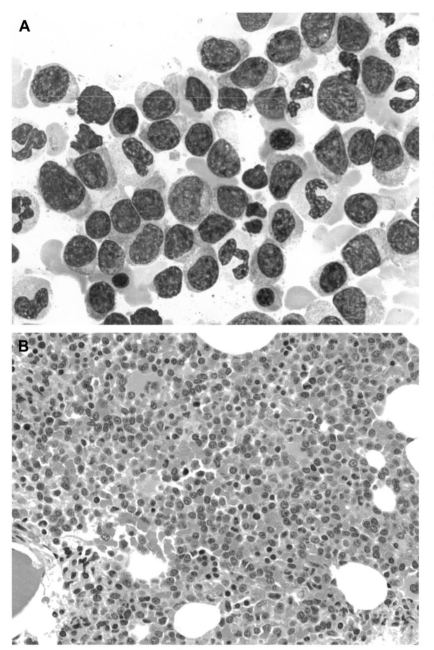

Fig. 3. PCM with small lymphocyte-like morphology. (*A*) In the bone marrow aspirate, the malignant PCs include many forms with relatively scant cytoplasm resembling a low-grade lymphoma. (*B*) The accompanying biopsy shows an interstitial infiltrate of lymphoid-appearing cells. FISH study confirmed the presence of the t(11;14) involving the *CCND1* locus (not shown).

Cases of PCM with blastic or anaplastic morphology may be morphologically indistinguishable from other malignancies, most notably DLBCL, plasmablastic lymphoma, AML, and, less commonly, metastatic carcinoma. This differential can be readily resolved in most instances by thorough immunophenotyping (**Fig. 6**).

Plasmablastic lymphoma may occasionally be associated with extensive bone marrow involvement. Because of the significant degree of morphologic and immunophenotypic overlap, distinction of this lymphoma subtype from plasmablastic myeloma can be difficult.[67] Epstein-Barr virus (EBV) positivity of the neoplastic cells,

Fig. 4. High-grade PCM. The marrow biopsy (*A*) and aspirate (*B*) are effaced by an infiltrate of neoplastic cells with plasmablastic morphology. Cytogenetics revealed a complex karyotype, with several abnormalities associated with an adverse prognosis, including mono-somy 13 and del(1p) (not shown). (*C*) PCM case with frequent large anaplastic myeloma cells.

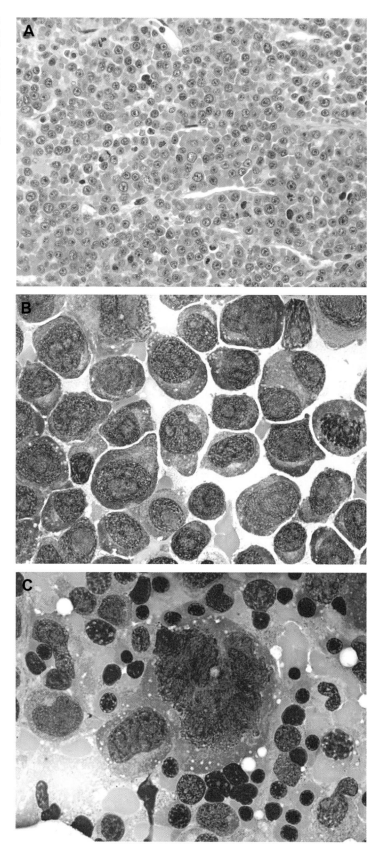

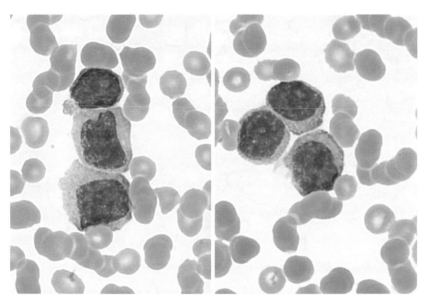

Fig. 5. PC leukemia. In the peripheral blood, circulating myeloma cells may be confused with monocytic cells, circulating large cell lymphoma cells or myeloid blasts, particularly in cases of plasmablastic morphology. (*Courtesy of* Marwan Yared, MD, Department of Pathology, University of Arkansas for Medical Sciences, Little Rock, AR.)

as assessed by EBV-encoded RNA ISH, strongly favors a diagnosis of plasmablastic lymphoma. In this setting, correlation with clinical findings, in particular, evaluation of the patient's HIV status, is helpful for appropriate diagnosis. A minority of PCMs have associated reticulin fibrosis, which may render an aspirate difficult or impossible to obtain and potentially mimicking primary myelofibrosis. Finally, PCMs with associated fibrosis and osteosclerosis are rarely encountered and may be a component of POEMS syndrome (*p*olyneuropathy, *o*rganomegaly, *e*ndocrinopathy, *m*onoclonal gammopathy, and *s*kin changes). This rare clinical

△△ *Differential Diagnosis*
PLASMA CELL MYELOMA INVOLVING THE BONE MARROW

Plasma Cell Myeloma Versus	Distinguishing Features
Monoclonal gammopathy of undetermined significance	• Light chain-restricted PCs but does not fulfill criteria for PCM • Lacks cytologically atypical PCs
Reactive bone marrow plasmacytosis[a]	• PCs are polyclonal
Lymphoplasmacytic lymphoma	• Presence of clonal B-cell component with surface light chain expression • Vast majority express IgM heavy chain (vs only 1% of PCM) • Cyclin D1 negative • CD138 only expressed in subset of neoplastic cells (vs uniform positivity in PCM)
Plasmablastic lymphoma	• EBV positive • Most affected patients are HIV+
Primary myelofibrosis	• Lacks light chain–restricted PCs
Metastatic malignancy	• Tumor cells are negative for light chains and MUM1/IRF4 and are usually CD138 negative[b]
Solitary osseous plasmacytoma	• Absence of clinical, laboratory, or radiologic evidence of disseminated disease

[a] Causes of reactive bone marrow plasmacytosis are listed in **Table 4**.
[b] Epithelial malignancies may express CD138.

Fig. 6. Lymphoma mimicking a high-grade PCM. (*A*) Biopsy of a large destructive iliac mass reveals an infiltrate of large neoplastic cells. By IHC, the tumor cells were weakly, focally CD138 positive (*B*), leading to an erroneous diagnosis of anaplastic PCM by the referring pathologist.

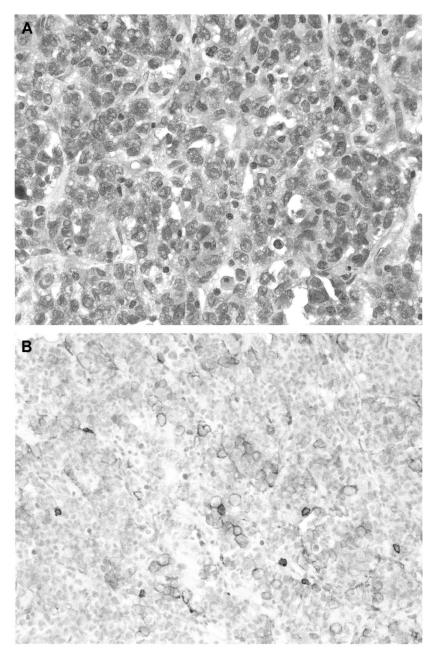

syndrome accounts for only approximately 1% of PCMs and is usually dominated clinically by peripheral neuropathic symptomatology. The serum paraprotein level is typically low, usually approximately 1 g/dL. Overexpression of vascular endothelial growth factor is believed to play a central pathogenetic role in POEMS syndrome.[68] When part of POEMS, the osseous myelomatous lesions are often multiple with only low-level involvement

outside of the confines of the osteosclerotic lesions. Due to the dense fibrosis, the neoplastic PCs may become distorted, making their recognition more difficult. PCM associated with POEMS is almost always λ light chain restricted.[69]

Nonsecretory PCM is an uncommon variant, comprising less than 5% of all myelomas. The availability of progressively more sensitive serum protein analytic techniques, such as immunofixation

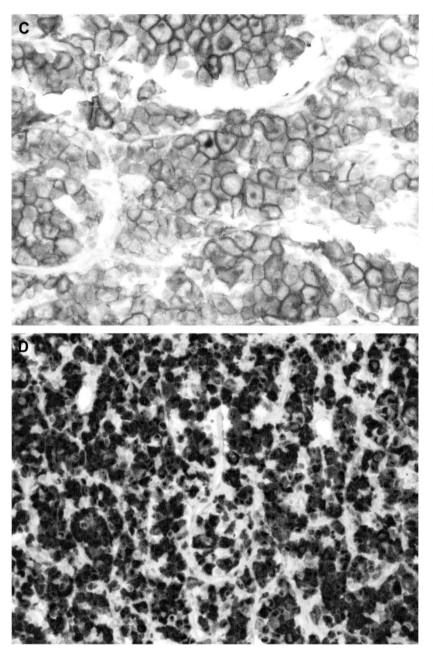

Fig. 6. Lymphoma mimicking a high-grade PCM. Additional IHC studies revealed that the tumor cells are strongly positive for CD30 (*C*) and anaplastic lymphoma kinase (ALK) (*D*), and are negative for CD20, CD79a, light chains, and T-cell markers (not shown), findings diagnostic of ALK-positive anaplastic large cell lymphoma.

electrophoresis and more recently the serum free light chain assay, has had an impact on both the definition and frequency of nonsecretory PCM. Under current WHO criteria, the nonsecretory variant is defined as a myeloma lacking a detectable serum or urine M protein by immunofixation electrophoresis. Approximately 70% of nonsecretory PCMs have abnormal ratios of free κ and λ serum light chains, indicating that many possess preserved, albeit low-level secretory activity.[70] Nonsecretory PCM is typically more of a diagnostic conundrum for clinicians than pathologists. Given the absence of a detectable paraprotein and the presence of osteolytic lesions, bone marrow biopsies and aspirates from patients with nonsecretory disease often come with a clinical diagnosis of "rule out metastatic malignancy". In at least a subset of nonsecretory PCMs, neither light mRNA nor protein expression by the neoplastic cells is detectable and thus reliance solely on light chain IHC or ISH may erroneously suggest a nonplasmacytic neoplasm (see Pitfalls: Plasma Cell Neoplasms box). Therefore, light chain studies in conjunction with CD138 or MUM1/IRF4 IHC are recommended for evaluation for nonsecretory PCM (**Fig. 7**).

PROGNOSIS

Cytogenetics is one of the most important determinants of prognosis in PCM. Several primary cytogenetic abnormalities, such as hyperdiploidy and the t(11;14), are associated with a favorable clinical outcome. By contrast, the t(4;14), t(14;16), and t(14;20) impart an unfavorable prognosis (reviewed by Kremer and colleagues[71] and Stewart and colleagues[72]). In addition, secondary genetic abnormalities, such as deletion of chromosome 13, p53 inactivation, and chromosome 1q amplification, are also associated with poor outcome. With the advent of newer therapeutics, such as proteasome inhibitors, the continued relevance of these genetic events with respect to clinical

Fig. 7. Nonsecretory PCM. (*A*) An infiltrate of neoplastic PCs is present, many with Dutcher bodies. (*B*) The neoplastic cells are strongly positive for CD138 by IHC.

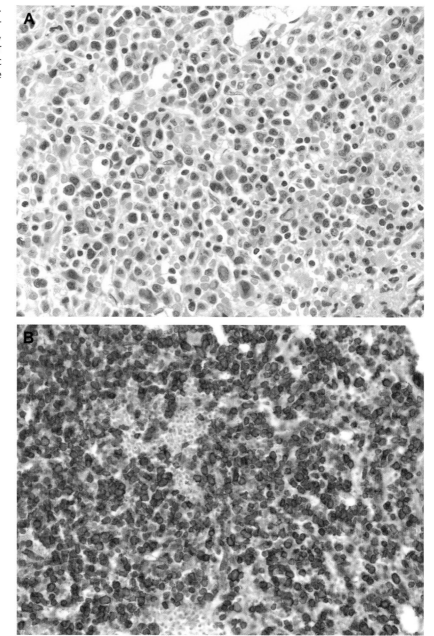

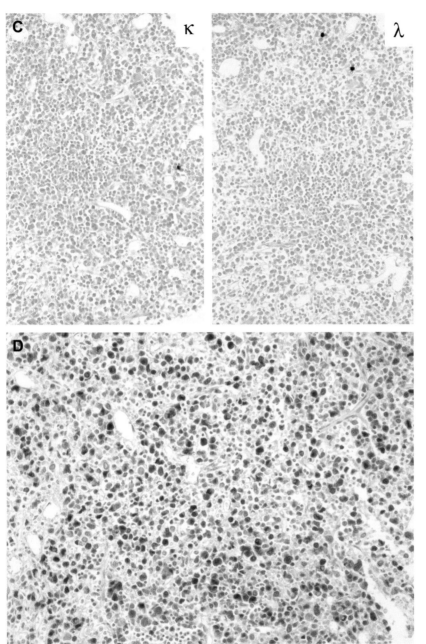

Fig. 7. Nonsecretory PCM. (*C*) ISH studies for κ (*left panel*) and λ (*right panel*) light chains show that the myeloma cells are negative, with scattered reactive PCs showing polytypic hybridization for light chains. (*D*) The myeloma cells are strongly positive for cyclin D1 by IHC. Cytogenetics confirmed the presence of the t(11;14).

outcome is the subject of ongoing clinical investigation.

PLASMA CELL MYELOMA WITH ASSOCIATED CRYSTAL-STORING HISTIOCYTOSIS

CLINICAL FEATURES

Although the clinical features are largely similar, PCM with crystal-storing histiocytosis (CSH) is associated with lower paraprotein levels than typical myelomas, probably reflecting a lower bone marrow burden of neoplastic PCs. Crystal deposition in the kidney has been associated with renal failure and rarely causes end-organ impairment secondary to formation of mass lesions.[73–75]

DIAGNOSIS: MICROSCOPIC FEATURES AND ANCILLARY STUDIES

These rare PCM cases are accompanied by a reactive histiocytic hyperplasia in which the histiocytes contain abundant cytoplasmic crystalline Ig inclusions.[76] In CSH-associated myelomas, the neoplastic PCs usually express κ light chain restriction and in many cases contain prominent Ig inclusions (**Fig. 8**). The molecular basis for the crystal formation is not well understood, because molecular or proteomic studies have been performed in only rare cases; in one study, a mutation in κ light chain was detected that was postulated to disrupt hydrophobic interactions within the light chain.[77] Although clonal Ig is usually detectable by IHC in the PC infiltrate, the Ig crystals may not be reactive, presumably because of epitope masking due to their crystalline nature.

DIFFERENTIAL DIAGNOSIS

The CSH in some cases may be so florid as to mimic a storage disorder, such as Gaucher disease. The histiocytes in Gaucher disease,

Fig. 8. PCM with CSH. (*A*) An infiltrate of histiocytic cells fills much of the intertrabecular marrow space, mimicking a storage disorder at low power. (*B*) The interstitial infiltrate of neoplastic PCs is masked to some extent by the prominent histiocytic infiltrate; the crystalline quality of the cytoplasmic contents is apparent, in contrast to the more fibrillary quality that characterizes Gaucher disease. In the aspirate, the neoplastic PC infiltrate is more apparent, with many of the neoplastic cells having prominent azurophilic crystals that resemble Auer rods (*inset*).

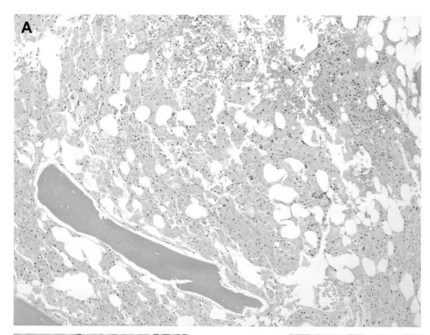

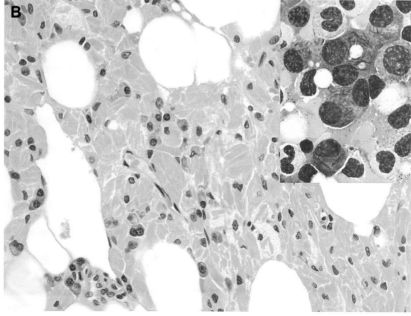

Pathologic Key Features
OF PLASMA CELL MYELOMA WITH ASSOCIATED CRYSTAL-STORING HISTIOCYTOSIS

- Crystal-storing histiocytosis (CSH) may be associated with PCM, lymphomas with plasmacytic differentiation, reactive disorders, and even nonhematopoietic neoplasms

- Most PC neoplasms associated with CSH are κ light chain restricted

- Bone marrow involvement by CSH may be florid, mimicking a storage disorder or masking an underlying plasmacytic neoplasm

Pathologic Key Features
OF AMYLOIDOSIS

- Typically a low burden of neoplastic PCs in primary amyloidosis

- Similar genetic features as PCM, although t(11;14) is more common in primary amyloidosis

- Definitive subtyping of amyloid deposits now possible using mass spectrometry

however, have the classical striated or crumpled tissue paper-appearing cytoplasm and do not contain the well-formed crystals characteristically seen in CSH (see **Fig. 8**). The presence of a CSH is not specific for myeloma, because it has been described in association with lymphoplasmacytic lymphoma and extranodal marginal zone lymphomas and rarely in association with reactive disorders or nonhematopoietic tumors, such as inflammatory myofibroblastic tumors. Thus, when confronted with suspected CSH, a thorough pathologic work-up must be performed, because the underlying disorder is not necessarily a PC dyscrasia. Finally, the histiocytic infiltrate can be so marked as to mask the PC infiltrate; therefore, a high index of suspicion in such cases is needed to avoid misdiagnosis.

PROGNOSIS

Other than end-organ damage which may be caused by the crystal deposition, PCM with CSH likely has a prognosis similar to that of typical PCM.

AMYLOIDOSIS AND PLASMA CELL MYELOMA WITH ASSOCIATED AMYLOIDOSIS

CLINICAL FEATURES

Primary amyloidosis involves middle-aged and older adults and is characterized by the extracellular deposition of Ig light chains or rarely heavy chains. These deposits assume an insoluble, β-pleated sheet structure, to which the dye Congo red binds, yielding the characteristic apple green birefringence under polarized light. These amyloid deposits induce end-organ damage at the anatomic sites where they form, most commonly kidney, heart, gastrointestinal tract, and peripheral

nerves, accounting for the protean clinical manifestations of amyloidosis. Light chain amyloidosis occurs in approximately 10% to 15% of patients with otherwise typical PCM; clinically occult deposits of amyloid may be detected in up to 40% of cases.[78,79] The new WHO classification has eliminated the diagnostic requirement for a minimum level of marrow plasmacytosis for symptomatic PCM; however, in the setting of low-level bone marrow clonal plasmacytosis (<10% of nucleated cells), end-organ impairment secondary to histopathologically confirmed amyloidosis does not qualify as myeloma-related damage and does not warrant a diagnosis of symptomatic myeloma. Therefore, if the clinical picture is dominated by the sequelae of amyloid deposition rather than the end-organ damage typical of PCM, a diagnosis of primary amyloidosis should be rendered.

DIAGNOSIS: MICROSCOPIC FEATURES AND ANCILLARY STUDIES

Although other organs, such as the gastrointestinal tract and kidney, may be involved, hematopathologists encounter amyloid most frequently in the bone marrow. The most common finding in primary amyloidosis is that of a mild plasmacytosis, although the marrow may appear normal by routine histologic evaluation; the frequency of clonal PCs is paradoxically low in most cases of primary amyloidosis, typically less than 10%.[80] Other than the amyloid deposits, the microscopic findings in cases of PCM with associated amyloidosis are similar to those of typical PCM. In cases with a low-level of deposition, amyloid may be inconspicuous on routine hematoxylin-eosin stains. When present, bone marrow amyloid deposits may be primarily vascular (either intramural or perivascular in location) or interstitial (**Fig. 9**). In some cases, extensive perivascular and interstitial amyloid deposition may be present, with occasional cases manifesting massive,

Fig. 9. PCM with amyloidosis. (*A*) There is both perivascular and interstitial amyloid deposition. (*B*) Higher magnification demonstrates an admixture of myeloma cells and interstitial amyloid deposits.

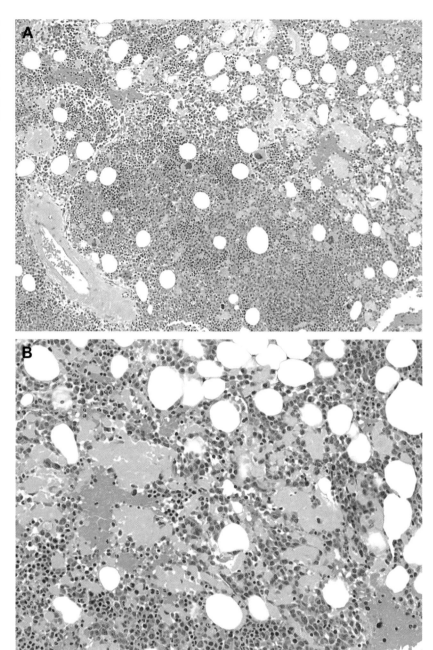

space-occupying amyloid deposition. These deposits may elicit a foreign-body giant cell reaction. The suspected presence of amyloid should be confirmed by Congo red staining.

DIFFERENTIAL DIAGNOSIS

Historically, amyloid deposits have been subtyped using IHC on fixed, paraffin-embedded tissues—a process not infrequently fraught with difficulty due to high background staining—or immunofluorescence on fresh frozen tissue. Amyloid deposits can now be definitively subtyped using mass spectrometry.[81] Amyloid deposits are not an exclusive feature of PC neoplasms and may rarely be seen in association with other lymphoid malignancies, including lymphoplasmacytic lymphoma and MALT (mucosa-associated lymphoid tissue) lymphoma, more commonly at extramedullary sites.[82,83]

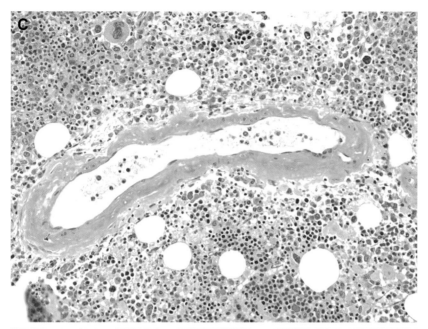

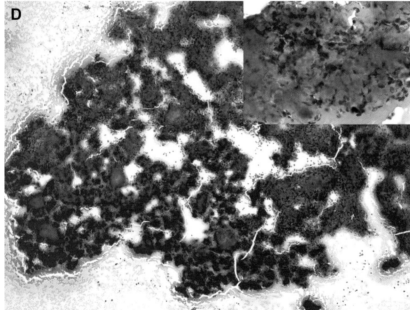

Fig. 9. PCM with amyloidosis. (*C*) PAS staining is useful for highlighting amyloid deposits. (*D*) In cases with significant amyloid deposition, the bone marrow particles often assume a "Chinese character" configuration in the bone marrow aspirate that is apparent at low magnification; amyloid characteristically has an amorphous basophilic or lightly eosinophilic appearance in the aspirate (*inset*).

PROGNOSIS

The median survival of patients with primary amyloidosis is approximately 2 to 4 years. Mortality is largely attributable to cardiac complications due to myocardial amyloid deposition.[80,84] Therapy for amyloidosis is focused on reducing the neoplastic PC burden, thereby suppressing the production of amyloidogenic Ig protein and minimizing end-organ dysfunction.

ASSOCIATION OF PLASMA CELL MYELOMA WITH OTHER MALIGNANCIES

PCM or MGUS may occasionally coexist with other malignancies. CLL is the hematologic

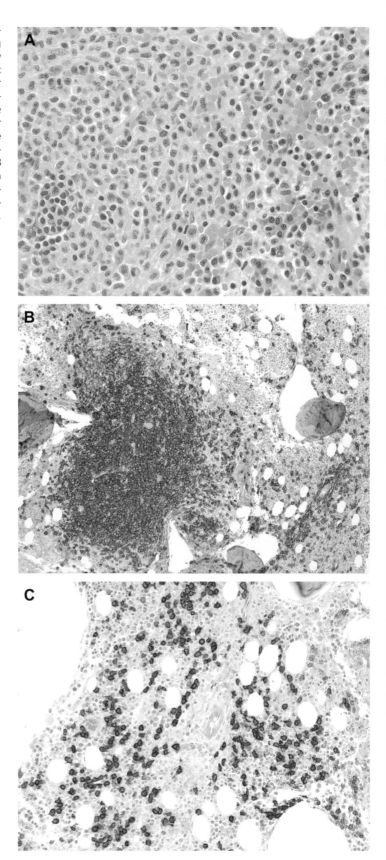

Fig. 10. PCM with systemic mastocytosis in an elderly man presenting with cachexia. (*A*) The bone marrow biopsy contains aggregates of mast cells as well as an increased number of mature-appearing PCs in the intervening marrow (*right*). (*B*) By IHC, the mast cells are strongly positive for CD117; PCR analysis confirmed the presence of a *KIT* Asp816Val mutation. (*C*) The plasma cells are CD138 positive. They were also κ light chain restricted by ISH (not shown). Subsequent serum protein analysis revealed an IgG κ paraprotein (2 g/dL).

malignancy most frequently coexisting with myeloma. These are typically metachronous and, as such, straightforward diagnostically. Rarely, the onset of myeloma may be synchronous with CLL or another lymphoid malignancy. In these instances, the differential diagnosis includes not only concurrent PC and lymphoid neoplasms but also single lymphoid neoplasms manifesting plasmacytic differentiation, such as CLL with plasmacytic differentiation, lymphoplasmacytic lymphoma, MALT lymphoma, and splenic marginal zone lymphoma. In this setting, FC is of great utility in characterizing both the lymphoid and plasmacytic components and distinguishing between these possibilities. As discussed previously, there are several immunophenotypic differences between the PCs of PCM or MGUS and those of a low-grade B-cell lymphoma with plasmacytic differentiation, which may aid in the distinction of these disorders. On morphology, the presence of nucleolated, cytologically malignant PCs favors a diagnosis of coexisting PC and lymphoid neoplasms, because the plasmacytic component of low-grade B-cell lymphomas with plasmacytic differentiation typically has mature features. Thorough pathologic characterization of both the lymphoid and plasmacytic components together with correlation with clinical, radiologic, and serum protein studies readily permits the distinction between these possibilities in most cases. In challenging cases, cell sorting with separate cytogenetic, fluorescence in situ hybridization (FISH), and gene rearrangement studies on each of the components may be required for final diagnosis. Recent studies indicate that concurrent PCM and CLL usually represent two distinct diseases that are clonally unrelated.[85]

PCM may rarely be associated with other non-lymphoid malignancies. Concurrent myeloma and metastatic carcinoma are occasionally encountered. As discussed previously, both PCM and most carcinomas express CD138; thus, when confronted with a suspected case of CD138-positive, anaplastic PCM, cytokeratin IHC is indicated to exclude metastatic carcinoma. Rarely, systemic mastocytosis may occur in association with PCM (**Fig. 10**).[86,87] In some instances, the mast cell infiltrate may be sufficiently prominent to mask the PC neoplasm.

Finally, myeloma patients frequently have extensive exposure to cytotoxic chemotherapy, including alkylating agents, such as melphalan. As such, these patients are at risk for the development of therapy-related myelodysplasia and AML. Thus, follow-up marrows should be thoroughly evaluated for the presence of dysplasia or increased blasts, particularly in those patients who have cytopenias unexplained by persistent PCM or recent chemotherapy.

SOLITARY OSSEOUS PLASMACYTOMA

CLINICAL FEATURES

Plasmacytoma is defined as a tumor-like proliferation of neoplastic PCs. According to the WHO criteria (see **Table 2**), two major types of plasmacytoma are recognized, namely solitary osseous plasmacytoma (SOP) and extramedullary plasmacytoma.[5] SOPs primarily affect middle-aged and older adults. They are skeletal-based lesions, comprise the majority of plasmacytomas, and predominantly involve the axial skeleton, most commonly the vertebrae.[88,89]

DIAGNOSIS: MICROSCOPIC FEATURES AND ANCILLARY STUDIES

Diagnosis of SOPs is usually straightforward, because most lesions are comprised of sheets of neoplastic cells with overt plasmacytic differentiation. A few routine immunohistochemical studies, including CD138 and Ig light chains, aid in confirming the diagnosis. High-grade plasmacytomas, in which the neoplastic cells have anaplastic or plasmablastic morphology, can be more problematic because these lesions may mimic a lymphoma or myeloid sarcoma. Fortunately, high-grade plasmacytomas most often arise in patients with a known history of myeloma and are less frequently encountered at initial clinical presentation. In patients lacking a history of PCM, immunophenotyping is often critical to confirming the diagnosis high-grade SOP (**Fig. 11**). Correlation with radiologic and other clinical data may also be required for appropriate diagnosis of plasmacytomas arising at unusual anatomic sites.

> ### Pathologic Key Features
> OF SOLITARY OSSEOUS PLASMACYTOMA
>
> - Diagnosis of solitary osseous plasmacytoma (SOP) should only be made in absence of clinical, radiologic, or pathologic evidence of disseminated disease
>
> - A sheet-like infiltrate of neoplastic PCs is typical
>
> - The cytologic spectrum and immunophenotype of SOP is similar to that of PCM

Fig. 11. Intraoral presentation of PCM at the site of a prior tooth extraction. (*A*) There is a diffuse infiltrate of malignant lymphoid cells, raising a differential of diffuse large B-cell or plasmablastic lymphoma. (*B*) The neoplastic cells have immature chromatin and scant cytoplasm; frequent mitoses are present. By IHC, the neoplastic cells were strongly and diffusely positive for CD138 and were negative for CD20 (not shown). Subsequent imaging studies demonstrated multiple osteolytic lesions with no evidence of lymphadenopathy, consistent with PCM.

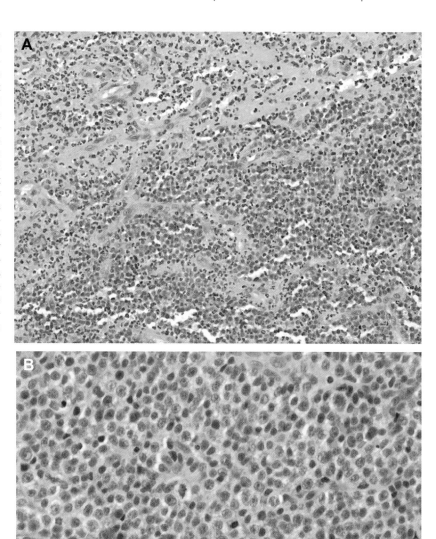

DIFFERENTIAL DIAGNOSIS

A diagnosis of SOP should only be rendered in the absence of any clinical, laboratory, or radiologic evidence of disseminated disease,[88] data that are frequently not available to pathologists. In this circumstance, a diagnosis of PC neoplasm is appropriate with a comment by the pathologist indicating that, although the lesion may represent a solitary plasmacytoma, correlation with radiologic and other clinical findings is required for final diagnosis. Finally, in so-called break out lesions, an osseous plasmacytoma may erode cortical bone and extend into adjacent soft tissue. These should not be misclassified as extramedullary plasmacytomas.

PROGNOSIS

SOP frequently progresses to PCM and is associated with an overall poorer survival than its extramedullary counterpart.[88,90,91] Some laboratory and pathologic findings are associated with progression of SOPs to PCM, for example,

increased angiogenesis and persistence of serum paraprotein after radiotherapy.[92,93]

PRIMARY EXTRAMEDULLARY PLASMACYTOMA

CLINICAL FEATURES

The most commonly encountered extraosseous plasmacytomas are those that develop in the setting of end-stage or widely disseminated

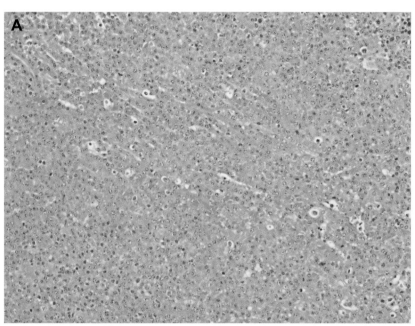

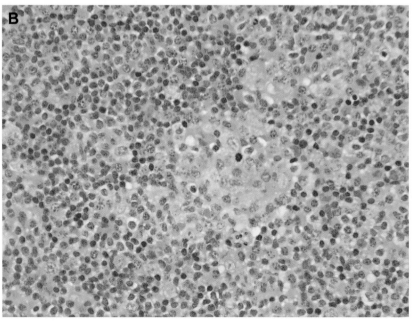

Fig. 12. Extranodal MALT lymphoma involving ocular adnexa mimicking a plasmacytoma. (*A*) At low magnification, most of the tumor is comprised of a diffuse infiltrate of plasmacytic cells. (*B*) Rare colonized germinal centers are a clue to the diagnosis of MALT lymphoma.

Fig. 12. Extranodal MALT lymphoma involving ocular adnexa mimicking a plasmacytoma. Immunohistochemical studies reveal only scattered islands of CD20 positive B cells (*C*), which coexpress BCL2 (*D*), whereas most of the neoplastic cells are strongly CD138 positive (*E*). CD21 immunostain highlights a colonized germinal center (*F*).

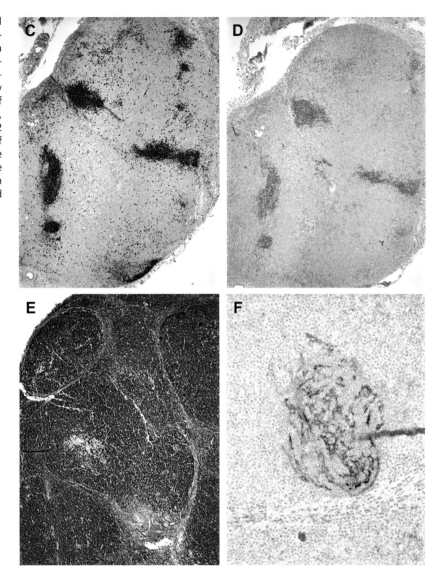

PCM. Primary extramedullary plasmacytoma (PEMP), defined as lesions developing in the absence of bone marrow involvement, is significantly less common, comprising less than 5% of all PC neoplasms. PEMPs primarily affect middle-aged and older adults. For unknown reasons, they have a striking proclivity for involvement of the upper aerodigestive tract, including the nasopharynx and oropharynx, where approximately 80% of these lesions occur; however, they may develop at a wide array of anatomic sites, including skin, gastrointestinal tract, and lymph nodes.

DIAGNOSIS: MICROSCOPIC FEATURES AND ANCILLARY STUDIES

PEMPs are comprised of sheets of PCs effacing the architecture of the involved organ or tissue. The cytology of the neoplastic cells is usually that of mature, Marschalko-type PCs, although atypical nucleolated forms occasionally predominate. In contrast to extramedullary manifestations of PCM, plasmablastic or anaplastic morphology is uncommon in PEMP. The neoplastic cells are CD138 positive and show light chain restriction.[71] The proliferative activity in PEMP is rather variable

Pathologic Key Features
OF PRIMARY
EXTRAMEDULLARY PLASMACYTOMA

- Diagnosis of primary extramedullary plasma-cytoma (PEMP) should only be made in absence of clinical, radiologic, or pathologic evidence of osseous or disseminated disease

- There is a sheet-like infiltrate of neoplastic PCs with light chain restriction

- Although immunophenotypically similar to its osseous counterpart, PEMP is only infrequently positive for CD56 and cyclin D1

and may be high in those tumors with more immature cytology. In contrast to extranodal marginal zone (MALT) lymphomas, PEMPs do not have a significant admixed nonplasmacytic B-cell component and do not form lymphoepithelial lesions when present at mucosal sites.

DIFFERENTIAL DIAGNOSIS

When confronted with an extramedullary plasmacytoma, there is a wide differential diagnosis that includes both reactive and neoplastic disorders (see boxes, Differential Diagnosis of Primary Extramedullary Plasmacytoma and Pitfalls: Plasma Cell Neoplasms). Analysis of light chain restriction is helpful in distinguishing extramedullary plasmacytomas from reactive or inflammatory lesions with a high content of PCs. The plasma cell variant of Castleman disease typically contains sheets of polytypic PCs with admixed reactive lymphoid follicles. Rarely, cases of histologic features of otherwise typical plasma cell variant Castleman disease may contain light chain-restricted PCs.[94,95] These unusual cases have not been immunophenotypically or genetically well characterized and may represent true PEMP.

Extranodal MALT lymphomas often manifest some degree of plasmacytic differentiation, which may be prominent in MALT lymphomas arising at certain anatomic sites, such as thyroid[96]; occasional MALT lymphomas manifest extreme plasmacytic differentiation (**Fig. 12**) and distinction from PEMP can be challenging in such cases. Identification of the characteristic features of MALT lymphoma (such as lymphoepithelial lesions and admixed secondary follicles) as well as detection of a clonal mature B-cell component by FC is particularly helpful for distinguishing MALT

Differential Diagnosis
PRIMARY EXTRAMEDULLARY PLASMACYTOMA

Primary Extramedullary Plasmacytoma Versus	Distinguishing Feature
Solitary osseous plasmacytoma	• Presence of associated osseous mass with extension into adjacent soft tissue (breakout lesion)
Extramedullary involvement by plasma cell myeloma	• Presence of clinical or radiologic evidence of disseminated disease • Tumor cells are often CD56 and/or cyclin D1 positive • Plasmablastic or anaplastic morphology may occur
Reactive (inflammatory) plasma cell infiltrate	• PCs are polyclonal
Inflammatory pseudotumor/ myofibroblastic tumor	• PCs are polyclonal • ALK1 may be positive
Plasma cell variant of Castleman disease	• PCs are usually polyclonal • Reactive lymphoid follicles are present
Extranodal marginal zone (MALT) lymphoma	• Neoplastic clonal B-cell component is present and detectable by flow cytometry • B cells infiltrate epithelium (lymphoepithelial lesions) and colonize germinal centers • Characteristic location (eg, ocular adnexa, stomach)
Plasmablastic lymphoma	• EBV positive • Plasmablastic morphology • Most affected patients are HIV+

Fig. 13. Extramedullary plasmacytoma of the maxillary sinus as the presenting feature of PCM. (*A*) There is an infiltrate of neoplastic PCs within the tissue with associated acute inflammation. (*B*) Many of the neoplastic cells contain prominent nucleoli and scattered mitoses are present. By IHC, the tumor cells express cyclin D1 (*inset*). They also expressed CD138 and showed κ light chain restriction, but were CD56 negative (not shown). Subsequent imaging studies revealed a focal thoracic vertebral lesion, consistent with disseminated involvement by PCM.

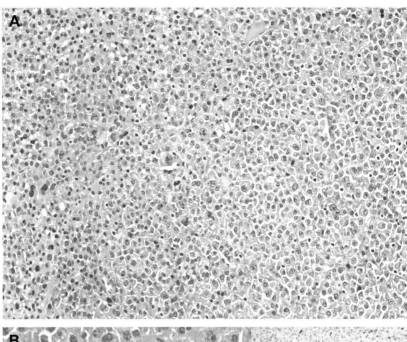

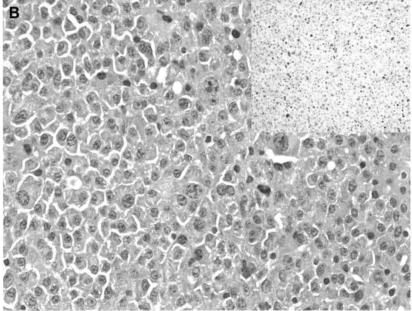

lymphoma from plasmacytoma. In addition, clinical features, such as anatomic site of involvement and lack of osteolytic lesions, can be helpful in the differential diagnosis. For example, the ocular adnexa and conjunctiva are well-recognized sites for MALT lymphoma, whereas involvement of these sites by PCM in the absence of adjacent bone involvement is uncommon. Although distinction of PEMP from extramedullary myelomatous involvement ultimately requires integration of the pathologic, clinical, and radiologic findings, there are immunophenotypic differences that may be

Pitfalls
PLASMA CELL NEOPLASMS

! PC neoplasms may be particularly challenging diagnostically when they initially manifest in an extramedullary site or as nonsecretory cases.

! PC neoplasms must be distinguished from lymphomas with extreme plasmacytic differentiation.

! Anaplastic PCM may simulate high-grade lymphomas, carcinomas, or other nonhematologic malignancies; appropriate use of IHC is critical in arriving at the correct diagnosis.

! PC leukemia may exhibit blastic features mimicking AML or the leukemic phase of a non-Hodgkin' lymphoma, particularly when it is the initial presentation of PCM.

! PCM not infrequently occurs together with an unrelated lymphoid malignancy.

diagnostically helpful in distinguishing PEMP from extramedullary PCM.[71,97] For example, PEMPs rarely express CD56 or cyclin D1, whereas extramedullary PCM is often CD56 positive and not infrequently cyclin D1 positive (**Fig. 13**).

PROGNOSIS

The diagnosis of PEMP is predicated on a thorough clinical evaluation to exclude systemic disease, which is lacking in many reported cases of PEMP. When disseminated disease (ie, PCM) is rigorously excluded, PEMP seems to rarely progress to PCM, in contrast to its osseous counterpart.[71] Radiotherapy with or without complete surgical excision seems to offer excellent local control.[98]

REFERENCES

1. Weiss BM, Abadie J, Verma P, et al. A monoclonal gammopathy precedes multiple myeloma in most patients. Blood 2009;113:5418–22.
2. Landgren O, Kyle RA, Pfeiffer RM, et al. Monoclonal gammopathy of undetermined significance (MGUS) consistently precedes multiple myeloma: a prospective study. Blood 2009;113:5412–7.
3. Chng WJ, Glebov O, Bergsagel PL, et al. Genetic events in the pathogenesis of multiple myeloma. Best Pract Res Clin Haematol 2007;20:571–96.
4. Bergsagel PL, Kuehl WM. Molecular pathogenesis and a consequent classification of multiple myeloma. J Clin Oncol 2005;23:6333–8.
5. Swerdlow SH, Campo E, Harris NL, et al. WHO classification of tumours of haematopoietic and lymphoid tissues. Lyon (France): IARC Press; 2008.
6. Mason DY, Cordell JL, Brown MH, et al. CD79a: a novel marker for B-cell neoplasms in routinely processed tissue samples. Blood 1995;86:1453–9.
7. Tedder TF, Tuscano J, Sato S, et al. CD22, a B lymphocyte-specific adhesion molecule that regulates antigen receptor signaling. Annu Rev Immunol 1997;15:481–504.
8. Ridley RC, Xiao H, Hata H, et al. Expression of syndecan regulates human myeloma plasma cell adhesion to type I collagen. Blood 1993;81:767–74.
9. Carbone A, Gloghini A, Gattei V, et al. Reed-Sternberg cells of classical Hodgkin's disease react with the plasma cell-specific monoclonal antibody B-B4 and express human syndecan-1. Blood 1997;89:3787–94.
10. Turley H, Jones M, Erber W, et al. VS38: a new monoclonal antibody for detecting plasma cell differentiation in routine sections. J Clin Pathol 1994;47:418–22.
11. Falini B, Fizzotti M, Pucciarini A, et al. A monoclonal antibody (MUM1p) detects expression of the MUM1/IRF4 protein in a subset of germinal center B cells, plasma cells, and activated T cells. Blood 2000;95:2084–92.
12. Chilosi M, Adami F, Lestani M, et al. CD138/syndecan-1: a useful immunohistochemical marker of normal and neoplastic plasma cells on routine trephine bone marrow biopsies. Mod Pathol 1999;12:1101–6.
13. Costes V, Magen V, Legouffe E, et al. The Mi15 monoclonal antibody (anti-syndecan-1) is a reliable marker for quantifying plasma cells in paraffin-embedded bone marrow biopsy specimens. Hum Pathol 1999;30:1405–11.
14. O'Connell FP, Pinkus JL, Pinkus GS. CD138 (syndecan-1), a plasma cell marker immunohistochemical profile in hematopoietic and nonhematopoietic neoplasms. Am J Clin Pathol 2004;121:254–63.
15. Ng AP, Wei A, Bhurani D, et al. The sensitivity of CD138 immunostaining of bone marrow trephine specimens for quantifying marrow involvement in MGUS and myeloma, including samples with a low percentage of plasma cells. Haematologica 2006;91:972–5.
16. Al-Quran SZ, Yang L, Magill JM, et al. Assessment of bone marrow plasma cell infiltrates in multiple myeloma: the added value of CD138 immunohistochemistry. Hum Pathol 2007;38:1779–87.
17. Reichard KK, McKenna RW, Kroft SH. ALK-positive diffuse large B-cell lymphoma: report of four cases and review of the literature. Mod Pathol 2007;20:310–9.
18. Chu PG, Arber DA, Weiss LM. Expression of T/NK-cell and plasma cell antigens in nonhematopoietic

epithelioid neoplasms. An immunohistochemical study of 447 cases. Am J Clin Pathol 2003;120: 64–70.

19. Kambham N, Kong C, Longacre TA, et al. Utility of syndecan-1 (CD138) expression in the diagnosis of undifferentiated malignant neoplasms: a tissue microarray study of 1,754 cases. Appl Immunohistochem Mol Morphol 2005;13:304–10.

20. Shaffer AL, Emre NC, Lamy L, et al. IRF4 addiction in multiple myeloma. Nature 2008;454:226–31.

21. Natkunam Y, Warnke RA, Montgomery K, et al. Analysis of MUM1/IRF4 protein expression using tissue microarrays and immunohistochemistry. Mod Pathol 2001;14:686–94.

22. Sulzbacher I, Fuchs M, Chott A, et al. Expression of VS38 in osteoblasts and stroma cells of bone tumors. Pathol Res Pract 1997;193:613–6.

23. Banham AH, Turley H, Pulford K, et al. The plasma cell associated antigen detectable by antibody VS38 is the p63 rough endoplasmic reticulum protein. J Clin Pathol 1997;50:485–9.

24. Shanks JH, Banerjee SS. VS38 immunostaining in melanocytic lesions. J Clin Pathol 1996;49:205–7.

25. Beck RC, Tubbs RR, Hussein M, et al. Automated colorimetric in situ hybridization (CISH) detection of immunoglobulin (Ig) light chain mRNA expression in plasma cell (PC) dyscrasias and non-Hodgkin lymphoma. Diagn Mol Pathol 2003;12:14–20.

26. de Tute RM, Jack AS, Child JA, et al. A single-tube six-colour flow cytometry screening assay for the detection of minimal residual disease in myeloma. Leukemia 2007;21:2046–9.

27. Morice WG, Hanson CA, Kumar S, et al. Novel multiparameter flow cytometry sensitively detects phenotypically distinct plasma cell subsets in plasma cell proliferative disorders. Leukemia 2007;21:2043–6.

28. Rawstron AC, Orfao A, Beksac M, et al. Report of the European Myeloma Network on multiparametric flow cytometry in multiple myeloma and related disorders. Haematologica 2008;93:431–8.

29. Paiva B, Vidriales MB, Perez JJ, et al. Multiparameter flow cytometry quantification of bone marrow plasma cells at diagnosis provides more prognostic information than morphological assessment in myeloma patients. Haematologica 2009;94:1599–602.

30. Lin P, Owens R, Tricot G, et al. Flow cytometric immunophenotypic analysis of 306 cases of multiple myeloma. Am J Clin Pathol 2004;121:482–8.

31. Mateo G, Castellanos M, Rasillo A, et al. Genetic abnormalities and patterns of antigenic expression in multiple myeloma. Clin Cancer Res 2005;11: 3661–7.

32. Lemoli RM, Fortuna A, Grande A, et al. Expression and functional role of c-kit ligand (SCF) in human multiple myeloma cells. Br J Haematol 1994;88:760–9.

33. Ocqueteau M, Orfao A, Garcia-Sanz R, et al. Expression of the CD117 antigen (c-Kit) on normal

and myelomatous plasma cells. Br J Haematol 1996;95:489–93.

34. Almeida J, Orfao A, Ocqueteau M, et al. High-sensitive immunophenotyping and DNA ploidy studies for the investigation of minimal residual disease in multiple myeloma. Br J Haematol 1999;107:121–31.

35. Van CB, Durie BG, Spier C, et al. Plasma cells in multiple myeloma express a natural killer cell-associated antigen: CD56 (NKH-1; Leu-19). Blood 1990;76:377–82.

36. Drach J, Gattringer C, Huber H. Expression of the neural cell adhesion molecule (CD56) by human myeloma cells. Clin Exp Immunol 1991;83:418–22.

37. Garcia-Sanz R, Gonzalez M, Orfao A, et al. Analysis of natural killer-associated antigens in peripheral blood and bone marrow of multiple myeloma patients and prognostic implications. Br J Haematol 1996;93:81–8.

38. Mateo G, Montalban MA, Vidriales MB, et al. Prognostic value of immunophenotyping in multiple myeloma: a study by the PETHEMA/GEM cooperative study groups on patients uniformly treated with high-dose therapy. J Clin Oncol 2008;26:2737–44.

39. Rawstron A, Barrans S, Blythe D, et al. Distribution of myeloma plasma cells in peripheral blood and bone marrow correlates with CD56 expression. Br J Haematol 1999;104:138–43.

40. Robillard N, vet-Loiseau H, Garand R, et al. CD20 is associated with a small mature plasma cell morphology and t(11;14) in multiple myeloma. Blood 2003;102:1070–1.

41. Cook JR, Hsi ED, Worley S, et al. Immunohistochemical analysis identifies two cyclin D1+ subsets of plasma cell myeloma, each associated with favorable survival. Am J Clin Pathol 2006;125:615–24.

42. Heerema MA, Waldron J, Hughes S, et al. Clinical, immunophenotypic, and genetic characterization of small lymphocyte-like plasma cell myeloma: a potential mimic of mature B-cell lymphoma. Am J Clin Pathol 2010;133:265–70.

43. Zojer N, Kirchbacher K, Vesely M, et al. Rituximab treatment provides no clinical benefit in patients with pretreated advanced multiple myeloma. Leuk Lymphoma 2006;47:1103–9.

44. Moreau P, Voillat L, Benboukher L, et al. Rituximab in CD20 positive multiple myeloma. Leukemia 2007;21: 835–6.

45. Raja KR, Kovarova L, Hajek R. Review of phenotypic markers used in flow cytometric analysis of MGUS and MM, and applicability of flow cytometry in other plasma cell disorders. Br J Haematol 2010;149: 334–51.

46. Grogan TM, Durie BG, Spier CM, et al. Myelomonocytic antigen positive multiple myeloma. Blood 1989; 73:763–9.

47. Robillard N, Wuilleme S, Lode L, et al. CD33 is expressed on plasma cells of a significant number of

myeloma patients, and may represent a therapeutic target. Leukemia 2005;19:2021–2.

48. Pellat DC, Bataille R, Robillard N, et al. Expression of CD28 and CD40 in human myeloma cells: a comparative study with normal plasma cells. Blood 1994;84: 2597–603.

49. Robillard N, Jego G, Pellat DC, et al. CD28, a marker associated with tumoral expansion in multiple myeloma. Clin Cancer Res 1998;4:1521–6.

50. Seegmiller AC, Xu Y, McKenna RW, et al. Immunophenotypic differentiation between neoplastic plasma cells in mature B-cell lymphoma vs plasma cell myeloma. Am J Clin Pathol 2007;127:176–81.

51. Morice WG, Chen D, Kurtin PJ, et al. Novel immunophenotypic features of marrow lymphoplasmacytic lymphoma and correlation with Waldenstrom's macroglobulinemia. Mod Pathol 2009;22:807–16.

52. Bartl R, Frisch B, Fateh-Moghadam A, et al. Histologic classification and staging of multiple myeloma. A retrospective and prospective study of 674 cases. Am J Clin Pathol 1987;87:342–55.

53. Carter A, Hocherman I, Linn S, et al. Prognostic significance of plasma cell morphology in multiple myeloma. Cancer 1987;60:1060–5.

54. Fritz E, Ludwig H, Kundi M. Prognostic relevance of cellular morphology in multiple myeloma. Blood 1984;63:1072–9.

55. Sukpanichnant S, Cousar JB, Leelasiri A, et al. Diagnostic criteria and histologic grading in multiple myeloma: histologic and immunohistologic analysis of 176 cases with clinical correlation. Hum Pathol 1994;25:308–18.

56. Larson RS, Sukpanichnant S, Greer JP, et al. The spectrum of multiple myeloma: diagnostic and biological implications. Hum Pathol 1997;28: 1336–47.

57. Greipp PR, Leong T, Bennett JM, et al. Plasmablastic morphology—an independent prognostic factor with clinical and laboratory correlates: Eastern Cooperative Oncology Group (ECOG) myeloma trial E9486 report by the ECOG myeloma laboratory group. Blood 1998;91:2501–7.

58. Peest D, Coldewey R, Deicher H, et al. Prognostic value of clinical, laboratory, and histological characteristics in multiple myeloma: improved definition of risk groups. Eur J Cancer 1993;29A:978–83.

59. Kyle RA, Therneau TM, Rajkumar SV, et al. Prevalence of monoclonal gammopathy of undetermined significance. N Engl J Med 2006;354:1362–9.

60. Singh J, Dudley AW Jr, Kulig KA. Increased incidence of monoclonal gammopathy of undetermined significance in blacks and its age-related differences with whites on the basis of a study of 397 men and one woman in a hospital setting. J Lab Clin Med 1990;116:785–9.

61. Landgren O, Weiss BM. Patterns of monoclonal gammopathy of undetermined significance and multiple myeloma in various ethnic/racial groups support for genetic factors in pathogenesis Leukemia 2009;23:1691–7.

62. Kyle RA, Therneau TM, Rajkumar SV, et al. A longterm study of prognosis in monoclonal gammopathy of undetermined significance. N Engl J Med 2002 346:564–9.

63. Horner MJ, Ries LAG, Krapcho M, et al. SEER cancer statistics review, 1975–2006. Surveillance Epidemiology and End Results (SEER). Bethesda (MD) National Cancer Institute; 2009. Available at: seer cancer.gov/csr/1975_2006. Accessed September 15, 2010.

64. Brunning RD, McKenna RW. Atlas of tumor pathology: tumors of the bone marrow. Washington DC: Armed Forces Institute of Pathology; 1994. p. 3

65. Garcia SR, Orfao A, Gonzalez M, et al. Primary plasma cell leukemia: clinical, immunophenotypic DNA ploidy, and cytogenetic characteristics. Blood 1999;93:1032–7.

66. Tiedemann RE, Gonzalez PN, Kyle RA, et al. Genetic aberrations and survival in plasma cell leukemia Leukemia 2008;22:1044–52.

67. Vega F, Chang CC, Medeiros LJ, et al. Plasmablastic lymphomas and plasmablastic plasma cel myelomas have nearly identical immunophenotypic profiles. Mod Pathol 2005;18:806–15.

68. Dispenzieri A. POEMS syndrome. Blood Rev 2007 21:285–99.

69. Dispenzieri A, Kyle RA, Lacy MQ, et al. POEMS syndrome: definitions and long-term outcome. Blood 2003;101:2496–506.

70. Drayson M, Tang LX, Drew R, et al. Serum free lightchain measurements for identifying and monitoring patients with nonsecretory multiple myeloma. Blood 2001;97:2900–2.

71. Kremer M, Ott G, Nathrath M, et al. Primary extramedullary plasmacytoma and multiple myeloma phenotypic differences revealed by immunohistochemical analysis. J Pathol 2005;205:92–101.

72. Stewart AK, Bergsagel PL, Greipp PR, et al A practical guide to defining high-risk myeloma for clinical trials, patient counseling and choice of therapy. Leukemia 2007;21:529–34.

73. Ionescu DN, Pierson DM, Qing G, et al. Pulmonary crystal-storing histiocytoma. Arch Pathol Lab Med 2005;129:1159–63.

74. Sailey CJ, Alexiev BA, Gammie JS, et al. Crystal-storing histiocytosis as a cause of symptomatic cardiac mass. Arch Pathol Lab Med 2009;133:1861–4.

75. Farooq U, Bayerl MG, Abendroth CS, et al. Renal crystal storing histiocytosis in a patient with multiple myeloma. Ann Hematol 2009;88:807–9.

76. Jones D, Bhatia VK, Krausz T, et al. Crystal-storing histiocytosis: a disorder occurring in plasmacytic tumors expressing immunoglobulin kappa light chain. Hum Pathol 1999;30:1441–8.

77. Lebeau A, Zeindl-Eberhart E, Muller EC, et al. Generalized crystal-storing histiocytosis associated with monoclonal gammopathy: molecular analysis of a disorder with rapid clinical course and review of the literature. Blood 2002;100:1817–27.

78. Desikan KR, Dhodapkar MV, Hough A, et al. Incidence and impact of light chain associated (AL) amyloidosis on the prognosis of patients with multiple myeloma treated with autologous transplantation. Leuk Lymphoma 1997;27:315–9.

79. Bahlis NJ, Lazarus HM. Multiple myeloma-associated AL amyloidosis: is a distinctive therapeutic approach warranted? Bone Marrow Transplant 2006;38:7–15.

80. Merlini G, Stone MJ. Dangerous small B-cell clones. Blood 2006;108:2520–30.

81. Vrana JA, Gamez JD, Madden BJ, et al. Classification of amyloidosis by laser microdissection and mass spectrometry-based proteomic analysis in clinical biopsy specimens. Blood 2009;114:4957–9.

82. Andriko JA, Swerdlow SH, Aguilera NI, et al. Is lymphoplasmacytic lymphoma/immunocytoma a distinct entity? A clinicopathologic study of 20 cases. Am J Surg Pathol 2001;25:742–51.

83. Dacic S, Colby TV, Yousem SA. Nodular amyloidoma and primary pulmonary lymphoma with amyloid production: a differential diagnostic problem. Mod Pathol 2000;13:934–40.

84. Wechalekar AD, Hawkins PN, Gillmore JD. Perspectives in treatment of AL amyloidosis. Br J Haematol 2008;140:365–77.

85. Pantic M, Schroettner P, Pfeifer D, et al. Biclonal origin prevails in concomitant chronic lymphocytic leukemia and multiple myeloma. Leukemia 2010; 24:885–90.

86. Pullarkat ST, Sedarat F, Paquette R, et al. Systemic mastocytosis with plasma cell dyscrasia: report of a case. Leuk Res 2008;32:1160–3.

87. Motwani P, Kocoglu M, Lorsbach RB. Systemic mastocytosis in association with plasma cell dyscrasias: report of a case and review of the literature. Leuk Res 2009;33:856–9.

88. Soutar R, Lucraft H, Jackson G, et al. Guidelines on the diagnosis and management of solitary plasmacytoma of bone and solitary extramedullary plasmacytoma. Br J Haematol 2004;124: 717–26.

89. Dores GM, Landgren O, McGlynn KA, et al. Plasmacytoma of bone, extramedullary plasmacytoma, and multiple myeloma: incidence and survival in the United States, 1992–2004. Br J Haematol 2009; 144:86–94.

90. Knobel D, Zouhair A, Tsang RW, et al. Prognostic factors in solitary plasmacytoma of the bone: a multicenter rare cancer network study. BMC Cancer 2006;6:118, 118.

91. Ramsingh G, Mehan P, Morgensztern D, et al. Prognostic factors influencing survival in solitary plasmacytoma. Br J Haematol 2009;145:540–2.

92. Wilder RB, Ha CS, Cox JD, et al. Persistence of myeloma protein for more than one year after radiotherapy is an adverse prognostic factor in solitary plasmacytoma of bone. Cancer 2002;94: 1532–7.

93. Kumar S, Fonseca R, Dispenzieri A, et al. Prognostic value of angiogenesis in solitary bone plasmacytoma. Blood 2003;101:1715–7.

94. Radaszkiewicz T, Hansmann ML, Lennert K. Monoclonality and polyclonality of plasma cells in castleman's disease of the plasma cell variant. Histopathology 1989;14:11–24.

95. Hall PA, Donaghy M, Cotter FE, et al. An immunohistological and genotypic study of the plasma cell form of castleman's disease. Histopathology 1989; 14:333–46.

96. Derringer GA, Thompson LD, Frommelt RA, et al. Malignant lymphoma of the thyroid gland: a clinicopathologic study of 108 cases. Am J Surg Pathol 2000;24:623–39.

97. Bink K, Haralambieva E, Kremer M, et al. Primary extramedullary plasmacytoma: similarities with and differences from multiple myeloma revealed by interphase cytogenetics. Haematologica 2008;93: 623–6.

98. Strojan P, Soba E, Lamovec J, et al. Extramedullary plasmacytoma: clinical and histopathologic study. Int J Radiat Oncol Biol Phys 2002;53: 692–701.

PEDIATRIC BONE MARROW INTERPRETATION

Mihaela Onciu, MD

KEYWORDS

- Bone marrow • Pediatric cancer • T cell • Marrow infiltrates • Genetic disorders

ABSTRACT

The evaluation of pediatric bone marrow poses specific challenges when compared with the general adult population. These challenges stem in part from the higher likelihood of congenital disorders with hematopoietic manifestations, some of which may give rise to hematologic malignancies. Familiarity with the spectrum of disorders seen in the pediatric age group allows for an appropriate and focused differential diagnosis. This review addresses the diagnostic workup of pediatric bone marrow samples, as directed by the peripheral blood and bone marrow findings in the context of the patient's clinical history. Recommendations for the appropriate use of ancillary studies in various scenarios are provided.

OVERVIEW

The evaluation of bone marrow samples obtained from children requires familiarity with the spectrum of hematologic diseases (including entities specific to this age group), as well as knowledge of the potential diagnostic pitfalls. First, it is important to realize that a large proportion of the benign and malignant disorders diagnosed during childhood are likely to be related to underlying genetic abnormalities, sometimes as the first manifestation of these defects. Another important consideration in children is that lymphoid progenitor cells (termed *hematogones*) normally present in the bone marrow are often increased in numbers as a reactive change to benign disorders or malignant neoplasms. These hematogone expansions overlap significantly with some of the most common leukemias seen in children, potentially misleading the observer toward an erroneous diagnosis of leukemia or the misclassification of a different neoplasm. Finally, certain types of malignant neoplasms with partially overlapping blastic morphologic features (so called "small blue-cell tumors"), but with vastly different biology requiring distinct therapeutic approaches, occur relatively frequently in young patients.

THE NORMAL PEDIATRIC BONE MARROW

The morphology of normal pediatric bone marrow overlaps significantly with that of adults. Two

> ### Pathologic Key Features
> #### OF PEDIATRIC BONE MARROW INTERPRETATION
>
> 1. Interpretation of pediatric bone marrow samples requires that the pathologist integrate clinical, morphologic, and ancillary study results to arrive at the correct diagnosis.
>
> 2. Congenital syndromes and florid reactive processes must always be considered in the differential diagnosis of hematologic malignancies in the pediatric population.
>
> 3. Recognition of the general pathologic pattern (hypercellular, hypocellular, or single-lineage defect) aids in narrowing the differential diagnosis when interpreting bone marrow samples from pediatric patients.

Department of Pathology, MS 250, St Jude Children's Research Hospital, 262 Danny Thomas Place, Memphis, TN 38105, USA
E-mail address: mihaela.onciu@stjude.org

Surgical Pathology 3 (2010) 1091–1125
doi:10.1016/j.path.2010.09.007

surgpath.theclinics.com

features are significantly different and may affect bone marrow interpretation: the overall cellularity and the presence of benign lymphoid precursors (hematogones), which may be markedly increased in some patients.

Most sources agree that bone marrow cellularity varies inversely with age, with a highly cellular marrow seen in very young patients and a gradual decrease seen with increasing age. Older studies using large wedge-shaped sections of bone obtained from sudden-death autopsy cases and the point-counting technique[1] reported an average cellularity of 78.8% (range 59% to 95%) in patients aged 1 to 9 years, and of 64.3% (range 41.5% to 86.6%) for patients in the second decade of life. More recent large-scale studies applied to biopsies obtained using a Jamshidi needle and direct visualization[2] have documented slightly lower marrow cellularities than previously accepted as normal values. In such studies, normal marrow cellularity was found to be about 80% in children younger than 2 years, declined to 60% to 70% by the age of 5 years, and remained relatively constant at about 60% in individuals aged 5 to 18 years.

Benign precursor B cells (also termed hematogones) are immature, often blastic-appearing lymphoid elements present in the marrow of all individuals, but particularly prominent in children.[3] These cells typically increase in number under a variety of reactive conditions, including both benign and malignant disorders. Hematogones encompass lymphoid cells with a spectrum of morphologic features, ranging from small lymphoblasts and larger blasts with homogeneous "smudgy" chromatin and cleaved nuclei, to mature-appearing lymphocytes; there are multiple intermediate forms with variable degrees of immaturity (**Fig. 1**A, B). When examined by flow cytometry, these cells show a characteristic pattern that mirrors their maturation sequence.[4] They include a minority of CD45dim+TdT+CD34+CD19+ CD10+CD20− early precursors, a majority of CD45stronger+ (but weaker than lymphocytes) TdT−CD34−CD19+CD10+CD20variably+ intermediate precursors, and a usually smaller subset of CD45 strong+CD20+ CD10+ more mature elements. These subsets vary in proportion depending on the clinical setting, with the early precursors predominating in the postchemotherapy recovery setting and the intermediate stage predominating in most other situations. These immunophenotypic profiles may also be demonstrated by immunohistochemical staining of biopsy samples. The spectrum of antigen expression in hematogones differs significantly from the strong and uniform pattern of antigen expression typically seen in B-lymphoblastic leukemia (B-ALL) (see **Fig. 1**C–F).

CLINICAL INDICATIONS FOR BONE MARROW EVALUATION IN CHILDREN

A variety of presenting clinical and laboratory findings, sometimes incidental in nature (such as extremely high, but asymptomatic leukocyte counts of chronic myeloid leukemia discovered on a routine blood examination in a primary physician's office) may trigger bone marrow evaluation in children. These findings are summarized in **Table 1**.

DIFFERENTIAL DIAGNOSIS: INTEGRATING CLINICAL AND MICROSCOPIC FEATURES AND ANCILLARY STUDIES

A combination of the clinical presenting features and peripheral blood and bone marrow morphology trigger specific diagnostic algorithms (including further ancillary studies). The following specific scenarios are discussed in the next sections, including the clinical and morphologic clues that help guide the use of ancillary studies and resolve the differential diagnosis particular to each scenario:

1. Hypercellular Bone Marrow
     Infiltration by blastic neoplastic cells
     Infiltration by histiocytic cells
     Expanded hematopoiesis (with or without fibrosis or increased blasts)
2. Hypocellular Bone Marrow
3. Selective Defects of Single Cell Lineages
     Erythroid
     Myeloid
     Megakaryocytic.

HYPERCELLULAR BONE MARROW

Much like in the adult population, the workup of a hypercellular bone marrow is guided by the morphologic features of the elements that accumulate to cause the observed increase in cellularity.

Infiltration by Blastic Neoplastic Cells

An increase in cellularity caused by sheets of blastic cells is typically related to one of the childhood hematopoietic blastic neoplasms. The distinction between these entities, which may be challenging at times, relies primarily on their morphologic and immunophenotypic features and to a lesser extent on their genetic features, as summarized in **Table 2**. Genetic features do play a major role in the subclassification of many of these neoplasms (most notably acute leukemias) into biologically

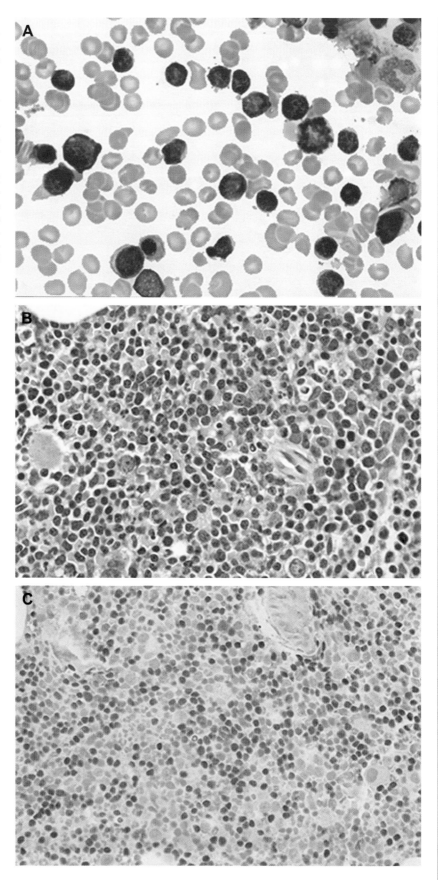

Fig. 1. Morphologic and immunohistochemical features of precursor B-cells (hematogones) in a bone marrow obtained 1 month following chemotherapy. Numerous immature lymphoid cells ranging from blastic elements to more mature lymphocytes are seen in the aspirate smear (*A*) (WG stain, ×100) and biopsy section (*B*) (H&E stain, ×40). On immunohistochemical staining, these cells are strongly positive for PAX-5 (*C*) (immunoperoxidase staining, hematoxylin counterstain ×40) and CD10 (not shown).

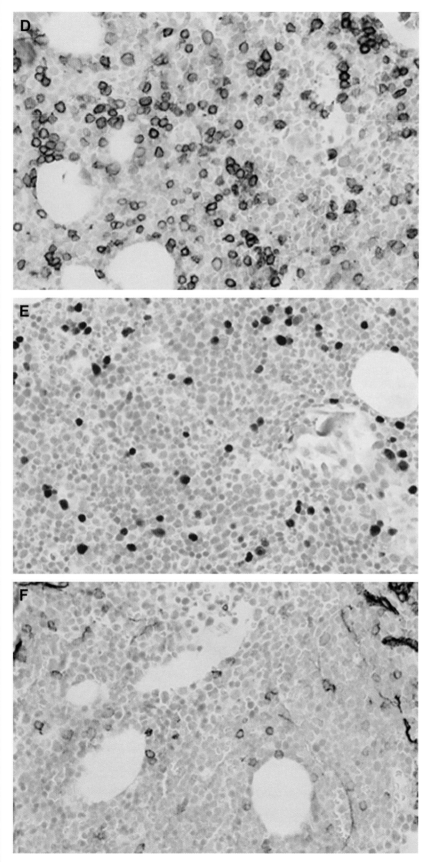

Fig. 1. Immunohistochemical features of precursor B-cells (hematogones) in a bone marrow obtained 1 month following chemotherapy. The hematogones are variably positive for CD20 (*D*), whereas only a very small subset expresses TdT (*E*) and CD34 (*F*) (*D–F*, immunoperoxidase staining, hematoxylin counterstain, ×40).

Table 1
Clinical abnormalities that may trigger bone marrow evaluation in children

Peripheral blood numerical abnormalities	Cytopenias (isolated or pancytopenia)
	    With or without dysplastic features
	    With or without circulating blasts
	Leukocytosis
	    Consisting of blasts
	    Consisting of neutrophilia and/or monocytosis with or without blasts

Systemic findings	Fever Lymphadenopathy and/or hepatosplenomegaly Bone pain Lytic bone lesions Masses suspicious for malignancy in anatomic sites that are difficult to sample; biopsy of bone marrow metastases may serve as the diagnostic sample Clinical manifestations of osteopetrosis

---

and clinically meaningful categories, each requiring a distinct therapeutic approach.[5] Therefore, every effort should be undertaken to secure tumor samples suitable for cytogenetics and molecular studies in this setting.

At a morphologic level, acute leukemias consist of neoplastic cells that are most often comparable in size to normal hematopoietic cells, are discohesive in the aspirate smears, and form diffuse sheets in the biopsy samples. One exception is that of acute megakaryoblastic leukemia (AMKL), which may yield clusters of cohesive cells mimicking metastatic solid tumors in some cases.[6] Some lymphoblastic leukemias with near-tetraploid DNA content may also show very large blasts reminiscent of solid tumor cells. Some leukemias (especially hyperdiploid B-ALL and AMKL) may be accompanied by significant marrow fibrosis, leading to a paucity of neoplastic cells available for ancillary studies in the aspirate samples. In such cases, the findings on the aspirate smears should be carefully correlated with the biopsy, as benign precursor cells (such as hematogones) may sometimes be mistaken for neoplastic elements and lead to an erroneous diagnosis of B-ALL in cases of AMKL or even aplastic anemia. Conversely, some B-ALL cases may be preceded by bone marrow aplasia and may present with markedly hypocellular marrows infiltrated by sparse neoplastic cells.[7] Immunophenotypic and genetic studies are crucial in the differential diagnosis with hematogones in all of these settings. Some acute leukemia patients may occasionally present with extensive marrow necrosis precluding a specific diagnosis; these cases may require repeat bone marrow sampling from a different anatomic site (ie, at a different iliac crest) to obtain viable diagnostic samples.

The age of the child should also be considered in the workup of all acute leukemias. In neonates and infants without Down syndrome (DS) the most common types of acute leukemia are B-ALL (**Fig. 2**A) with *MLL* gene rearrangement resulting from a t(4;11)(q21;q23) and acute monoblastic leukemias (see **Fig. 2**B) associated with *MLL* gene rearrangement, typically as a result of the t(9;11) (p22;q23). In neonates and infants with DS, a spontaneously resolving type of AMKL, the transient myeloproliferative disorder of DS, is most common.[8] In older children (including those with DS) the most common type of acute leukemia is B-ALL. Although virtually any subtype of acute myeloid leukemia (AML) may be encountered in older children, certain subtypes are particularly common. Acute monocytic/monoblastic leukemias (typically associated with 11q23 *MLL* abnormalities), AMKL (see **Fig. 2**C, D), and AML with t(8;21) occur more commonly in children than in adults.[9] In children with DS, the most common AML subtype is AMKL, which appears to be biologically distinct from AMKL in non-DS patients and is typically associated with excellent therapeutic outcomes.[8,10]

The non-Hodgkin lymphomas most commonly encountered in pediatric bone marrows are high-grade lymphomas, such as Burkitt lymphoma and anaplastic large lymphoma; these lymphomas may involve the marrow in a patchy fashion or extensively (leukemic phase) and often need to be considered in the differential diagnosis of acute leukemias. Leukemic Burkitt lymphoma (**Fig. 3**A) may overlap with B-ALL. Conversely, some cases of B-ALL, often with a hypodiploid karyotype, may feature large blasts with abundant, deeply basophilic, and even vacuolated cytoplasm reminiscent of Burkitt lymphoma. However, these cases usually show the typical precursor B immunophenotype and

Table 2
Morphologic, immunophenotypic, and genetic features of the most common blastic neoplasms encountered in pediatric bone marrow

Neoplasm Type	Morphologic Features in Bone Marrow	Immunophenotype (Antigens Commonly Expressed)	Recurring Genetic Abnormalities
B-ALL	Diffuse growth pattern Small blasts with scanty cytoplasm, homogeneously dispersed nuclear chromatin, small or absent nucleoli	*Hematopoietic:* CD43+, CD45± *B-lineage:* CD19+, CD20±, CD22+, CD79a+, PAX-5+ *Other:* CD10±, CD34±, TdT+, HLA-DR+ *Myeloid:* CD13−/+, CD15−/+, CD33−/+	t(12;21)(p13;q22); *TEL-AML1 (ETV6-RUNX1)* Hyperdiploidy (50+ chromosomes) 11q23 abnormalities; *MLL* gene rearrangements t(9;22)(q34;q11.2); *BCR-ABL* t(1;19)(q23;p13.3); *E2A-PBX1 (TCF3-PBX1)* Hypodiploidy (<46 chromosomes)
T-ALL	Diffuse or nodular growth pattern Blasts similar to B-ALL	*Hematopoietic:* CD43+, CD45+ *T-lineage:* CD2+, cytoplasmic CD3+, CD4±, CD5±, CD7+, CD8±, TCRα/β or γ/δ, CD56−/+ *Other:* CD1a+, CD10±, CD34±, HLA-DR−/+, TdT+ *Myeloid:* CD11b−/+, CD13−/+, CD33−/+, CD117−/+	t(10;11)(p13;q14); *CALM-AF10* Translocations involving *TCRα, β or γ* loci at 14q11.2, 7q35, and 7p14-15 11q23 abnormalities; *MLL* gene rearrangements
AML	Diffuse growth pattern Large blasts, with moderate to abundant cytoplasm, oval or indented nuclei, finely dispersed chromatin, prominent nucleoli, Auer rods Surface blebs in AMKL May be accompanied by dysplastic maturing myeloid cells	*Hematopoietic:* CD43+, CD45+ *Myeloid:* CD11b±, CD13+, CD14−/+, CD15−/+, CD33+, CD64±, CD117+, MPO± *Other:* CD4−/+, CD7−/+, CD19−/+, CD56−/+, HLA-DR+, CD34±, TdT−/+	Inv(16)(p13.1q22); *CBFB-MYH11* 11q23 abnormalities; *MLL* gene rearrangements t(8;21)(q22;q22); *AML1-ETO (RUNX1-RUNX1T1)* t(15;17)(q22;q12); *PML-RARA* t(1;22)(p13;q13); *RBM15-MKL*
Mixed-lineage acute leukemia	Diffuse growth pattern Blasts may resemble lymphoid or myeloid blasts Bilineal leukemias may contain distinct lymphoid and myeloid blast populations	*Hematopoietic:* CD43+, CD45+ *B-lineage:* strong CD19+, CD79a+, cytoplasmic CD22+ OR *T-lineage:* cytoplasmic CD3+ AND *Myeloid lineage:* MPO+	11q23 abnormalities; *MLL* gene rearrangements t(9;22)(q34;q11.2); *BCR-ABL*
Burkitt lymphoma	Diffuse growth pattern Large blastic cells with deeply basophilic cytoplasm, vacuoles, coarse chromatin and 1–3 nucleoli	*Hematopoietic:* CD43+, CD45+ *B-lineage:* CD19+, CD20strong+, CD22+, CD24+, surface Ig+ with light chain restriction *Other:* CD10+, BCL6+, EBV±	t(8;14)(q24;q32); *MYC-IGH* t(8;22)(q24;q11); *MYC-IGL* t(2;8)(p12;q24); *IGK-MYC*

	Morphology	Immunophenotype	Genetics
Hepatosplenic T-cell lymphoma	Intrasinusoidal growth pattern Large blastic cells with abundant pale cytoplasm, fine chromatin, prominent nucleoli HLH	CD2+, CD3+, CD4−, CD5−, CD7+, CD8−/+, CD30-, CD45+, CD56+, TCRγδ+ (rarely TCRαβ+), TIA1+, granzyme M+, granzyme B−, perforin−, EBV−	i(7)(q10)
Anaplastic large cell lymphoma, ALK+	Interstitial or diffuse growth pattern Small lymphocytes with markedly cleaved nuclei or large immunoblastic cells with basophilic granulated or vacuolated cytoplasm and/or giant bizarre Reed-Sternberg-like multinucleated cells	CD2+, CD3±, CD4+, CD5±, CD7+, CD8−, CD30+, CD43+, CD45±, ALK+, EMA+, EBV− *Myeloid antigens:* CD11c−/+, CD13−/+, CD33−/+	t(2;5)(p23;q35); *NPM-ALK* Other translocations involving the *ALK* gene
EBV+ T-cell LPD of childhood	Interstitial or diffuse growth pattern Small cells without atypia; rarely medium to large atypical lymphoid cells with irregular nuclear outlines HLH	CD2+, CD3+, CD8+, CD4−, CD56−, TIA1+, EBV+ (in acute primary EBV infection); CD8−, CD4+ (in chronic active EBV infection)	No known recurrent abnormalities
Neuroblastoma	Patchy or diffuse growth, sometimes intravascular Cohesive variably sized blastic cells with scanty cytoplasm Neuropil and rosette formation Ganglion cells and Schwannian stroma post-therapy	Chromogranin+, synaptophysin+, NSE+, NB84+ Myogenin−, desmin−, CD99−, WT1−, keratins−, TdT−, CD45−	N-MYC amplification (subset of cases)
Rhabdomyosarcoma	Patchy or diffuse growth Large cohesive and discohesive blastic cells with abundant cytoplasm; typically alveolar subtype	Myogenin+, MyoD1+, desmin+. Synaptophysin−, NSE−, chromogranin−, CD99−, TdT−, CD45−	t(2;13)(q35;q14);PAX3-FKHR (FOXO1) (70%) t(1;13)(p36;q14); PAX7-FKHR (FOXO1) (10%−15%) t(2;2)(q35;p23); PAX3-NCOA1 (<1%)
Ewing sarcoma family	Patchy or diffuse growth Small blastic cells with variable cytoplasm, often cohesive forming clusters Sometimes rosettes	CD99+ (strong membrane staining), synaptophysin+ (weak/focal). Myogenin−, MyoD1−, TdT−, CD45−, chromogranin−	EWS gene rearrangements t(11;22)(q24;q12); EWS-FLI1(85%) t(21;22)(q22;q12); EWS-ERG (10%)

Abbreviations: ALK, anaplastic lymphoma kinase; AMKL, acute megakaryoblastic leukemia; AML, acute myeloid leukemia; B-ALL, B lymphoblastic leukemia; EBV, Epstein-Barr virus; HLH, hemophagocytic lymphohistiocytosis; LPD, lymphoproliferative disease; T-ALL, T lymphoblastic leukemia.

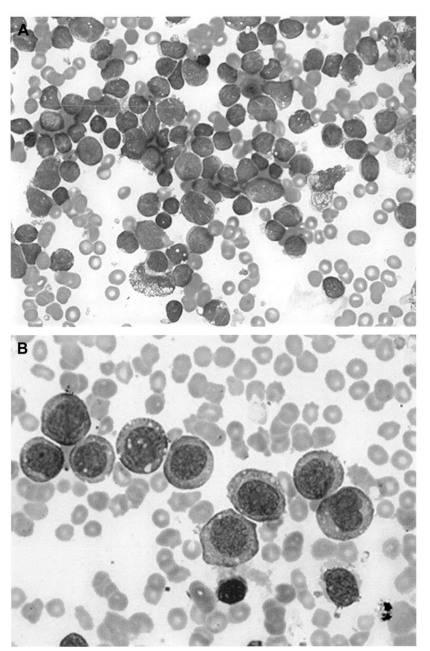

Fig. 2. Acute leukemias most commonly encountered in children. (*A*) Acute lymphoblastic leukemia in bone marrow aspirate (WG stain, ×60). (*B*) Acute monoblastic leukemia in bone marrow aspirate (WG stain, ×100).

cytogenetic abnormalities of B-ALL. Some cases of ALL with classic morphology may express complete surface immunoglobulin with light chain restriction, similar to mature B-cell neoplasms; many of these cases have *MLL* gene rearrangements.[11,12] The lymphoblastic morphology, otherwise typical precursor B immunophenotype (including expression of CD34, CD133, and/or TdT), and lack of Burkitt-type chromosomal translocations (see

Table 1) are helpful in this context. Last, some B-lymphoid neoplasms may present with extensive marrow involvement, often lacking significant extramedullary involvement, and show mixed lymphoblastic and Burkitt-type morphology as well as mixed precursor and mature B-cell immunophenotypic features (eg, expression of TdT and CD34 with strong CD20 and monotypic surface immunoglobulin).[13,14] In such cases, correlation with

Fig. 2. Acute leukemias most commonly encountered in children. (*C*) Acute megakaryoblastic leukemia (AMKL) in bone marrow aspirate, with surface "blebs" on the blasts (WG stain, ×100). (*D*) Appearance of AMKL in bone marrow biopsy section, mimicking a solid tumor (H&E stain, ×60).

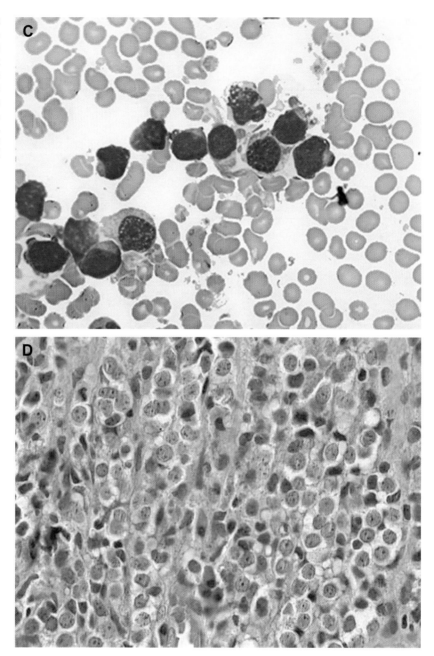

cytogenetics is essential, as the presence of a Burkitt-type chromosomal translocation involving *MYC* is typically associated with successful treatment of these leukemias with Burkitt-type therapies. At the present time, the World Health Organization (WHO) classification for such cases is controversial.

T lymphoblastic leukemia (T-ALL) should be distinguished from mature peripheral T-cell lymphomas, especially cases of that resemble more mature thymocytes, lack CD34 and TdT expression, and show strong expression of surface CD3, T-cell receptor, and CD4 or CD8. Correlation with the clinical presentation and morphologic features are essential in this context: the presence of a mediastinal mass and lymphoblastic morphology are typical of T-ALL. Conversely, in a patient with significant hepatosplenomegaly and peripheral blood cytopenias (especially thrombocytopenia) but no lymphadenopathy, the marrow should be searched for

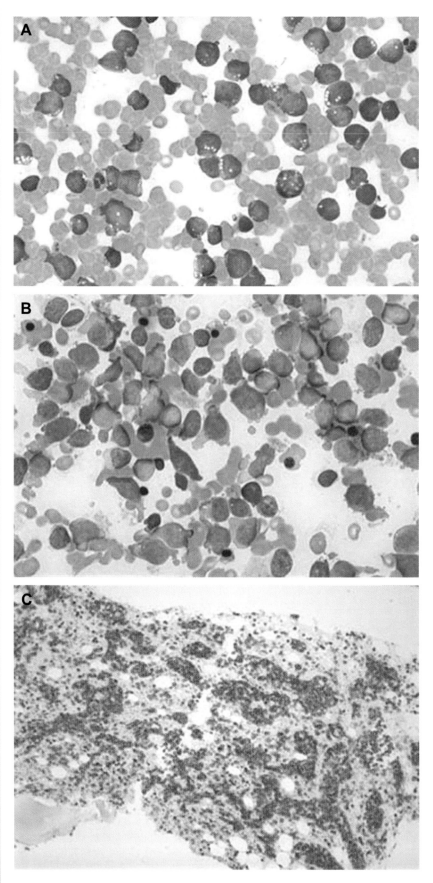

Fig. 3. High-grade lymphomas most often seen in pediatric bone marrow. (*A*) Burkitt lymphoma in bone marrow aspirate (WG stain, ×60). (*B*) Hepatosplenic T-cell lymphoma in bone marrow aspirate (WG stain, ×60). (*C*) Hepatosplenic T-cell lymphoma in bone marrow biopsy, with immunohistochemical stain for CD3 highlighting the intrasinusoidal growth pattern.

Fig. 3. High-grade lymphomas most often seen in pediatric bone marrow. (*D*) EBV+ T-cell lymphoproliferative disorder of childhood in bone marrow biopsy, with in situ hybridization for EBER (H&E stain, ×40) (*E*) demonstrating EBV expression in the lymphoma cells. (*F*) Anaplastic large cell lymphoma with leukemic involvement of peripheral blood (WG stain, ×60).

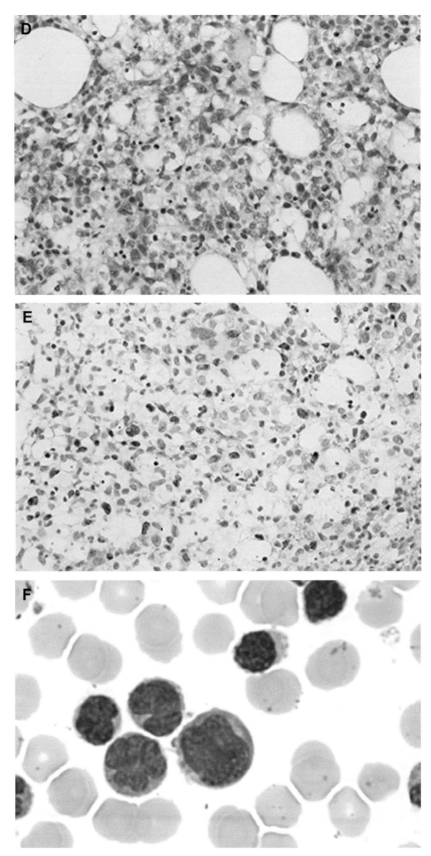

involvement by hepatosplenic T-cell lymphoma, which may be subtle. In the aspirate smears, the neoplastic cells appear large and blastic, often with surface cytoplasmic projections, resembling AML blasts (see **Fig. 3**B, C). Presentation with a hemophagocytic syndrome should also prompt careful evaluation for an associated mature T-cell lymphoma, most notably hepatosplenic T-cell lymphoma and the EBV+ T-cell lymphoproliferative disorder of childhood (see **Fig. 3**D, E). Hemophagocytic syndrome may also be encountered in children with subcutaneous panniculitis-like T-cell lymphoma, but this neoplasm does not typically involve the bone marrow. In a young patient presenting with systemic illness, leukocytosis, and diffuse lung infiltrates mimicking infection, the peripheral blood and bone marrow smears should be carefully evaluated for the presence of small, markedly atypical lymphocytes of leukemic anaplastic large cell lymphoma (see **Fig. 3**F), which may be masked in the bone marrow by florid myeloid hyperplasia and in the blood by neutrophilia.[15] In all of these cases, the use of confirmatory ancillary studies (including immunophenotype and cytogenetics) are of great help in establishing a correct diagnosis.

The "small blue cell tumors" that most often present in pediatric bone marrow include high-stage neuroblastoma and rhabdomyosarcoma (typically alveolar subtype, ARS). Less frequently, Ewing sarcoma tumors and, very rarely, advanced-stage retinoblastoma or brain tumors such as medulloblastoma and glioblastoma multiforme may extensively infiltrate the marrow, and cause a pancytopenic presentation. The pathologist examining the bone marrow may be faced with the task of establishing a primary diagnosis in patients where the marrow biopsy has been performed in lieu of sampling a more deeply seated tumor: an example would include an adrenal mass detected on imaging studies along with elevated urine catecholamines, raising the clinical suspicion of neuroblastoma. The aforementioned solid tumors are typically composed of blastic-appearing cells that may approximate or exceed the size of hematopoietic cells and usually form at least some tridimensional clusters in the aspirate smears. Occasionally, some of these tumors (especially ARS) may present as widely metastatic disease with an inconspicuous primary site. In such cases, the marrow may be extensively involved by cells that morphologically resemble monoblasts and are highly discohesive (**Fig. 4**A). Although the immunophenotypic and genetic features are typically necessary for a final diagnosis in such cases, some morphologic clues may be helpful in focusing the ancillary workup. For instance, tumor cell rosettes are typically

associated with neuroblastoma and Ewing sarcoma tumors, but not ARS, whereas neuropil, appearing as pale, eosinophilic, finely fibrillary "tails" associated with clusters of tumor cells in aspirate smears, appears to be unique to neuroblastoma (see **Fig. 4**B, C). Because of some immunophenotypic overlap, the morphologic and immunophenotypic features should always be integrated in the workup of all blastic tumors of childhood. For example, a significant percentage of pediatric B-ALL (especially hyperdiploid cases, which represent 25% to 30% of ALL cases occurring in children) may be CD45− and CD20− by immunohistochemistry on paraffin-embedded tissue sections. These features, combined with frequent strong membrane expression of CD99 in ALL, may lead to a misdiagnosis of Ewing sarcoma. As these B-ALL cases are always strongly positive for CD79a, PAX-5, and TdT, markers that are not expressed in Ewing sarcoma, it is recommended to include at least two of these markers in the immunohistochemical panels used to evaluate blastic neoplasms in such instances.

Infiltration by Histiocytic Cells

A variety of reactive, benign, and malignant entities, as well as entities of indeterminate malignant potential, may manifest as infiltrates of cells with a histiocytic appearance in pediatric bone marrow; these entities are more common in children than in adults. Their salient morphologic, immunophenotypic, and, as applicable, genetic features are summarized in **Table 3**. Because of significant morphologic and immunophenotypic overlap between a variety of entities included in this category, integration with clinical and laboratory features is critical in the workup of such cases.[16] The diagnosis of Langerhans cell histiocytosis is typically quite straightforward, because of its unique immunophenotypic profile (**Fig. 5**A, B).

Diagnosis of hemophagocytic lymphohistiocytosis (HLH) may be more difficult, as the infiltrating macrophages are often admixed with abundant T lymphocytes and have no distinctive immunophenotypic features. Often, patients with HLH are very ill, adding to the urgency of the diagnostic workup. Moreover, the hemophagocytic cells (macrophages containing erythrocytes as well as nucleated hemopoietic elements, **Fig. 5**C) may not be always present in the marrow of patients with HLH, and are not, by themselves, specific for this diagnosis. It is important to remember that, although most commonly occurring as a result of viral infection or as idiopathic/familial cases, HLH may also accompany lymphoid neoplasms, especially those of T-cell lineage.

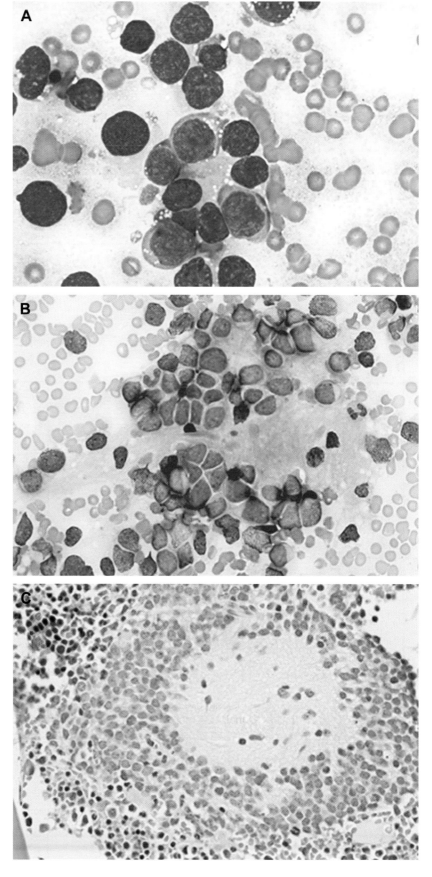

Fig. 4. Metastatic small blue cell tumors most often seen in the bone marrow. (*A*) Alveolar rhabdomyosarcoma in the bone marrow aspirate (WG stain, ×60). (*B*) Neuroblastoma in bone marrow aspirate (WG stain, ×60). (*C*) Neuroblastoma seen in bone marrow biopsy, illustrating a rosette (H&E stain, ×40).

Table 3
Clinical and pathologic features of histiocytic disorders involving pediatric bone marrow

Entity	Clinical Features	Laboratory Features	Characteristic Morphologic Features	Immunophenotype of Histiocytic Cells	Other
LCH	One or multiple lytic bone lesions Diabetes insipidus Skin rash Multisystem disease, including HSM and fever	Cytopenias Increased LFTs and inflammatory markers (in multisystem disease)	Large histiocytes with grooved nuclei; eosinophilia	CD1a+, langerin (CD207)+, S-100+, CD68+, CD11c+, CD13+, CD14±, CD15+, CD33+, CD64+, CD163+, CD4 dim+, CD45 dim+	EM: Birbeck granules
HLH	Fever HSM (may be marked)	Cytopenias Increased serum triglycerides ferritin, LFTs Coagulopathy (DIC), Decreased/absent NK cell activity Increased serum/CSF CD25	Hemophagocytic cells	CD45+, CD68+, CD163+, S-100±, CD4 dim+, CD13+, CD14+, CD15+, CD33+, CD1a−, langerin−	Germline homozygous mutations in perforin (*PRF1*) or *hMunc13-4* genes (in familial cases) Some cases associated with EBV
AMoL	Fever, pallor, weakness, fatigue, weight loss, bone pain Gingival hypertrophy, bleeding Solitary or multiple skin lesions, lung infiltrates HSM (usually not marked)	Leukocytosis with leukemic cells on blood smears Coagulopathy (DIC) Abnormal electrolytes suggesting renal tubular dysfunction	Monoblasts, promonocytes and atypical monocytes in blood and bone marrow	CD45+, CD68+, CD163+, CD11b+, CD13+, CD14±, CD15±, CD33±, CD64±, CD65±, HLA-DR+; CD34−/+, MPO−/+, S-100−, CD1a−, langerin−	Genetics: 11q23/*MLL* gene rearrangements
Infections	Symptoms depending on patient's immune status and affected organ system	Leukocytosis or leucopenia, other cytopenias Elevated inflammatory markers Positive blood, bone marrow or tissue cultures	Diffuse infiltrates or granulomata (necrotizing or non-necrotizing)	CD45+, CD68+, CD163+, S-100−/+, CD1a−, langerin−	Special stains for microorganisms (fungi, mycobacteria) may be positive
Metabolic storage disorders	HSM Neurologic deficits	Variable with disease	Gaucher cells, foamy histiocytes, PAS+/−	CD45+, CD68+, CD163+, S-100−/+, CD1a−, langerin−	Appropriate metabolic or genetic testing positive

Abbreviations: AMoL, Acute monocytic/monoblastic leukemia; CSF, cerebrospinal fluid; DIC, disseminated intravascular coagulation; EM, electron microscopy; HLH, hemophagocytic lymphohistiocytosis; HSM, hepatosplenomegaly; LCH, Langerhans cell histiocytosis; LFTs, liver function tests; MPO, myeloperoxidase.

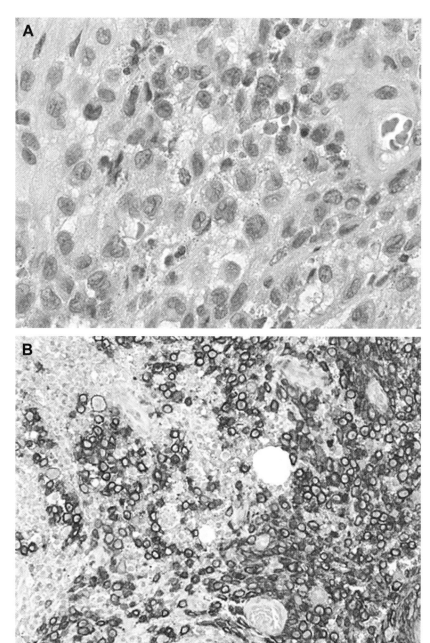

Fig. 5. Histiocytic infiltrates presenting in pediatric bone marrow. (*A*) Langerhans cell histiocytosis in the bone marrow biopsy (H&E stain, ×60). (*B*) CD1a immunohistochemistry strongly stains the Langerhans cells.

These lymphomas may involve the marrow to varying degrees concurrently with the HLH. Such an association may be seen with anaplastic large cell lymphoma, hepatosplenic T-cell lymphoma (in our experience more commonly in adolescents than younger children), and the systemic EBV+ T-cell lymphoproliferative disease of childhood (occurring in pediatric patients of any age). Careful morphologic examination of the bone marrow combined with flow cytometric and molecular studies will ensure that the diagnosis of lymphoma is not missed. Indeed, although HLH is often responsible for the characteristically fulminant clinical presentation in such cases, the appropriate therapy also includes treating the underlying lymphoma. Flow cytometric studies from the bone

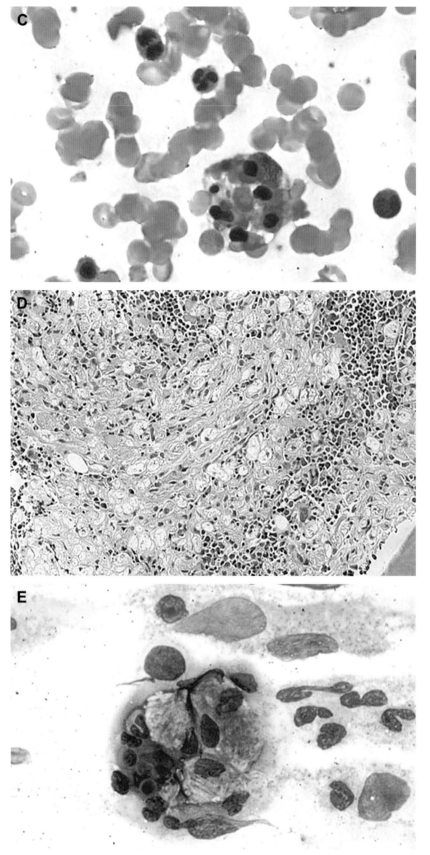

Fig. 5. Histiocytic infiltrates presenting in pediatric bone marrow. (C) Hemophagocytic cell in the bone marrow aspirate from a patient with hemophagocytic lymphohistiocytosis (WG stain, ×60). (D) Abundant Gaucher cells seen in bone marrow biopsy in a patient with Gaucher disease (H&E stain, ×20). (E) A cluster of Gaucher cells in the bone marrow aspirate from the same patient.

marrow and blood of patients with HLH should be interpreted with caution, as increased populations of cytologically atypical and immunophenotypically aberrant, but polyclonal, CD8+ lymphocytes that lack perforin expression have been described.[17] Notably, a rare report of one familial HLH case documented the prolonged presence of expanded peripheral blood populations of mature monocytes that correlated with the HLH disease activity. These cells expressed dim CD14; bright CD16; and lower levels of CD11b, CD64, and CD35, suggesting differentiation toward macrophages.[18] Thus, HLH should be considered in the differential diagnosis of acute monocytic/monoblastic leukemia (AMoL). In most cases of AMoL, correlation with the clinical presentation, peripheral blood findings, and immunophenotype allows for a relatively straightforward diagnosis. In addition, most AMoL cases in children are associated with chromosome 11q23 abnormalities and *MLL* gene rearrangements. However, it should be kept in mind that in tissue sections, some AMoL infiltrates may appear deceptively well differentiated and may mimic infiltrates of mature macrophages. Also, AMoL cells are often CD34−, adding difficulty to the diagnosis of a precursor monocytic neoplasm. Finally, bone marrow infiltrates of histiocytes with foamy or striated cytoplasm should prompt an adequate diagnostic workup for a glycogen storage disorder (such as Niemann-Pick syndrome or Gaucher disease) (see **Fig. 5**D, E).

Expanded Hematopoiesis With or Without Increase in Blasts and With or Without Fibrosis

The disorders most commonly associated with hypercellular bone marrow in children are summarized in **Table 4**. Expansion of one or several lines of hematopoietic cells may be present in association with increased peripheral blood counts, such as in myeloproliferative neoplasms (MPN), autoimmune diseases, reactive conditions, or secondary to administration of hematopoietic growth factors; decreased peripheral counts, such as in myelodysplastic syndromes (MDS) and some nutritional deficiencies; or a combination of mechanisms, such as in myelodysplastic/myeloproliferative neoplasms (MDS/MPN) or toxic agents. Some of these conditions may be associated with marrow fibrosis, typically seen as an increase in reticulin fibers and, less commonly, as collagen fibrosis detected by trichrome stain.

Integration of the clinical data with the morphologic findings and genetic features is critical in the evaluation of such hypercellular bone marrows. The clinical findings are often the strongest clues

in establishing if the findings are likely to be reactive in nature or caused by a primary marrow process. A recent history of hematopoietic growth factor (eg, granulocyte colony stimulating factor [G-CSF] or granulocyte/macrophage colony stimulating factor [GM-CSF]) administration for primary or chemotherapy-induced neutropenia will suffice to explain a hypercellular (often 100% cellular) marrow with marked myeloid hyperplasia, left-shifted myeloid maturation, toxic granulation, Döhle bodies, and even dysplastic changes in granulocytes. These changes overlap closely with those seen in bacterial sepsis occurring in immunocompetent children. Clinical and laboratory data consistent with an autoimmune disorder (juvenile rheumatoid arthritis or, in older teenagers, systemic lupus) can explain a hypercellular bone marrow that may feature reticulin fibrosis, one or more expanded cell lines, and cytopenia(s) owing to peripheral destruction. Although dyserythropoiesis may be seen if the disease manifests with hemolytic anemia, dysplasia in other cell lines would not be expected in such a context. A similar picture may be encountered in disorders that exhibit increased peripheral destruction of select cell lines, which will be discussed later. Nutritional deficiencies, especially vitamin B12 deficiency, can be associated with hypercellularity (most prominently attributable to erythroid expansion) and megaloblastic and/or dysplastic changes in erythroid and myeloid elements. Association with peripheral cytopenias should be helpful in the differential diagnosis from an MPN, but excluding MDS may still be problematic, especially because transient clonal chromosomal abnormalities have been reported in this context.[19] Thus, correlation with serum vitamin B12 levels remains critical in the workup of any suspected MDS. Bone marrow samples are rarely obtained in children with iron deficiency, as the characteristic abnormalities in red cell indices and iron studies typically confirm that diagnosis. However, we have rarely encountered iron deficiency as an incidental finding in patients being staged for a malignant tumor associated with occult gastrointestinal bleeding. Iron deficiency is typically associated with erythroid expansion and often with megakaryocytic hyperplasia in the bone marrow. The absence of stainable storage iron in the marrow is helpful in this context. We have also encountered a rare case of peripheral blood cytopenias with marrow hypercellularity and dysplastic changes associated with severe rickets, corrected with vitamin D supplementation.

The MPN entity most commonly encountered in children is chronic myelogenous leukemia (CML). Other major categories of MPN are virtually absent in children; rare cases of idiopathic polycythemia

Table 4
Disorders associated with increased bone marrow cellularity due to expanded hematopoiesis most common in children

Disorder	Clinical/Laboratory Features	Peripheral Blood Abnormalities	Bone Marrow Morphologic Features	Other
Chronic myelogenous leukemia	Asymptomatic (incidental leukocytosis) or Fatigue, weight loss, night sweats Splenomegaly	Marked leukocytosis with neutrophilia, basophilia, eosinophilia, thrombocytosis Myeloid left shift with myeloblasts present	Markedly hypercellular with myeloid and megakaryocyte hyperplasia Predominance of promyelocytes and myelocytes Basophilia, eosinophilia No significant myeloid or erythroid dysplasia Many small hypolobulated megakaryocytes Variable increase in myeloblasts Pseudo-Gaucher cells Increased reticulin	t(9;22)(q34;q11.2); *BCR-ABL1*
Juvenile myelomonocytic leukemia	Fevers Hepatosplenomegaly, skin rash Bleeding History of NF1 in some patients	Leukocytosis with neutrophilia and immature myeloid elements Marked monocytosis Anemia, thrombocytopenia	Markedly hypercellular with myeloid hyperplasia Variable increase in monocytes Rarely basophilia with abnormal basophils, eosinophilia Variable degrees of dysplasia Variable increase in myeloblasts Increased reticulin fibers	Increased HbF Hypersensitivity to GM-CSF Cytogenetic abnormalities (monosomy 7)
Myelodysplastic syndrome[a]	Manifestations of cytopenia(s) De novo or therapy-related	Selective cytopenias or pancytopenia	Hypercellular or hypocellular with variable increase or aplasia of cell lines Dysplastic features Increased blasts Increased reticulin	Cytogenetic abnormalities (-5, del 5q; -7, del 7q, other)

Condition	Clinical features	Blood findings	Bone marrow findings	Other
Hypereosinophilic syndrome	Skin rash, mucosal ulcerations, congestive heart failure, neurologic deficits, Family history of eosinophilia	Eosinophilia (>1.5 × 10⁹/L).	Hypercellular with marked eosinophilia, Increased reticulin, Increased lymphoblasts if associated with lymphoblastic leukemia/lymphoma	Evaluate for *FGFR1, PDGFRA* abnormalities or a t(5;14), *IL3-IGH* abnormality
Autoimmune disorders (JRA, SLE)	Fevers, Skin rash, arthralgias, LAD, Renal dysfunction, Coagulation abnormalities	Leukocytosis or leukopenia, anemia, thrombocytopenia	Hypercellular, Reticulin fibrosis, Hyperplasia of all or selected cell lines	Autoantibodies present; Hemolytic anemia
Infection in immunocompetent patient	Fevers, Skin rash, LAD, Site-specific manifestations	Leukocytosis, neutrophilia, Immature myeloid elements, Monocytosis, Toxic granulation, vacuoles and Döhle bodies in granulocytes	Hypercellular with myeloid hyperplasia and increased immature myeloid elements	Microorganisms (bacteria) identified on special stains or cultures
Growth factors (G-CSF, GM-CSF, EPO)	History of cytopenias, or post-chemotherapy, or post HSCT	Similar to infection for G-CSF and GM-CSF, Prominent monocytosis for GM-CSF, Many immature myeloid and monocytic cells present, Myeloblasts often present	*G-CSF/GM-CSF:* Hypercellular with myeloid hyperplasia, increased immature myeloid elements, toxic changes in granulocytes; no abnormalities in other cell lines. Increased immature monocytes and eosinophilia for GM-CSF. *EPO:* No myeloid abnormalities; erythroid hyperplasia, with or without dysplastic changes in erythroid precursors	None
Nutritional deficiencies (vitamin B12, folate, iron, vitamin D)	Anemia	Macrocytic or microcytic anemia, Thrombocytosis	Expansion of one or several cell lines (mainly erythroid, megakaryocytic) with or without dysplastic/ megaloblastic changes Absent stainable marrow iron in iron deficiency.	Decreased iron studies Decreased vitamin B12 or red cell folate levels

Abbreviations: EPO, erythropoietin; G-CSF, granulocyte colony stimulating factor; GM-CSF, granulocyte/macrophage colony stimulating factor; HbF, Hemoglobin F; HSCT, hematopoietic stem cell transplantation; JRA, juvenile rheumatoid arthritis; LAD, lymphadenopathy; NF1, neurofibromatosis type 1; SLE, systemic lupus erythematosus.
[a] See also **Table 6.**

or thrombocytosis are more likely to be caused by constitutional abnormalities in specific receptor or receptor signaling pathway genes. A CML diagnosis is relatively straightforward in cases presenting in chronic phase. However, cases presenting in accelerated phase (typically with increased blasts and some peripheral blood cytopenias) may present a challenge owing to partial overlap with MDS/MDN entities such as juvenile myelomonocytic leukemia (JMML). Features that help with this differential diagnosis are the identification of the BCR-ABL1 fusion that can be detected in blood and bone marrow by conventional cytogenetics, fluorescent in situ hybridization (FISH) or reverse-transcriptase polymerase chain reaction (RT-PCR) in CML. Megakaryoblastic differentiation of blasts is present in many of the accelerated and blastic CML cases that occur in children, but is not expected in JMML. In our experience, the initial diagnosis of JMML is often very challenging, primarily because of its significant clinical and pathologic overlap with a variety of infectious and autoimmune disorders. The diagnostic criteria established for JMML[20,21] are, with the exceptions of clonal cytogenetic abnormalities and in vitro hypersensitivity to GM-CSF, nonspecific. In addition to nonspecific clinical features, JMML cases often lack significant morphologic dysplasia, whereas the peripheral blood count abnormalities that constitute diagnostic criteria for JMML (leukocytosis with myeloid left shift, monocytosis, anemia, thrombocytopenia) can be encountered in reactive conditions. Conventional cytogenetics demonstrate clonal abnormalities such as monosomy 7 in less than half of patients with JMML. In vitro hypersensitivity to GM-CSF is a helpful diagnostic test, but it is offered only by a limited number of reference laboratories and results may not be immediately available. Last, elevated levels of fetal hemoglobin may be seen in any disorder associated with stress-erythropoiesis (including hypersplenism, which may be present in many myeloid disorders and reactive conditions, and hemoglobinopathies). Moreover, measurements of hemoglobin F may be noncontributory because of recent red cell transfusions administered to these sometimes severely anemic patients. In cases of suspected JMML where clonal cytogenetic abnormalities are lacking, careful exclusion of all possible infectious and autoimmune causes is critical for establishing a diagnosis of MDS/MPN most consistent with JMML.

Although children may develop a form of hypocellular MDS, designated as refractory cytopenia of childhood in the 2008 WHO Classification of Hematopoietic Neoplasms,[5] a hypercellular,

"adult-type" MDS may also occur in this age group, both as a de novo and as a therapy-related disease. This type of MDS is often easier to diagnose than the hypocellular subtype. It typically features persistent cytopenias associated with striking multilineage dysplasia, often with increased myeloblasts and even Auer rods. Clonal cytogenetic abnormalities may or may not be present. Therapy-related MDS (t-MDS) usually has a similarly dramatic morphologic appearance, often with ring sideroblasts and characteristic clonal cytogenetic abnormalities involving chromosomes 5 and 7. Notably, it is not unusual for t-MDS in children to develop after a much shorter latency period than the 5 to 10 years typically described for adults treated with alkylating agents and/or ionizing radiation; this may reflect a genetic background predisposing to neoplastic disorders seen in some pediatric patients. The most extreme example seen in our practice was that of a patient who developed t-MDS while still receiving chemotherapy for a solid tumor.

Last, marrow hypercellularity may be associated with hypereosinophilic syndrome/chronic eosinophilic leukemia. Although this entity does not typically constitute a challenge from a morphologic standpoint, it is important to remember the differential diagnosis of a different and sometimes subtle hematopoietic neoplasm. In children, this is most commonly B-lymphoblastic leukemia with t(5;14) and IL3-IGH fusion (Fig. 6). T lymphoblastic leukemia/lymphoma with rearrangements of PDGFRA (such as the FIPIL1-PDGFRA fusion)[22] or FGFR1 may also occur in children. Systemic mastocytosis may occur in children and manifest with a hypercellular marrow and blood and marrow eosinophilia; recognition of the dense aggregates of atypical mast cells are critical at establishing this diagnosis.

HYPOCELLULAR BONE MARROW

Examination of hypocellular bone marrow samples poses distinct challenges: one has to differentiate between secondary myelosuppression, aplastic anemia (AA), a congenital bone marrow failure syndrome, and hypoplastic MDS (Table 5). Secondary myelosuppression is often relatively straightforward to establish through correlation with the clinical history and spontaneous resolution after a relatively brief (3- to 4-week) follow-up. Clues to secondary myelosuppression in the bone marrow biopsy appearance are stromal changes (accumulation of lightly basophilic glycosaminoglycan ground substance) that suggest recent injury to the marrow leading to cell drop-out (Fig. 7A, B). In contrast, completely

Fig. 6. Acute lymphoblastic leukemia with eosinophilia and t(5;14). (*A*) Bone marrow aspirate smear shows blasts amid numerous eosinophils (WG stain, ×100). (*B*). The prominent eosinophilia is also evident on the bone marrow biopsy (H&E stain, ×40).

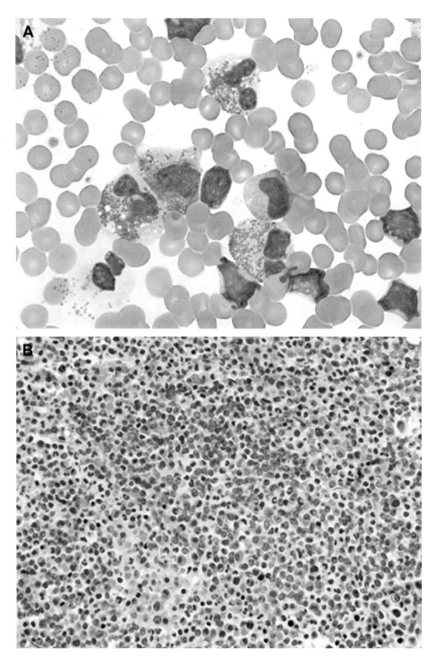

fatty marrows are usually seen in established aplastic anemia and bone marrow failure syndromes (see **Fig. 7**C). A recent history of a respiratory or gastrointestinal viral infection can often be elicited in cases of hypocellular marrow because of secondary myelosuppression. A particularly dramatic presentation may be seen in patients with sickle cell disease or other congenital red cell disorders who develop a sudden aplastic crisis, usually related to parvovirus B19 infection.

A wide variety of drugs and nutritional deficiencies may also lead to hypoplastic bone marrow. An example of the latter is anorexia nervosa, typically occurring in teenage girls, which has been associated with pancytopenia, macrocytosis and marrow hypoplasia.[22,23]

Acquired AA may be difficult to distinguish from the aforementioned secondary myelosuppression. However, unlike the latter, acquired AA shows persistence or progression of the cytopenias and

Table 5
Disorders associated with decreased bone marrow cellularity encountered in children

Disorder	Clinical Features	Peripheral Blood Findings	Bone Marrow Findings	Genetics
Secondary myelosuppression (viral, drugs)	Cytopenias develop after viral syndrome, other acute illness, drug administration	Variable cytopenias May show dysplastic features	Hypocellular with fat and "empty" basophilic stroma (serous atrophy) Variable lineage involvement Changes resolve spontaneously within 3–4 weeks	No clonal abnormalities; serologic or molecular testing may be positive for a specific virus
Myelodysplastic syndrome (refractory cytopenia of childhood)	None or fatigue, fever, infection, bleeding	Variable cytopenias Macrocytosis Dysplastic granulocytes Blasts (<2%)	Normocellular or hypocellular Variable decrease in individual cell lines Dysplasia in at least 2 lineages (at least 10% of cells) Blasts <5%	Clonal cytogenetic abnormalities (monosomy 7, complex karyotypes, trisomy 8)
Aplastic anemia	Fatigue, infections, bruising May have exposure to drugs, pesticides, solvents or prior hepatitis May have PNH	Variable cytopenias (thrombocytopenia consistently present) Decreased reticulocytes Macrocytosis	Hypocellular marrow with panhypoplasia or selective hypoplasia (megakaryocytes markedly decreased or absent) Erythroid elements may show megaloblastic dyserythropoiesis Increased mast cells Decreased iron in patients with PNH No reticulin fibrosis	N/A

Syndrome	Clinical features	Peripheral blood	Bone marrow	Genetics
Fanconi anemia	Skin hyperpigmentation, short stature, upper limb malformations	Pancytopenia (thrombocytopenia develops first) Macrocytosis Increased HgbF and i antigen	Similar to aplastic anemia	Increased chromosomal fragility; mutations in genes of the Fanconi anemia complex (FANC, including biallelic mutations of FANCD1/BRCA2)
Dyskeratosis congenita (DKC)	Reticulated skin hyperpigmentation, dystrophic nails, tooth decay, hair loss, leukoplakia	Pancytopenia	Similar to aplastic anemia	Short telomeres (flow-FISH assay of blood leukocytes); mutations in DKC pathway genes (including DKC1, TERT, TERC, NOLA2, NOLA3, TINF1)
Shwachman-Diamond syndrome	Exocrine pancreas insufficiency, skeletal abnormalities, endocrinopathies, cardiomyopathy, neurocognitive defects	Pancytopenia (neutropenia may be mild or "cyclic") Decreased reticulocytes Increased HgbF	Variably cellular, Dysplastic features seen in all cell lines No increase in blasts Some cases may evolve to aplastic marrow	Chromosomal abnormalities: del (20q), inv (7q); Mutations in SDBS gene
Dubowitz syndrome	Craniofacial abnormalities, eczema, growth retardation, mental retardation, frequent infections	Variable cytopenias	Similar to aplastic anemia	No specific known genetic abnormalities; a clinical diagnosis.
Reticular dysgenesis	SCID and sensorineural deafness present at birth	Markedly decreased or absent granulocytes and lymphocytes	Hypocellular marrow with selective decrease in lymphoid elements Myeloid elements decreased and blocked at promyelocyte stage	Mutations in AK2 gene

Abbreviations: AK2, adenylate kinase 2 gene; *BRCA2*, breast/ovarian cancer susceptibility gene (monoallelic mutations result in increased breast and ovarian cancer susceptibility); *SBDS*, Schwachman-Bodian-Diamond syndrome gene; SCID, severe combined immunodeficiency; PNH, paroxysmal nocturnal hemoglobinuria.

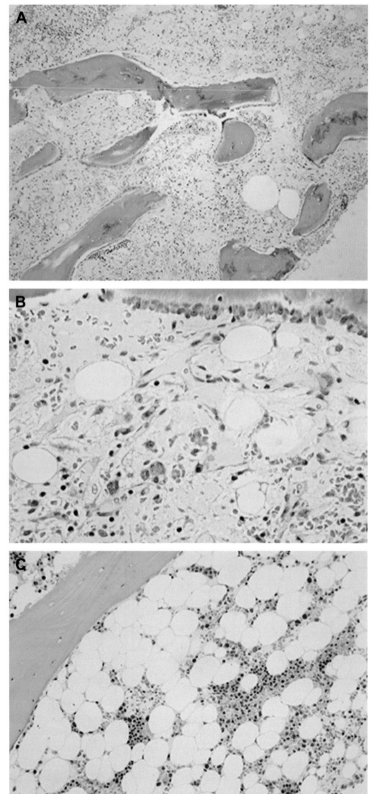

Fig. 7. Hypocellular bone marrow examples. (*A*) Profound secondary myelosuppression in a 2-month-old infant who developed severe pancytopenia shortly after a diarrheal illness. (*B*) High-power view from the same case, showing lightly basophilic stroma indicating acute marrow injury. (*C*) Bone marrow biopsy sample from a 12-year-old girl with persistent, severe aplastic anemia (H&E stain, ×20).

marrow hypocellularity on follow-up. Although the degree of marrow hypocellularity in AA can be variable, it is notable that significant thrombocytopenia associated with megakaryocyte hypoplasia is a consistent feature. As previously mentioned, the rare presentation of B lymphoblastic leukemia following an aplastic marrow episode should be considered in the differential diagnosis of AA: such a presentation has been reported to occur in about 2% of patients with B-ALL. The leukemia typically follows the aplastic episode within a few months.[22,23]

The distinction between acquired AA in a child and an inherited bone marrow failure (BMF) syndrome may be very difficult if not impossible based only on the bone marrow morphology. In fact, in practice this distinction is typically left to the treating clinician, who must incorporate a variety of clinical and laboratory features, including genetic testing, to diagnose and correctly classify these disorders. The classic developmental abnormalities associated with the various BMF syndromes may not be manifest at the time of the bone marrow evaluation in a significant percentage of these patients; this is why approximately 20% of the children thought to have a BMF syndrome remain without a specific subclassification of their disease.[22,23] There is significant overlap between the morphologic findings in disorders such as acquired AA, Fanconi anemia (FA), and dyskeratosis congenita (DKC). However, the distinction between these entities is clinically critical, as the management of patients with FA and DKC is markedly different from that of patients with AA: FA and DKC do not respond to immunosuppressive therapy used to treat AA and these patients require upfront bone marrow transplantation. Because of congenital defects in DNA repair and telomere length, bone marrow transplantation in these patients uses modified conditioning regimens and a different sibling donor screening strategy from transplantation in AA patients. FA and DKC patients must also be screened for secondary malignancies.[22,24,25] Thus, upfront evaluations for these disorders using appropriate testing (see **Table 5**) is becoming a standard of care in children with presumed AA. In some cases of hypoplastic bone marrow in infants, the pathologist may be able to detect morphologic clues associated with particular entities. This is often the case in Shwachman-Diamond syndrome, where the presence of characteristic multilineage dysplasia (**Fig. 8**) and chromosomal abnormalities in the context of the typical skeletal abnormalities can lead to the correct diagnosis.[26]

Another important challenge in hypoplastic marrow in pediatric patients is posed by the distinction between AA, a congenital BMF syndrome, and hypoplastic MDS. The latter entity may arise de novo or in the background of AA or a congenital BMF syndrome, both of which carry an increased risk of myeloid malignancies. These diagnostic challenges result from the fact that the marrow aspirates in all of these entities tend to be hypocellular, allowing for evaluation of a relatively small number of cells for dysplasia and often rendering cytogenetic studies very difficult. In addition, AA and the BMF syndromes may be associated with dyspoietic changes, especially megaloblastic dyserythropoiesis, even in the absence of MDS. The difficulty is further complicated by the fact that FISH studies of AA have uncovered small clones harboring abnormalities such as monosomy 7 and trisomy 8 in marrows without any morphologic or conventional cytogenetic evidence of MDS. It appears that whereas AA and hypoplastic MDS harboring trisomy 8 can be responsive to immunosuppressive therapy, the presence of a monosomy 7 renders this therapy insufficient, and requires consideration of bone marrow transplantation as a therapeutic option.[23,27,28] The bone marrow of patients with FA may also harbor transient clones that appear and disappear on consecutive evaluations, suggesting that stringent criteria should be used when diagnosing an emerging MDS in this context. With all of these caveats in mind, the criteria for diagnosing hypoplastic/hypocellular MDS remain the combination of persistent, unexplained peripheral blood cytopenias, dysplasia present in at least 2 cell lines (and involving at least 10% of the cells of each lineage), and often persistent clonal cytogenetic abnormalities. The importance of integrating all of these findings is underscored by the fact that, in some MDS cases (especially those associated with monosomy 7), the marrow may not show significant abnormalities of cellularity or morphology for a very long follow-up period, whereas the persistent clonal abnormality can be consistently demonstrated by cytogenetics. Last, one should evaluate all patients with AA, BMF syndromes, and hypocellular MDS for the presence of paroxysmal nocturnal hemoglobinuria (PNH) clones, which has been reported in approximately 20% of children with AA[22,23] and 18% of patients with low-grade MDS (refractory anemia).[29] In the latter, it appears to portend a better prognosis and is associated with a benign course and responsiveness to immunosuppressive therapy. In both of these settings, the PNH clones may be clinically and biochemically apparent as mild to moderate disease (typically associated with <30% glycosyl-phosphatidylinositol-anchored protein-deficient granulocytes in peripheral blood, as detected by

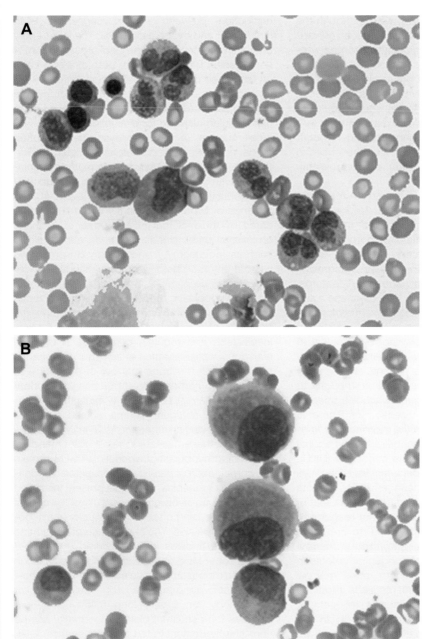

Fig. 8. Morphologic abnormalities in the bone marrow aspirate from an infant with Shwachman-Diamond syndrome. (*A*) Dysplastic granulocytes. (*B*) Predominance of small, hypolobulated megakaryocytes (WG stain, ×60).

flow cytometry) or even as subclinical disease, with no apparent intravascular hemolysis and less than 1% abnormal granulocytes in peripheral blood.[29] Among the latter patients, only 10% to 15% may develop clinically apparent PNH, typically after several years of immunosuppressive therapy.[29]

SELECTIVE DEFECTS OF SINGLE CELL LINEAGES

Bone marrow samples from children with peripheral blood abnormalities may show a selective increase or decrease of a single cell lineage, with or without morphologic or maturation abnormalities, whereas the other cell lines appear relatively unaffected. These abnormalities may be associated with decreased, normal, or variably increased marrow cellularity. The most common disorders and their etiologies are summarized in **Table 6**. As with other bone marrow abnormalities, corroboration with the clinical and laboratory findings is critical in establishing the significance of these findings. The presence of peripheral blood abnormalities since birth or early infancy (and persistence past the neonatal period) is generally suggestive of a congenital rather then an acquired disorder. In most of such cases, the hematologic abnormalities are associated with developmental abnormalities, which offer very important clues as to the specific diagnosis and/or may suggest further appropriate ancillary studies and genetic testing. Conversely, reactive etiologies underline most acquired single cell lineage defects. In some of these disorders, particular morphologic abnormalities seen in the affected cell lines may offer additional clues as to the etiology.

Erythroid Abnormalities

Evaluation of the erythroid lineage should include an assessment of cell numbers, morphology, and iron staining (with evaluation for iron stores and ring sideroblasts). Reactive expansions of erythroid precursors may be florid and are often associated with variable degrees of dyserythropoiesis, even in the absence of MDS or a nutritional deficiency. Therefore, such abnormalities should be interpreted with caution, especially when they are limited to this cell line. Congenital red cell aplasias are almost always associated with Diamond-Blackfan anemia.[30] Outside this context, secondary causes of pure red cell aplasia should be considered, such as parvovirus B19 infection or paraneoplastic pure red cell aplasia.[31] The presence of ring sideroblasts associated with anemia should raise a differential diagnosis that includes congenital disorders (especially in infants) as well as acquired disorders (especially in older children). Possible etiologies for the latter include drugs, toxins, copper deficiency, zinc excess, and MDS. Congenital disorders include the rare X-linked and autosomal dominant congenital sideroblastic anemia; pathologic clues to this diagnosis include the presence of dimorphic (microcytic and macrocytic) red cells in the peripheral smear and numerous ring sideroblasts in the bone marrow aspirate. One should also consider Pearson syndrome, in which prominent vacuolization in red cell precursors (and sometimes in myeloid elements and lymphocytes) are important clues (**Fig. 9**A). Normoblast expansions accompanied by anemia and not explained by a nutritional deficiency or other extrinsic factors may be caused by congenital dyserythropoietic anemia (CDA). In most cases of CDA, the suspicion arises after excluding other factors. The diagnosis may be confirmed by genetic testing in the case of CDA subtype 1. Electron microscopy of the marrow shows abnormalities characteristic for one of the CDA subtypes 1 through 3 (see **Fig. 9**B).[32] Although electron microscopy is still considered by many

as the "gold standard" test required for diagnosing CDA, it has been increasingly considered obsolete by many clinicians, who favor the use of other clinical and laboratory features (such as the Ham test) as acceptable.[32] One important entity to be considered in the differential diagnosis of CDA is parvovirus B19 infection occurring in the background of sickle cell disease or other chronic hemolytic conditions. In immunodeficient patients, rather than the classic red cell aplasia accompanied by giant proerythroblasts (see **Fig. 9**C), one can see a marked erythroid expansion with prominent dyserythropoiesis (see **Fig. 9**D) and sometimes numerous inclusions in normoblasts.[33,34] Finally, patients with undiagnosed hemoglobinopathies may present with stress erythropoiesis, with marked erythroid hyperplasia and dysplastic changes in erythroid elements (see **Fig. 9**E). Correlation with patient ethnicity, family history, and hemoglobin electrophoresis are helpful in diagnosing this cause of anemia and erythroid hyperplasia.

Bone marrow erythroid expansions associated with polycythemia are virtually never attributable to an MPN such as polycythemia vera in the pediatric age group. Most often these are secondary polycythemias related to environmental factors (such as smoking in teenagers) or defects in oxygen transport by erythrocytes attributable to high-oxygen affinity hemoglobins, 2,3-DPG deficiency, or methemoglobinemia. Such secondary polycythemias are associated with appropriately high levels of erythropoietin (EPO). Rarely, when all of these causes have been excluded, one may consider familial polycythemias associated with increased sensitivity to EPO owing to mutations in the receptor gene; these patients show normal or decreased levels of EPO.[35] Whether reactive or congenital, pediatric polycythemias are typically associated with minimal dyserythropoiesis, lack other cell line abnormalities, and show no evidence of marrow fibrosis.

Myeloid Abnormalities

Isolated myeloid abnormalities—whether associated with increase or decrease in myeloid precursors—are most often reactive in the pediatric age group. Reactive increases may often be associated with changes such as toxic granulation and Döhle bodies in the granulocytes and a shift toward immature myeloid precursors. Myelosuppression, commonly caused by drugs or recent viral infections, is usually associated with decreases in other cell lines. One should be extremely cautious in interpreting the extreme left-shift and even apparent dysplastic changes

Table 6
Pediatric bone marrow abnormalities selectively involving individual cell lineages

Affected Lineage	Numerical Abnormality	Mechanism of Numerical Abnormality	Disorder	Etiology
Myeloid	Increase	Reactive[a]	Infection, inflammation, acute stress, corticosteroid therapy; autoimmune destruction	Specific to each disorder
		Ineffective myelopoiesis	Myelokathexis (WHIM syndrome)	*CXCR4* mutations
			Chediak-Higashi syndrome	*CHS1* mutations
			Idiopathic chronic neutropenia	Increased apoptosis (mechanism unknown)
	Decrease	Defect in production	Secondary myelosuppresion (drugs, infection)	Variable mechanisms
			Kostman syndrome	*ELA2, HAX1* or *G6PC3* mutations; secondary *CSF3R* mutations
			Cyclic neutropenia	*ELA2* mutations
Erythroid	Increase	Reactive[a] (appropriate response to endogenous EPO)	Hemolysis (autoimmune, trauma, PNH), hypersplenism, high-affinity hemoglobin, 2,3-DPG deficiency, methemoglobinemia, hypoxia, red cell defects (spherocytosis, thalassemia).	Specific to each disorder
		EPO hypersensitivity	Familial polycythemia	*EPOR* mutations
		Inefficient erythropoiesis	Nutritional deficiencies	Vitamin B12, folate, iron deficiency
			Congenital dyserythropoietic anemias (I-VIII)	*CDAN1* mutations in CDA type 1
			Congenital sideroblastic anemias (ring sideroblasts present)	*ALAS*, ferrochelatase and COPRO-oxidase mutations (in X-linked form); autosomal forms; porphyrias.
			Low-grade MDS (refractory anemia)	Known or unknown acquired clonal genetic abnormalities

			Disorder	Cause / Genetics
	Decrease	Defect in production	Transient erythroblastopenia of childhood	Infection with parvovirus B19
			Other acquired pure red cell aplasia	Viral infections, drugs, neoplasms (lymphoma, thymoma), autoimmune (antibodies or T-cell mediated)
			Diamond-Blackfan anemia (congenital)	RPS19 mutations
			Pearson syndrome (congenital)	Mitochondrial DNA deletions
Megakaryocytes	Increase	Reactive[a]	Acquired: Immune platelet destruction (ITP, auto-antibodies), hypersplenism, TTP/HUS, DIC, trauma, iron deficiency Constitutional: platelet dysfunction/giant platelet syndromes (Bernard-Soulier, May-Hegglin)	Specific to each disorder
		Defect in regulation of platelet homeostasis	Hereditary thrombocythemia	TPO gene mutations leading to increased TPO levels; Activating mutations in c-MPL
	Decrease	Defect in production	Secondary (drugs, viral infections, autoimmune)	Specific to each disorder
			X-linked amegakaryocytic thrombocytopenia	Mutations of c-MPL resulting in decreased or absent receptor function
			Thrombocytopenia absent radii (congenital)	Specific genetic defect unknown (microdeletion on chromosome 1q)
			Cyclic thrombocytopenia (congenital or acquired)	Unknown etiology

Abbreviations: ALAS, aminolevulinate synthase; c-MPL, thrombopoietin receptor; CHS1, Chediak-Higashi syndrome 1 (LYST) gene; CSF3R, gene coding for the intracytoplasmic domain of the G-CSF receptor; CXCR4, C-X-C motif chemokine receptor 4; DIC, disseminated intravascular coagulation; ELA2, neutrophil elastase 2 gene; EPO, erythropoietin; EPOR, erythropoietin receptor gene; G6PC3, glucose-6-phosphate catalytic subunit 3 gene; HAX1, HS-1-associated protein X-1 gene; ITP, idiopathic thrombocytopenic purpura; TTP/HUS, thrombotic/thrombocytopenic purpura/hemolytic-uremic syndrome; TPO, thrombopoietin; WHIM, warts, hypogammaglobulinemia, infectious, myelokathexis.

[a] Marrow reacting appropriately to increased extramedullary destruction or other increased demand, via physiologic regulatory mechanisms.

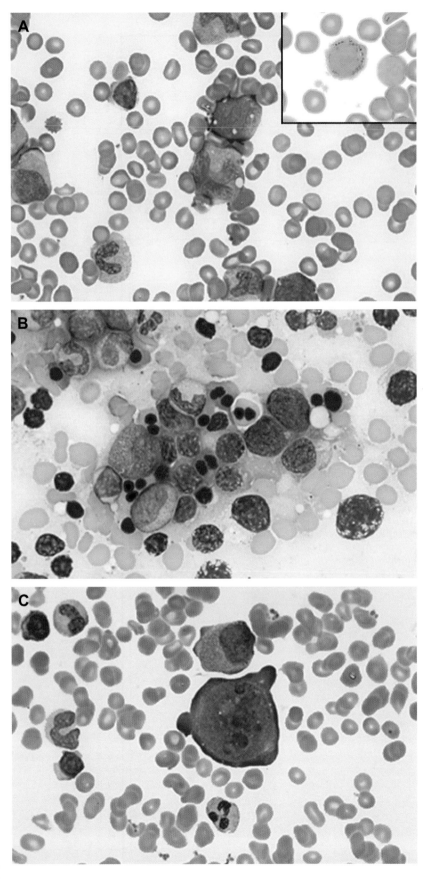

Fig. 9. Abnormalities affecting the erythroid lineage in pediatric bone marrow aspirates. (*A*) Pearson syndrome is characterized by vacuolization of erythroid precursors (not seen here) and myeloid precursors (center of image), with ring sideroblasts demonstrated on iron stain (*inset*). (*B*) Congenital dyserythropoietic anemia type 2, showing expanded erythroid elements, many of which are binucleated. (*C*) Classic findings in parvovirus B19 infection, with erythroid hypoplasia and giant proerythroblasts (*A–C*, WG stain, ×100).

Fig. 9. Abnormalities affecting the erythroid lineage in pediatric bone marrow aspirates. (*D*) Unusual presentation of parvovirus B19 infection, with marked erythroid expansion and dyserythropoiesis. (*E*) Stress erythropoiesis in a case of beta-thalassemia, with dyspoiesis in erythroid elements mimicking myelo dysplasia (*D, E,* WG stain, ×100).

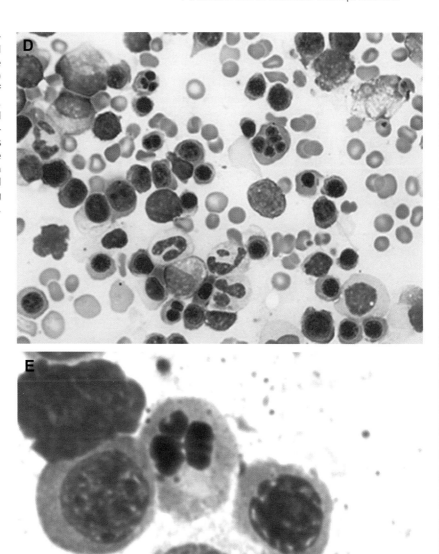

in the myeloid series that can occur after drug administration or in patients suffering from severe infections. The rare congenital neutropenias are typically associated with very characteristic morphologic changes: Kostman syndrome features a block in maturation at the promyelocyte/myelocyte stage, associated with a decrease in the number of myeloid elements and an overall decreased marrow cellularity (**Fig. 10**). Patients with Kostman syndrome should undergo yearly surveillance bone marrow examinations for emerging myeloid malignancies, because of their increased susceptibility to secondary MDS or AML while on chronic G-CSF therapy.[36] Patients

with the Chediak-Higashi syndrome have peripheral neutropenia and show prominent salmon-colored, myeloperoxidase-positive inclusions in both peripheral granulocytes and marrow myeloid precursors. Some of these patients may develop a HLH-like "accelerated phase" during their clinical course. Myelokathexis, as a part of the WHIM (Wart, Hypogammaglobulinlemia, Infection, Myelokathexis) syndrome[37,38] (see **Table 6**), is associated with neutropenia. Granulocytic elements in the bone marrow and blood show characteristic pyknotic nuclear lobes connected by long strands of DNA. Clinical follow-up is essential for the diagnosis of cyclic neutropenia,

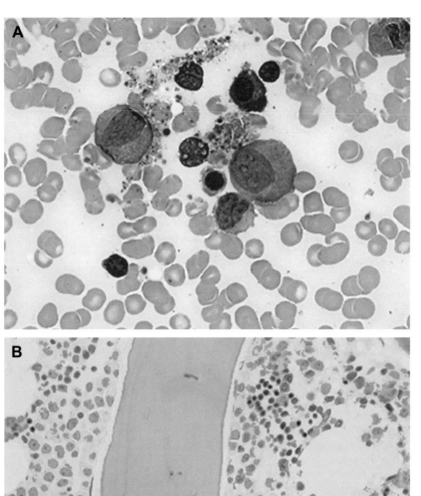

Fig. 10. Bone marrow abnormalities in Kostman syndrome. (*A*) In the aspirate smear, maturation is blocked at promyelocyte/myelocyte stage (WG stain, ×100). (*B*) The biopsy is mildly hypocellular, with myeloid elements limited to immature nucleolated forms localized adjacent to the bony trabeculae (H&E stain, ×40).

which may be associated with a decrease or increase in marrow myeloid precursors, depending on the phase of the cycle when the marrow sample is obtained.

Megakaryocyte Abnormalities

Most isolated megakaryocyte abnormalities of the pediatric bone marrow are related to an altered number (increase or decrease) of megakaryocytes. However, increased megakaryocyte proliferations in reactive conditions are often associated with a shift toward immature megakaryocytes, which are typically small and hypolobulated, potentially mimicking those seen in MDS. Thus, a careful investigation of the clinical history to search for a possible reactive cause of such a megakaryocyte "left shift" is important when considering a diagnosis of MDS based on megakaryocyte morphologic abnormalities. Thrombocytopenia associated with increased megakaryocytes is most often attributable to extramedullary destruction of platelets (usually immune thrombocytopenia) and is rarely attributable to congenital disorders associated with

Fig. 11. Idiopathic congenital thrombocythemia in a child, associated with increased numbers of morphologically normal mature megakaryocytes in the bone marrow biopsy (H&E stain, ×60).

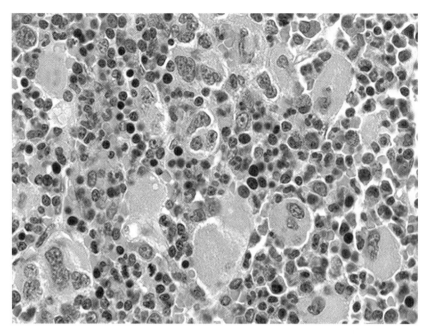

platelet dysfunction (Bernard-Soulier, May-Hegglin, or gray platelet syndrome). Thrombocytopenia associated with decreased megakaryocytes may be congenital, most often presenting in early infancy, or acquired. Although acquired forms are most often secondary to drug or infection-related myelosuppression, evolving AA should also be considered, as thrombocytopenia with decreased megakaryocytes may be the first manifestation of that disease. Congenital forms are related to two rare disorders: X-linked amegakaryocytic thrombocytopenia and thrombocytopenia absent radii (TAR) syndrome.[39] Both of these disorders may present initially with normocellular marrows and selective megakaryocyte hypoplasia or aplasia. Depending on the patient age at the time of initial evaluation, the bone marrow of these patients typically shows a steady decline in overall cellularity and may harbor emerging clones of MDS bearing a monosomy 7 or other cytogenetic abnormality even in the absence of overt dysplasia. Therefore, careful correlation with cytogenetic findings is important in this setting.

Thrombocytosis associated with increased megakaryocytes is most likely reactive in children, where trauma, recovery after recent myelosuppression (whether because of infection or chemotherapy), or iron deficiency may all be associated with vigorous increases in platelet counts. Essential thrombocythemia is exceedingly rare in children. Rare cases of hereditary thrombocythemia do occur. Some of these remain unexplained (**Fig. 11**), whereas others are caused by mutations in thrombopoietin or thrombopoietin receptor genes.[40,41] These latter cases are typically

---

Pitfalls
OF PEDIATRIC BONE MARROW INTERPRETATION

! Benign B-cell precursors (hematogones) can occur in significant numbers in the bone marrow of children with cytopenias of non-neoplastic causes and may be mistaken for involvement by B-lymphoblastic leukemia.

! Benign B-cell precursors (hematogones) often represent a significant proportion of the cells in hypocellular marrow aspirates from acute megakaryoblastic leukemia (with marrow fibrosis) potentially leading to a misdiagnosis of B lymphoblastic leukemia.

! B-lymphoblastic leukemias with a CD45−, CD20−, CD99+ immunophenotype may be mistaken for Ewing sarcoma, especially in small bone or bone marrow biopsies.

! Hemophagocytic syndromes may be associated with peripheral T-cell lymphomas; diagnostic lymphoma cells are sometimes present in small numbers in the bone marrow aspirates and may be missed.

! Variably prominent populations of polyclonal CD8+ T lymphocytes with immunophenotypic aberrancies may be present in familial hemophagocytic histiocytosis; they may be mistaken for peripheral T-cell lymphoma.

! Parvovirus B19 infections occurring in patients with constitutional red cell disorders may cause erythroid hyperplasia and significant dyserythropoiesis, resembling congenital dyserythropoietic anemia.

characterized by normocellular or mildly hypercellular bone marrow with megakaryocyte hyperplasia, a predominance of mature, morphologically normal megakaryocytes, and variable increases in bone marrow reticulin fibers.

REFERENCES

1. Hartsock RJ, Smith EB, Petty CS. Normal variations with aging of the amount of hematopoietic tissue in bone marrow from the anterior iliac crest. A study made from 177 cases of sudden death examined by necropsy. Am J Clin Pathol 1965;43:326−31.

2. Friebert SE, Shepardson LB, Shurin SB, et al. Pediatric bone marrow cellularity: are we expecting too much? J Pediatr Hematol Oncol 1998;20:439−43.

3. McKenna RW, Washington LT, Aquino DB, et al. Immunophenotypic analysis of hematogones (B-lymphocyte precursors) in 662 consecutive bone marrow specimens by 4-color flow cytometry. Blood 2001;98:2498−507.

4. Kroft SH. Role of flow cytometry in pediatric hematopathology. Am J Clin Pathol 2004;122(Suppl): S19−32.

5. Swerdlow SH, Campo E, Harris NL, et al, editors. WHO classification of tumours of haematopoietic and lymphoid tissues. Lyon (France): IARCPress; 2008. p. 109−76.

6. Pui CH, Rivera G, Mirro J, et al. Acute megakaryoblastic leukemia. Blast cell aggregates simulating metastatic tumor. Arch Pathol Lab Med 1985;109:1033−5.

7. Matloub YH, Brunning RD, Arthur DC, et al. Severe aplastic anemia preceding acute lymphoblastic leukemia. Cancer 1993;71:264−8.

8. Zwaan CM, Reinhardt D, Hitzler J, et al. Acute leukemias in children with Down syndrome. Hematol Oncol Clin North Am 2010;24:19−34.

9. Rubnitz JE, Razzouk BI, Ribeiro RC. Acute myeloid leukemia. In: Pui CH, editor. Childhood leukemias. 2nd edition. Cambridge (UK): Cambridge University Press; 2006. p. 499−539.

10. Ribeiro RC, Oliveira MS, Fairclough D, et al. Acute megakaryoblastic leukemia in children and adolescents: a retrospective analysis of 24 cases. Leuk Lymphoma 1993;10:299−306.

11. Kansal R, Deeb G, Barcos M, et al. Precursor B lymphoblastic leukemia with surface light chain immunoglobulin restriction: a report of 15 patients. Am J Clin Pathol 2004;121:512−25.

12. Li S, Lew G. Is B-lineage acute lymphoblastic leukemia with a mature phenotype and l1 morphology a precursor B-lymphoblastic leukemia/lymphoma or Burkitt leukemia/lymphoma? Arch Pathol Lab Med 2003;127:1340−4.

13. Komrokji R, Lancet J, Felgar R, et al. Burkitt's leukemia with precursor B-cell immunophenotype and atypical morphology (atypical Burkitt's leukemia/lymphoma): case report and review of literature. Leuk Res 2003;27:561−6.

14. Navid F, Mosijczuk AD, Head DR, et al. Acute lymphoblastic leukemia with the (8;14)(q24;q32) translocation and FAB L3 morphology associated with a B-precursor immunophenotype: the Pediatric Oncology Group experience. Leukemia 1999;13:135−41.

15. Onciu M, Behm FG, Raimondi SC, et al. ALK-positive anaplastic large cell lymphoma with leukemic peripheral blood involvement is a clinicopathologic entity with an unfavorable prognosis. Report of three cases and review of the literature. Am J Clin Pathol 2003;120:617−25.

16. Onciu M. Histiocytic proliferations in childhood. Am J Clin Pathol 2004;122(Suppl):S128−36.

17. Karandikar NJ, Kroft SH, Yegappan S, et al. Unusual immunophenotype of CD8 + T cells in familial hemophagocytic lymphohistiocytosis. Blood 2004;104:2007−9.

18. Emminger W, Zlabinger GJ, Fritsch G, et al. CD14 (dim)/CD16(bright) monocytes in hemophagocytic lymphohistiocytosis. Eur J Immunol 2001;31:1716−9.

19. Wollman MR, Penchansky L, Shekhter-Levin S. Transient 7q- in association with megaloblastic anemia due to dietary folate and vitamin B12 deficiency. J Pediatr Hematol Oncol 1996;18:162−5.

20. Hasle H, Niemeyer CM, Chessells JM, et al. A pediatric approach to the WHO classification of myelodysplastic and myeloproliferative diseases. Leukemia 2003;17:277−82.

21. Arico M, Biondi A, Pui CH. Juvenile myelomonocytic leukemia. Blood 1997;90:479−88.

22. Metzgeroth G, Walz C, Score J, et al. Recurrent finding of the FIP1L1-PDGFRA fusion gene in eosinophilia-associated acute myeloid leukemia and lymphoblastic T-cell lymphoma. Leukemia 2007;21:1183−8.

23. Guinan EC. Acquired aplastic anemia in childhood. Hematol Oncol Clin North Am 2009;23:171−91.

24. Green AM, Kupfer GM. Fanconi anemia. Hematol Oncol Clin North Am 2009;23:193−214.

25. Savage SA, Alter BP. Dyskeratosis congenita. Hematol Oncol Clin North Am 2009;23:215−31.

26. Burroughs L, Woolfrey A, Shimamura A. Shwachman-Diamond syndrome: a review of the clinical presentation, molecular pathogenesis, diagnosis, and treatment. Hematol Oncol Clin North Am 2009; 23:233−48.

27. Kojima S, Ohara A, Tsuchida M, et al. Risk factors for evolution of acquired aplastic anemia into myelodysplastic syndrome and acute myeloid leukemia after immunosuppressive therapy in children. Blood 2002;100:786−90.

28. Sloand EM. Hypocellular myelodysplasia. Hematol Oncol Clin North Am 2009;23:347−60.

29. Parker CJ. Bone marrow failure syndromes: paroxysmal nocturnal hemoglobinuria. Hematol Oncol Clin North Am 2009;23:333−46.

30. Lipton JM, Ellis SR. Diamond-Blackfan anemia: diagnosis, treatment, and molecular pathogenesis. Hematol Oncol Clin North Am 2009;23:261–82.

31. Sawada K, Hirokawa M, Fujishima N. Diagnosis and management of acquired pure red cell aplasia. Hematol Oncol Clin North Am 2009;23:249–59.

32. Renella R, Wood WG. The congenital dyserythropoietic anemias. Hematol Oncol Clin North Am 2009;23:283–306.

33. Carpenter SL, Zimmerman SA, Ware RE. Acute parvovirus B19 infection mimicking congenital dyserythropoietic anemia. J Pediatr Hematol Oncol 2004;26:133–5.

34. Crook TW, Rogers BB, McFarland RD, et al. Unusual bone marrow manifestations of parvovirus B19 infection in immunocompromised patients. Hum Pathol 2000;31:161–8.

35. Huang LJ, Shen YM, Bulut GB. Advances in understanding the pathogenesis of primary familial and congenital polycythaemia. Br J Haematol 2010; 148:844–52.

36. Welte K, Zeidler C. Severe congenital neutropenia. Hematol Oncol Clin North Am 2009;23:307–20.

37. Gorlin RJ, Gelb B, Diaz GA, et al. WHIM syndrome, an autosomal dominant disorder: clinical, hematological, and molecular studies. Am J Med Genet 2000;91:368–76.

38. Kawai T, Malech HL. WHIM syndrome: congenital immune deficiency disease. Curr Opin Hematol 2009;16:20–6.

39. Geddis AE. Congenital amegakaryocytic thrombocytopenia and thrombocytopenia with absent radii. Hematol Oncol Clin North Am 2009;23:321–31.

40. Ding J, Komatsu H, Wakita A, et al. Familial essential thrombocythemia associated with a dominant-positive activating mutation of the c-MPL gene, which encodes for the receptor for thrombopoietin. Blood 2004;103:4198–200.

41. Graziano C, Carone S, Panza E, et al. Association of hereditary thrombocythemia and distal limb defects with a thrombopoietin gene mutation. Blood 2009; 114:1655–7.

DIAGNOSIS OF MYELODYSPLASTIC SYNDROMES IN CYTOPENIC PATIENTS

Sa A. Wang, MD

KEYWORDS

- Cytopenia • Myelodysplastic syndromes • Flow cytometry • Aplastic anemia • Cytogenetics
- Algorithm • Diagnostic criteria

ABSTRACT

Sustained clinical cytopenia is a frequent laboratory finding in ambulatory and hospitalized patients. For pathologists and hematopathologists who examine the bone marrow (BM), a diagnosis of cytopenia secondary to an infiltrative BM process or acute leukemia can be readily established based on morphologic evaluation and flow cytometry immunophenotyping. However, it can be more challenging to establish a diagnosis of myelodysplastic syndrome (MDS). In this article, the practical approaches for establishing or excluding a diagnosis of MDS (especially low-grade MDS) in patients with clinical cytopenia are discussed along with the current diagnostic recommendations provided by the World Health Organization and the International Working Group for MDS.

OVERVIEW

Sustained ($\geq$6 months) clinical cytopenia involving one or more hematopoietic lineages (erythrocytes, neutrophils, or platelets) is a frequent laboratory finding in patients treated at ambulatory clinics and in hospitalized patients.[1–4] The first question to be addressed (usually by a clinician, before considering sampling the BM) is whether or not the cytopenia is due to decreased production of hematopoietic cells or increased destruction, consumption, or loss of blood cells. For cytopenia attributed to decreased production of hematopoietic cells, the underlying causes can be attributed to either an intrinsic hematopoietic stem cell disorder or secondary etiology. Increased destruction or consumption can be due to blood loss, hemolysis, hypersplenism, mechanical cardiac valve placement, and other factors. The

Pathologic Key Features
OF MYELODYSPLASTIC SYNDROMES

1. Myelodysplastic syndromes (MDS) are hematopoietic stem cell neoplasms that involve the blood and bone marrow (BM) and manifest with varying degrees of peripheral cytopenias and morphologic dysplasia.

2. The BM in MDS is often hypercellular with disturbed topography, but 15% of cases are hypocellular.

3. Morphologic dysplasia must be present in more than 10% of cells in at least one hematopoietic lineage; in the absence of significant dysplasia, MDS can only be diagnosed if characteristic cytogenetic abnormalities are present in the clinical setting of unremitting cytopenia.

4. Accurate enumeration of myeloblasts in MDS is critical for classification and risk stratification

5. Flow cytometry immunophenotyping can be useful in differentiating a reactive process versus a neoplastic stem cell process, such as MDS.

Department of Hematopathology, University of Texas, MD Anderson Cancer Center, Unit 72, 1515 Holcombe Boulevard, Houston, TX 77030-4009, USA
E-mail address: swang5@mdanderson.org

Surgical Pathology 3 (2010) 1127–1152
doi:10.1016/j.path.2010.09.006

current recommended guidelines for the initial clinical evaluation of patients with cytopenia generally include a review of the patient's medical history and a thorough laboratory work-up (complete blood count and assessment of iron, folate, and vitamin B_{12} levels). BM biopsies and aspirates are subsequently performed in some cases because of an unrevealing laboratory work-up or to rule out an infiltrative BM process.[3,4]

For pathologists who examine the BM, a diagnosis of cytopenia secondary to an infiltrative process (such as lymphoma, myeloma, or metastatic carcinoma) or an acute leukemia can usually be easily established based on morphologic evaluation and flow cytometry immunophenotyping (FCI). It can be more challenging, however, to establish a diagnosis of MDS, a clonal BM disorder characterized by peripheral cytopenia, ineffective hematopoiesis, morphologic dysplasia, and recurrent cytogenetic abnormalities. Traditionally, the gold standard for diagnosing MDS has been BM morphology and cytogenetic studies in conjunction with a clinical presentation of persistent and unexplained cytopenia.[5,6] Not all patients with clinically suspected MDS evince definitive morphologic dysplasia,[7–9] and some non-MDS-related cytopenias may mimic MDS on morphologic evaluation.[10] Moreover, cytogenetic abnormalities are infrequent in patients with MDS cases lacking excess blasts.[11] The 2008 World Health Organization (WHO) classification subcategorizes MDS into several different diseases, based on the types of cytopenias, morphology, and specific cytogenetic abnormalities. These disease categories have different clinical behaviors and prognosis. The MDS entities defined in the 2008 WHO classification and their abbreviations are listed in **Box 1**. Although there is no recognized pathologic grading scheme for MDS, for the purposes of this topic, lower-grade MDS cases are defined as blasts greater than 5%, including refractory cytopenia with unilineage dysplasia (RCUD), refractory cytopenia with multilineage dysplasia (RCMD), and MDS with del(5q), whereas higher-grade MDS cases are defined as blast greater than or equal to 5%, including refractory anemia with excess blasts (RAEB).

Diagnosing MDS can be particularly challenging in patients who have received chemotherapy for primary malignancies and developed prolonged cytopenia. In such patients, a question to answer is whether the cytopenia is attributed to BM injury due to exogenous factors or if MDS has developed secondary to the chemotherapy. Morphologic dysplasia is a frequent finding in postchemotherapy BM samples and becomes less reliable in making the distinction between MDS and

Box 1
Myelodysplastic syndrome entities according to the WHO 2008 classification
Refractory cytopenia with unilineage dysplasia (RCUD)
Refractory neutropenia
Refractory anemia
Refractory thrombocytopenia
Refractory anemia with ring sideroblasts (RARS)
Refractory cytopenia with multilineage dysplasia (RCMD)
Refractory anemia with excess blasts (RAEB)
RAEB-1
RAEB-2
MDS with isolated del(5q) abnormality
MDS, unclassified
Therapy-related MDS (t-MDS)

postchemotherapy BM injury. A similarly challenging situation exists in the differential diagnosis between aplastic anemia (AA) and hypoplastic MDS cases. Although the BM of patients with AA exhibits hypocellularity and usually lacks significant dysplasia,[12] in some cases the distinction between hypocellular MDS and AA may not be possible.[9,13] Morphologic evaluation can be further hampered by suboptimal BM material. For example, core biopsy samples may be of inadequate length, consist predominantly of cortical bone, or exhibit obscuring crush artifact. In addition, aspirate smears may be inadequate because of hemodilution, air drying, or poor staining.

This content addresses the diagnostic challenges faced by pathologists interpreting BM samples taken to evaluate cytopenic patients. The morphologic and clinical features that distinguish MDS from cytopenias secondary to non-MDS causes are described, in particular, the appropriate interpretation of cytogenetic findings and application of ancillary testing (mainly FCI). An algorithm based on the WHO and International Working Group (IWG) guidelines for diagnosis of MDS is also provided.

CLINICAL FEATURES

As defined by the International Prognostic Scoring System (IPSS) for MDS, cytopenia is characterized by a hemoglobin level less than 10 g/dL, absolute neutrophil count less than 1.8×10^9/L, and platelet count less than 100×10^9/L.[14] The IWG defines cytopenia as a hemoglobin level less than 11 g/dL, absolute neutrophil count less than 1.5×10^9/L, and platelet count less than 100×10^9/L.[15] Cytopenia in MDS is often unremitting or progressive. In some patients, however, cytopenia can be less severe at presentation or have less than a 6-month duration due to early detection. A diagnosis of MDS can still be rendered in such settings if definitive morphologic and/or cytogenetic findings are present (**Box 2**).[15,16]

Most patients with MDS present with cytopenia-related symptoms. Symptoms related to anemia, such as fatigue and malaise, with eventual transfusion dependence, are most common. Patients can also present with petechiae, ecchymoses, and nose and gum bleeding due to thrombocytopenia. Fever, cough, or septic shock may be manifestations of serious bacterial or fungal infections secondary to neutropenia. Hepatosplenomegaly or lymphadenopathy is uncommon in MDS patients. Therapy-related MDS (t-MDS) and other therapy-related myeloid neoplasms secondary to alkylating agents and/or ionizing radiation most commonly occur 5 to 10 years after exposure. Patients often present with t-MDS and evidence of BM failure, although a minority may present with t-MDS/myeloproliferative neoplasm (MPN) or with overt therapy-related acute myeloid leukemia (AML). Therapy-related myeloid neoplasms after treatment with topoisomerase II inhibitors have a latency period of approximately 1 to 5 years; most of these patients do not develop MDS but instead present with overt AML. In practice, many patients have received chemotherapeutic regimens that include both alkylating agents and topoisomerase II inhibitors and the clinicopathologic features may not be clear-cut. In addition, in elderly patients who receive cytotoxic therapy, cytopenias may be due to coincidental primary MDS or concurrent MDS due to genetic predisposition to cancer.

Box 2
Minimal diagnostic criteria for patients with myelodysplastic syndromes, as recommended by the International Working Conference (2007)

(A) Prerequisite criteria (both 1 and 2 required)

  1. Constant cytopenia in one or more of the following cell lineages:

   - Erythroid (hemoglobin <11 g/dL[a])
   - Neutrophilic (absolute neutrophil count <1.5×10^9/L[b]) or
   - Megakaryocytic (platelets <100×10^9/L)

  2. Exclusion of all other hematopoietic or nonhematopoietic disorders as the primary reason for cytopenia/dysplasia

(B) MDS-related decisive criteria (at least one required)

   - Dysplasia in ≥10% of all cells in at least one of the following lineages in the BM smear: erythroid, neutrophilic, or megakaryocytic, or >15% ringed sideroblasts (iron stain)
   - 5%−19% Blast cells in the BM or PB
   - Typical chromosomal abnormality (by conventional karyotyping or fluorescence in situ hybridization [FISH])

(C) Co-criteria (for patients fulfilling "A" but not any of the "B" criteria above and who otherwise show typical clinical features [eg, transfusion-dependent macrocytic anemia]) (at least one required)

   - Abnormal phenotype of BM cells clearly indicative of a monoclonal population of erythroid and/or myeloid cells, determined by flow cytometry,
   - Clear molecular signs of a monoclonal cell population on X-inactivation assay, gene chip profiling, or point mutation analysis (eg, *RAS* mutations),
   - Markedly and persistently reduced colony formation (±cluster formation) of BM and/or circulating progenitor cells by colony-forming unit assay.

[a] The WHO 2008 classification recommends using a hemoglobin level of <10 g/dL.
[b] The WHO 2008 classification recommends using an absolute neutrophil count level of <1.8×10^9/L.

Nevertheless, because they are difficult or impossible to distinguish from t-MDS, according to the WHO classification such cases are considered by default to represent t-MDS.

DIAGNOSIS: MICROSCOPIC FEATURES

PERIPHERAL BLOOD

The peripheral blood (PB) in patients with MDS nearly always shows some evidence of cytopenia. In addition, the anemia is often macrocytic and the red cell distribution width is often increased. Patients with significant ring sideroblasts (RS) in the marrow may show a dimorphic red cell appearance due to a combination of macrocytes and hypochromic microcytes. Granulocytic dysplasia may be more visible in the PB than in the BM. Recognizing and reporting circulating blasts are important, because the presence of these blasts can change the disease classification and predict patients' clinical outcomes. Circulating immature cells, including blasts, can also be seen in patients who have received growth factor treatment, in those with an actively regenerating BM, in those with an acute marrow stress such as sepsis, or in those who have undergone recent stem cell transplantation.

BONE MARROW BIOPSY

Bone marrow biopsy is important for assessing cellularity, relative lineage proportions, fibrosis, stromal alterations, and megakaryocytic dysplasia. Normal BM usually shows a cellularity appropriate for a patient's age, with orderly maturation and a normal cellular distribution: the myeloid precursors are generally found along the bone trabeculae, whereas the erythroid and megakaryocytic precursors are located more centrally (**Fig. 1**A). In MDS, the BM is usually hypercellular, and the BM topography is disrupted (see **Fig.** 1B). Altered stroma is common, including markedly uneven distribution of fat cells with alteration of adipocyte size, increased histiocytes, increased small blood vessels, and increased reticulin fibrosis. Significant differences in the size of hemopoietic islands are often present and the erythroid islands may be disrupted or poorly delineated. Abnormal localization of immature precursors (ALIPs), defined as clusters or aggregates of myeloblasts and promyelocytes located away from bone trabeculae (see **Fig.** 1C), is an adverse prognostic feature in MDS and is an uncommon finding in lower-grade MDS cases.[17] However, ALIPs are not unique to MDS and can be seen in active BM regeneration or after growth factor treatment.[18,19]

Immunohistochemistry (IHC) can be useful in assessing for MDS, especially in a case of fibrotic or hypocellular BM. The expression of CD34, a marker of early progenitor cells, is positive in most MDS blasts, regardless of the MDS subtype.[20] The presence of increased and/or clustered CD34+ blasts not only helps confirm a diagnosis of MDS but also assists in identifying ALIPs that are correlated with increased risk of transformation to AML.[21] CD34 is also present on endothelium and sinus lining cells, highlighting the increased angiogenesis characteristic of MDS. In rare cases, blasts in MDS are negative for CD34 and CD117 (c-KIT) may be used as an alternative blast marker; however, CD117 also stains some early erythroid precursors (pronormoblasts), some promyelocytes, and mast cells. Megakaryocytic markers, such as CD61, CD42b, and von Willebrand factor-associated protein, are useful for highlighting micromegakaryocytes and abnormal groupings or clusterings of megakaryocytes. These markers are also helpful in differentiating MDS from acute megakaryocytic leukemia (M7), where the megakaryoblasts have an immature phenotype, most commonly CD61+ but with partial or negative staining for CD42 and von Willebrand factor-associated protein.

BONE MARROW ASPIRATE

High-quality BM aspirate smears are critical for diagnosing and classifying MDS. BM aspirate evaluation includes recording the percentage of blasts and the degree of unilineage or multilineage dysplasia. Dysplasia must be present in at least 10% of the cells of any lineage, and the particular dysplastic changes seen may be relevant in predicting the biology and specific cytogenetic abnormalities of MDS.

Dysgranulopoiesis includes nuclear hypolobation, such as the pseudo-Pelger-Huët anomaly, hypersegmentation of the nuclei at an inappropriate stage, and abnormal cytoplasm ix granularity (agranularity, hypogranularity, hypergranularity or large, irregularly shaped eosinophilic pseudo-Chédiak-Higashi granules). Abnormally large or small granulocytes are also evidence of dysplasia, but giant neutrophils with nuclear hypersegmentation can also be seen in patients with vitamin B_{12} or folate deficiency. Dysplastic features present at earlier stages of myeloid lineage include hypogranulation, abnormally shaped (eg, elongated) granules, abnormal nuclear lobation, and nuclear/cytoplasmic dyssynchrony (**Fig. 2**A, B). Recognization of dysplastic features in early myeloid cells is

Fig. 1. Morphologic features of BM biopsies in MDS. (*A*) Topography of normal BM shows a normal cellular distribution, with preserved erythroid islands and normal appearing megakaryocytes. (*B*) Altered BM topography in a patient with MDS: the marrow is hypercellular, with altered cellular distribution, increased histiocytes, and increased vasculature. Dysplastic megakaryocytes are present, and appreciated at this power. (*C*) Abnormal localization of immature precursors (ALIPs), clusters of large immature cells (*arrows*) located away from the bone trabecula are present. The cellular components of ALIPs are mainly composed of myeloblasts and promyelocytes.

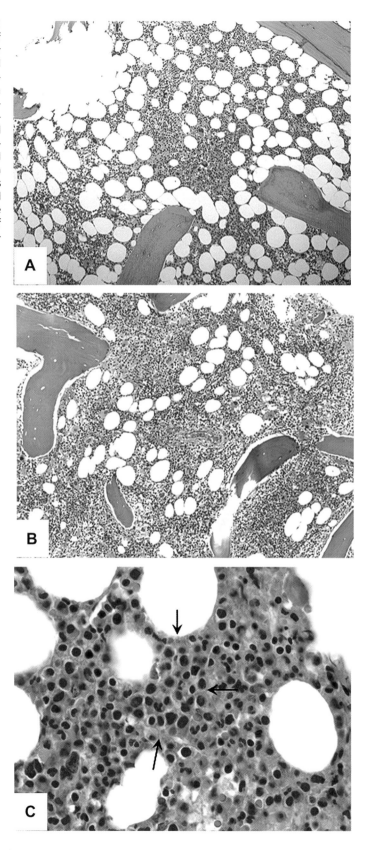

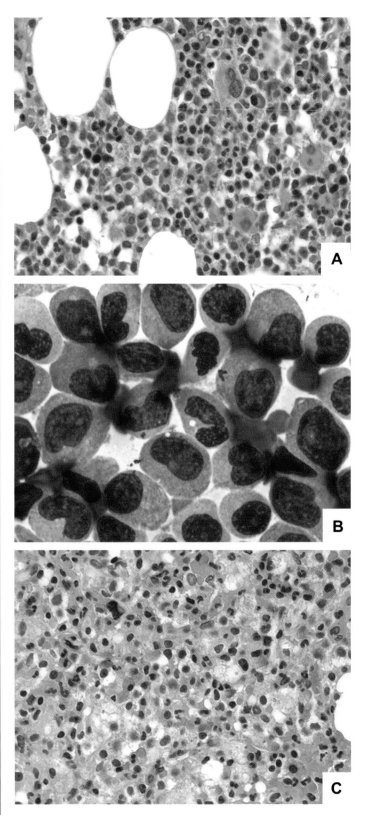

Fig. 2. Unusual features that can be seen in some cases of MDS. (*A*) MDS with myeloid hyperplasia and left-shifted myeloid maturation in the bone marrow biopsy; also present in the field are dysplastic megakaryocytes. (*B*) Myeloid lineage dysplasia can be observed in early and intermediate stage myeloid cells in the bone marrow aspirate. (*C*) MDS with pure red cell aplasia (BM biopsy).

Fig. 2. Unusual features that can be seen in some cases of MDS. (*D*) MDS with erythroid hypoplasia. The rare erythroid cells present are mainly immature forms (BM aspirate). (*E, F*) Erythroid-predominant MDS case with left-shifted erythroid maturation on the bone marrow biopsy (*E*) and numerous RS on iron stain (*F*); such cases should not be misdiagnosed as pure erythroidleukemia (AML M6B).

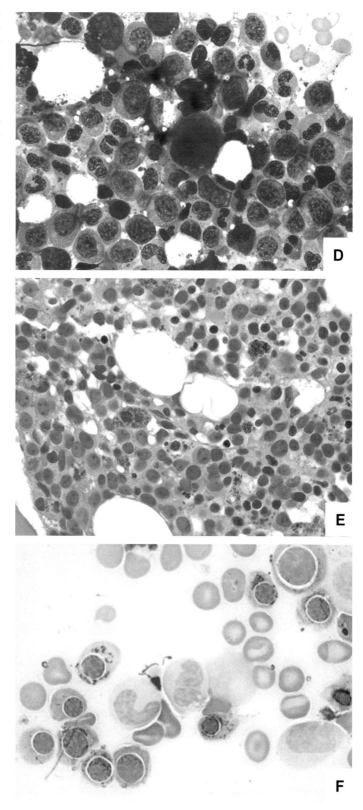

important, especially in cases of MDS with left-shifted myeloid maturation.

Dyserythropoietic features include nuclear budding, internuclear bridging, karyorrhexis, multinuclearity, nuclear hyperlobation, cytoplasmic basophilic stippling, and vacuoles. Megaloblastoid change (nuclear-cytoplasmic dyssynchrony) is nonspecific and is common in non-MDS BM samples, thus should not be overinterpreted. RS, another manifestation of dyserythropoiesis, should have at least five siderotic granules present, covering at least one-third of the circumference of the nucleus.[5,22] Erythroblasts with less than five granules or with granules that are not in a perinuclear location should not be counted as RS. The presence of 15% RS or greater in a BM with less than 5% blasts classify patients as having refractory anemia with RS (RARS) if dysplasia is confined to the erythroid lineage. The presence of RS in MDS with multilineage dysplasia, cases with specific cytogenetic abnormalities, or those with increased blasts (5% or greater) do not change the MDS subcategorization. RS may occur in non-neoplastic conditions, such as alcoholism, hereditary sideroblastic anemia, and due to effects of certain drugs.

Marked erythroid hyperplasia (50% or greater) with or without left-shifted erythroid maturation (see **Fig. 2**C) can be seen in approximately 15% of patients with MDS. RS are frequently present (see **Fig. 2**D). In these patients, myeloblasts should be assessed as a proportion of nonerythroid cells: if myeloblasts are 20% or greater of nonerythroid cells, the case would meet criteria for acute erythroid leukemia, erythroid/myeloid subtype (FAB: AML-M6A); if myeloblasts are less than 20% of nonerythroid cells, the current recommendation is to enumerate the blasts as a proportion of total cells for subcategorization. Recent studies have shown that in erythroid-predominant MDS, however, blast calculation as a proportion of BM nonerythroid cells may be better than total nucleated cells for stratifying patients into prognostically relevant groups,[23,24] and MDS with erythroid predominance and M6A may be a biologic continuum that is arbitrarily divided by a blast cut-off.[23] Conversely, erythroid hypoplasia or aplasia is observed in approximately 5% of MDS cases (see **Fig. 2**E, F) and is often associated with an oligo- or monoclonal T-cell proliferation,[25] suggesting immune-mediated destruction of erythroid precursors. Some of these patients may respond to cyclosporine treatment.[26]

Dysmegakaryopoiesis in MDS is characterized by micromegakaryocytes with hypolobated nuclei; megakaryocytes of all sizes with monolobated nuclei; or megakaryocytes with multiple, widely separated nuclei (pawn-ball appearance). However, the latter forms can be seen in non-MDS conditions, such as paraneoplastic syndrome. Megakaryocytes can be increased, decreased, or normal in number. In evaluating megakaryocyte dysplasia, the best approach is to make the initial evaluation based on BM biopsy and then verify the findings on the BM aspirate smears. Commenting on dysmegakaryopoiesis should be based on an assessment of at least 20 to 30 megakaryocytes, ideally including evaluation of megakaryocytes in both the biopsy sections and aspirate smears.

Blast recognition and enumeration are critical in the diagnosis, risk stratification, and assessment of treatment response in MDS. A 500-cell differential count is required for accurate blast enumeration. The presence of Auer rods shifts the classification to RAEB-2, regardless of the blast percentage. Myeloblasts in MDS often show marked heterogeneity in size and can be classified into two morphologic types: agranular and granular. Promyelocytes in MDS can be misinterpreted as granular blasts due to dysplastic changes. Normal promyelocytes have a visible Golgi zone, uniformly dispersed azurophilic granules, and, in most instances, basophilic cytoplasm, whereas dysplastic promyelocytes may have reduced or irregular cytoplasmic basophilia, a poorly developed Golgi zone, hyper- or hypogranularity, or irregular distribution (clumps) of granules. Unlike most blasts in MDS, however, dysplastic promyelocytes should still contain an oval or indented nucleus that is often eccentric with somewhat coarse chromatin and at least a faintly visible Golgi zone. Dysplastic promyelocytes are also often larger than myeloblasts.[22] Some myeloblasts can have deeply basophilic cytoplasm and can be confused with early erythroid precursors (**Fig. 3**). Erythroid precursors have relatively mature clumped chromatin and often larger than myeloblasts at early stages.

DIAGNOSIS: ANCILLARY STUDIES

FLOW CYTOMETRIC IMMUNOPHENOTYPING

Flow cytometric immunophenotyping (FCI) is a highly sensitive and reproducible method for quantitatively and qualitatively evaluating hematopoietic cell abnormalities. FCI abnormalities in MDS have been shown to be highly correlated with morphologic dysplasia and cytogenetic abnormalities.[27–29] In addition, FCI is less subjective and may be more sensitive and less affected by specimen quality than morphologic evaluation

Fig. 3. Myeloblasts in MDS can be difficult to differentiate from dysplastic promyelocytes and dysplastic erythroid elements (*A, B*). Long thick arrows point to blasts. Note that one blast panel shows basophilic cytoplasm reminiscent of a pronormoblast, but contains a single centrally located nucleolus and dispersed chromatin and is smaller than a pronormoblast. Short thick arrows point to dysplastic promyelocytes with ill-defined Golgi zones and round or indented nuclei. Thin arrows point to dysplastic monocytes.

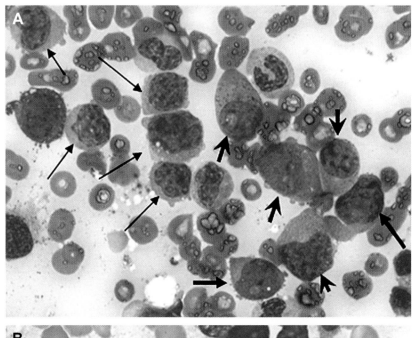

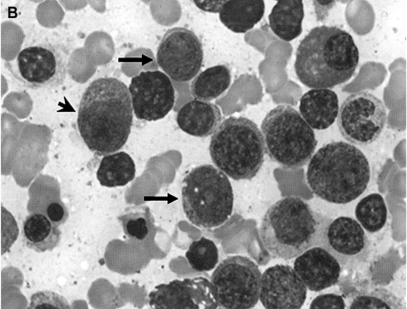

of dysplasia on smears. In particular, FCI demonstrates usefulness in supporting or ruling out MDS in the most diagnostically challenging BM samples obtained from patients with chronic, persistent cytopenia with no significant morphologic dysplasia or cytogenetic abnormalities.[30,31] A positive FCI result is more indicative of MDS or MDS/MPN whereas a negative FCI result is more frequently associated with non-MDS-related cytopenia. The use of FCI as an ancillary test in diagnosing MDS is gradually gaining acceptance by most pathologists. Given the wide range of findings observed in MDS thus far, however, FCI is only recommended for experienced laboratories, because some of the changes seen in FCI overlap with the changes seen in reactive and recovering BM samples.

Recently, the European LeukemiaNet has published standardization of FCI in diagnosis of MDS, providing guidelines on panel design and data interpretation.[32] Most published studies using FCI for diagnosing MDS are based on interpreting altered myelomonocytic differentiation or maturation patterns, using antigen combinations, such as CD13/CD16, CD11b/CD16, CD64/CD10, CD33/HLA-DR, CD65, and CD15. These approaches are sensitive, and MDS cases have demonstrated multiple abnormalities on FCI. However, myelomonocytic maturation patterns on FCI can show alterations in patients with reactive conditions, such as in patients with regenerating BM, those who have received growth factor treatment, and those with acute BM injury, severe infection, HIV, or autoimmune conditions. In addition, specimen quality such as hemodilution, or aged samples as well as increased eosinophils, can alter some normal patterns and the expression levels of some markers (eg, CD16, CD11b, and CD10). Moreover, abnormalities of some markers, such as decreased

CD33 expression, can be attributed to genetic polymorphism and are not necessarily indicative of dysplasia. Although these nonspecific changes can be recognized,[28] the pattern recognition methodology requires that pathologists have extensive knowledge and experience in normal myelomonocytic maturation patterns and understand the immunuphenotypic mimics.

In contrast, a focus on myeloblast phenotype seems to be a better approach.[20,31,33] Changes in myeloblasts more reliably indicate a stem cell neoplasm and are uncommonly seen in reactive conditions. These findings are easier for pathologists to interpret and report. This type of FCI analytic approach is focused on CD34+ cells, which in a reactive BM should show diverse differentiation and maturation patterns (Fig. 4). On side scatter versus CD45, normal myeloid precursors are scattered, showing a normal level of CD45

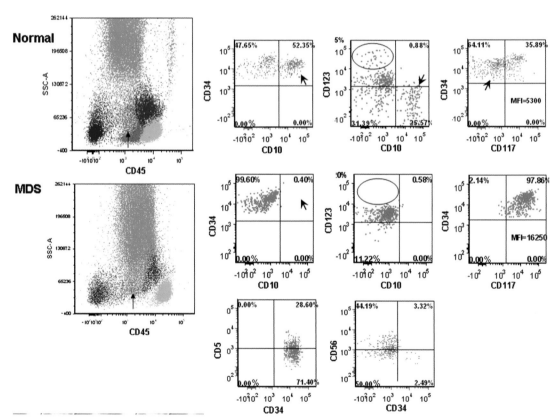

Fig. 4. FCI of MDS using an approach focusing on CD34+ cells. The upper row shows a normal marrow (lymphoma staging). Side scatter versus CD45 shows normal granularity of myeloid cells, well-separated myeloid (*light green*) and monocytic (*dark blue*) populations, with many hematogones and normal CD45 expression level of CD34+ myeloid precursors (red, *arrow*). The CD34+ cells contain many CD10+ hematogones (*short arrow*), CD123+ plasmacytoid dendritic precursors (*circled*), and myeloblasts with a normal CD117 expression level. The lower rows show BM from a patient with MDS. Side scatter versus CD45 shows hypogranulation of maturing myeloid cells (*light green*) and decreased CD45 expression on CD34+ blasts (*arrow*) and monocytes (*dark blue*). The CD34+ compartment is devoid of hematogones (*short arrow*) and plasmacytoid dendritic precursors (*circled*), and shows increased CD117 expression as well as aberrant expression of CD5 and CD56 (*bottom panels*).

expression (often at the same level of granulocytes and side scatter). The normal CD34+ stem cells are able to produce hematogones (normal CD19+, CD10+ immature B-cell precursors), plasmacytoid dendritic precursors (CD123bright+, HLA-DR+), differentiating myeloid precursors (CD34+, CD15+, CD65+), and monocytic precursors (CD34+, CD64+, CD4+). In contrast, the CD34+ blasts in MDS appear to be clonal, forming a discrete population on side scatter versus CD45 and lacking evidence of differentiation toward hematogones, plasmacytoid dendritic cells, or monocytes. Alterations of antigenic expression levels, such as decreased or increased CD45 expression, increased CD34 or CD117 expression (see **Fig. 4**), increased CD33 or CD13 expression, or decreased CD38 expression, are often observed. Aberrant expression of lymphoid antigens (eg, CD2, CD5, CD7, and CD56) can also be observed.

The FCI analysis based on CD34+ blasts can be combined with significant changes in myelomonocytic cells to improve detection sensitivity and specificity. These changes include marked hypogranulation of granulocytes, significant alterations or asynchronous maturation of myelomonocytic cells, and substantial expression of CD56 on maturing granulocytes or monocytes. Examples of the markers and antibody combinations for MDS on FCI are shown in **Table 1**. Changes observed in CD34+ blasts and myelomonocytic cells from MDS cases are shown in **Box 3**. A positive FCI result does not distinguish MDS from MDS/MPN or some cases of MPN: some MPN, especially chronic idiopathic myelofibrosis, can exhibit similar changes as MDS. FCI abnormalities alone are not considered sufficient to diagnose MDS in the 2008 WHO Classification of Tumours of Haematopoietic and Lymphoid Tissue; however, it is recommended that cases with borderline dysplasia and no cytogenetic abnormalities but FCI results highly suggestive of MDS be re-evaluated over several months for definitive morphologic or cytogenetic evidence of MDS.

Although FCI is useful at demonstrating aberrant phenotypes of blasts and differentiating cells in MDS, it is not recommended as a method of enumerating blasts. Not all myeloblasts express CD34, and not all CD34+ cells are myeloblasts (for example, early hematogones are CD34+). Furthermore, the number of blasts enumerated on FCI can be affected by hemodilution, incomplete red blood cell lysis, lysis of late-stage nucleated red blood cells, suboptimal cell viability due to sample aging, and cell loss due to sample processing. Often, FCI underestimates the blasts compared with morphologic counting or IHC performed on the BM biopsy. When a BM sample shows marked erythroid hyperplasia, the blasts detected on FCI may be overestimated because of erythroid lysis.

CYTOGENETICS

Conventional karyotyping remains an essential component of the diagnostic work-up of any

---

Table 1
Examples of flow cytometric panels for myelodysplastic syndromes (focusing on the blast population)

4-Color Panel	5-Color Panel	6- and 7-Color Panel
Chromogens: FITC, PE, PerCPCy5.5, APC	Chromogens: FITC, PE, ECD, PEcy5.5, PEcy7	Chromogens: FITC, PE, PerCPCy5.5, PEcy7, APC, V500, V450
CD45, CD10, CD34, CD117	CD38, CD10, CD45, CD117, CD34	CD65, CD64, CD34, CD10, CD2, CD45, CD14
CD15, CD56, CD34, CD33	CD15, CD56, CD45, CD33, CD34	
CD7, CD2, CD34, CD5	CD7, CD2, CD45, CD5, CD34	CD7, CD5, CD34, CD38, CD45, CD19
HLA-DR, CD38, CD34, CD123	HLA-DR, CD38, CD45, CD123, CD34	HLA-DR, CD123, CD34, CD10, CD184, CD45, CD56
CD16, CD11b, CD45, CD13	CD16, CD11b, CD45, CD13, CD34	CD16, CD11b, CD34, CD33, CD13, CD45, CD15
CD14, CD64, CD45, HLA-DR	CD14, CD64, CD45, HLA-DR, CD34	
Kappa, Lambda, CD45, CD19	Kappa, Lambda, CD19, CD45, CD5	Kappa, Lambda, CD19, CD20, CD5, CD45
CD8, CD4, CD45, CD3	CD8, CD57, CD45, CD3, CD4	CD57, CD4, CD3, CD8, CD45, CD56

Box 3
Antigenic abnormalities detected on flow cytometry in patients with myelodysplastic syndromes

CD34+ blasts

- Decreased numbers or absence of hematogones and plasmacytoid dendritic precursors
- Discrete population formed
- Increased CD117 and CD34 expression
- Decreased or increased CD45 expression
- Increased CD33 and CD13 expression
- Increased CD123 expression
- Aberrant expression of CD2, CD5, CD7, and CD56
- Decreased CD38 expression
- Absent or markedly increased CD15, CD64, and CD65 expression
- Aberrant CD10 and CD19 expression (make sure they are not hematogones)
- Increased in numbers ($\geq$3%)

Maturing myeloid cells[a]

- Hypogranulation
- CD11b/CD13/CD16 abnormalities
- Decreased CD33, CD15, and CD65 expression
- Decreased CD38 expression and increased HLA-DR expression
- Decreased CD64 expression on relative immature population (no granulocytes)
- Decreased or absence of CD10 expression on granulocytes
- CD56 expression (>15%)
- Aberrant expression of CD2, CD5, CD7, and CD56

Monocytes[a]

- Decreased CD45 expression
- Decreased or increased CD64 expression, decreased CD14 expression
- Decreased HLA-DR expression, increased CD184 expression
- Decreased CD13 expression
- Decreased CD11b expression
- Loss of CD16 expression
- Increased CD15 and CD65 expression
- CD56 expression (>25%)
- Aberrant CD2, CD5, and CD7 expression

[a] Abnormalities identified in CD34+ blasts are more specific for a stem cell neoplasm whereas changes on maturing myelomonocytic cells are relatively nonspecific, especially in patients who have received chemotherapy and growth factor treatment and who have acute illness.

---

patient with suspected MDS, but these results need to be interpreted with caution. Isolated (nonclonal) cytogenetic abnormalities are commonly observed in BM samples and may represent an artifact of short-term culture before harvesting. To avoid false-positive results, a standardized definition for clonality, such as finding the same chromosomal gain or structural aberration in at least two BM cells and the same chromosome loss in at least three BM cells, is essential. In borderline cases or in the post-treatment setting where low numbers of metaphases are obtained, confirmation of the suspected chromosome changes by FISH on interphase (noncultured) cells is recommended. Clonal cytogenetic abnormalities are observed in approximately 50% of MDS cases and include many different alterations: a recent multicenter study showed 684 different types of chromosome abnormalities among 1080 patients with MDS who had abnormal karyotypes.[34] The IPSS uses cytogenetic abnormalities to define three risk categories: (1) good, which includes a normal karyotype, isolated interstitial del(5q), isolated del(20q), and $-$Y; (2) poor, which includes a complex karyotype with more than three abnormalities, as well as del(7q) and $-$7, either alone or in combination with other anomalies; and (3) intermediate, which includes all other abnormalities.[14] Recent studies have shown that some of the less common cytogenetic abnormalities seen in MDS may have different roles in terms of clinical outcome from their IPSS assignment, suggesting that a more sophisticated classification scheme is needed.[34–36] In addition, as therapy shifts, additional evaluations of these cytogenetic risk associations will be required. One such attempt at improving the IPSS scoring identified additional favorable cytogenetic results as del(12 p), del(9 p), +21, $-$21, del(11 p), del(15 p), and del(11q); reclassified sole del(7q) as intermediate risk; and added i(17q) and other forms of 17p loss as poor-risk changes.[37]

FLUORESCENCE IN SITU HYBRIDIZATION

FISH has also been used to evaluate MDS cases for recurring genetic abnormalities.[36–38] MDS FISH panels include probes for detection of $-$5/del(5q), $-$7/del(7q), del(20q), and trisomy 8. The major advantage of FISH is its relatively high sensitivity with regard to the number of scorable cells as compared with the routine analysis of only 20 cells by conventional cytogenetics. FISH can be informative in MDS cases with karyotype failure as well as in cases of RAEB and RCMD showing a normal G-band karyotype.[38] FISH has been shown to have only limited usefulness in cases of RCUD and in MDS cases that have abnormal karyotypes by conventional cytogenetics.[39] In addition, the clinical relevance of low percentages of abnormal cells which are near the cut-off value in FISH assays remains unclear, apart from residual disease detection in patients with a previously characterized abnormality. In particular, the precision for detecting deletions varies with the probe used, and small populations that represent less than 6% to 8% of the total number of cells may fall beneath the threshold of detection for the assay.[40]

COMPARATIVE GENOMIC HYBRIDIZATION ARRAYS AND SINGLE-NUCLEOTIDE POLYMORPHISM ARRAYS

Comparative genomic hybridization arrays[41,42] and single-nucleotide polymorphism arrays[43,44] are potential complementary techniques that can be applied to detect unbalanced chromosomal rearrangements in MDS interphase cells. When applied and interpreted together with conventional karyotyping and FISH, these arrays can improve the diagnostic yield for identifying genetic abnormalities in MDS and can better describe abnormal karyotypes. The clinical impact of alterations found by single-nucleotide polymorphism array or comparative genomic hybridization array, however, is still a subject of intense research.

MOLECULAR TESTING

Molecular clonality assays (such as G6PD isoenzymes, restriction-linked polymorphisms, and X-linked DNA polymorphisms of the androgen receptor gene) have helped to define MDS as a clonal disorder but are rarely used in clinical practice. In contrast, molecular genetic analyses looking for mutations and copy number changes in oncogenes and tumor suppressor genes are more informative as to the pathogenesis of MDS. Following the model used for AML, such mutations have been grouped as class I, where they target genes involved in signal transduction (commonly FLT3, RAS genes, and KIT), or as class II, where they involve transcription factors affecting differentiation (eg, RUNX1/AML1, EVI1, or WT1).[45] In early-stage MDS, class I mutations are usually absent, but a variety of class II mutations may be observed.

Tumor suppressors are regulatory genes whose loss promote growth and cell cycle progression in many neoplasms. These genes can be lost by mutation, deletion, promoter methylation silencing, transcriptional regulation, or post-transcriptional mechanisms, such as microRNA targeting. Because large chromosomal deletions and chromosomal losses are common features of de novo MDS, loss of tumor suppressors by gene deletion is likely an extremely important disease mechanism in these neoplasms. To date, however, with the exception of 17p deletion that leads to the loss of TP53 function,[46,47] tumor suppressor gene loss has not been clearly implicated in the most common MDS-associated chromosomal alterations. Instead, recent data have implicated copy number loss of genes involved in cell metabolism, such as ribosome biogenesis, protease function, and cytoskeleton regulation, in MDS pathogenesis.[46] Microarray-based gene expression profiling may help to define which gene levels are most critical and establish prognostically relevant gene signatures that correlate with French America British (FAB), WHO, or IPSS subtypes.[48,49] These studies, however, have shown considerable overlap in gene expression profiles between high-risk MDS and AML as well as between low-risk MDS and non-neoplastic conditions.

AN ALGORITHM FOR DIAGNOSING MYELODYSPLASTIC SYNDROMES

Establishing a diagnosis of MDS, particularly lower-grade MDS types, in clinical cytopenia patients can be challenging. It requires that pathologists be aware of other, non-MDS causes of cytopenia and their associated changes that may mimic MDS. FCI is particularly useful in diagnostically equivocal cases. Moreover, a FCI analytic approach based mainly on CD34+ cells is highly specific for identifying stem cell neoplasms and is more straightforward for pathologists in various practice settings to interpret. When pathologists assess BM samples obtained from clinical cytopenia patients, it is recommended to follow the minimal diagnostic criteria recommended by MDS IWG and the criteria of the 2008 WHO classification. The recommended diagnostic approach for MDS is summarized in **Box 2** and a suggested diagnostic aligorithm is shown in **Fig. 5**.

For many patients, diagnosing MDS using the 2008 WHO criteria is straightforward. Diagnosis can be challenging, however, when (1) there is no detectable cytogenetic abnormality and only mild cytopenia; (2) there are both a karyotypic abnormality and cytopenia but only minimal morphologic dysplasia; or (3) there is isolated persistent thrombocytopenia, neutropenia, or transfusion-dependent macrocytic anemia but no karyotypic abnormality or overt morphologic dysplasia. Therefore, an international working conference composed of representatives from the National Comprehensive Cancer Network, the International MDS Working Group, and the European Leukemia-Net proposed consensus guidelines for the minimal diagnostic criteria for MDS (see **Box 2**). A MDS

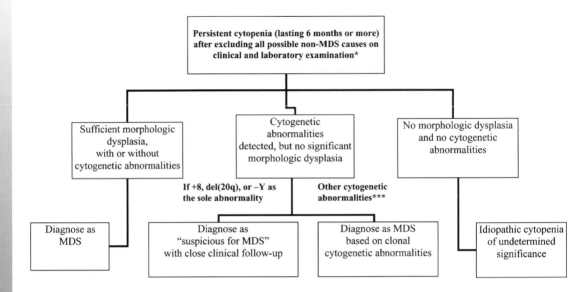

* A diagnosis of MDS can be made if cytopenia lasts <6 months but other MDS criteria are met.
** Flow cytometry immunophenotyping is particularly helpful in these cases: if abnormal results, favors MDS; if normal results, favors a benign process of cytopenia.
***Clonal cytogenetic abnormalities, including -7, -5, del(7q), del(5q), del(11q), i(17q), -13, del(13q), del(11q), del(12p), del(9q), t(6;9)(p23;q34), and/or any translocation involving 3q, 11q, 12p, or 17p.

Fig. 5. Diagnostic algorithm for evaluating cytopenia patients to establish or exclude a diagnosis of MDS.

diagnosis can be established when both prerequisite criteria and at least one decisive criterion are fulfilled. If no decisive criterion is fulfilled, the co-criteria should be applied. Some patients may have MDS coexisting with another hematologic or nonhematologic disease; therefore, detection of another disease potentially causing cytopenia does not exclude a diagnosis of MDS.

Patients presenting with persistent cytopenia (lasting 6 months or more) that cannot be explained by any other disease but lacking the full diagnostic criteria for MDS may be classified as idiopathic cytopenia of undetermined significance (ICUS), a newly coined term.[15,50] ICUS is a diagnosis of exclusion requiring careful BM examination, chromosome analysis and a thorough search of underlying causes. Careful follow-up is advised: approximately 20% to 50% of patients with ICUS eventually progress to MDS or AML.[50,51] FCI may be helpful in distinguishing a stem cell neoplasm versus reactive cytopenia in such cases.[30] A recent study has showed that stem cell clonality is detected in a significant subset of ICUS patients by human androgen receptor gene-based assay.[51]

In patients with persistent cytopenia, BM may show a clonal karyotypic abnormality but minimal (less than 10%) morphologic dysplasia. The 2008 WHO classification suggests handling these cases based on the type of cytogenetic change seen. When the sole aberration is −Y, +8, or del(20q), the recommendation is to diagnose these cases as suspicious for MDS, because such changes can occasionally be encountered in metaphases analysis of non-neoplastic BM, such as aplastic anemia (AA) or idiopathic thrombocytopenic purpura (ITP).[52] The finding of any other cytogenetic abnormality is regarded as presumptive evidence for MDS.

DIFFERENTIAL DIAGNOSIS

NON-MDS CAUSES OF CYTOPENIA

Common reactive causes of cytopenia are often diagnosed clinically by hematologists through a detailed history, physical examination, and laboratory tests to exclude iron, vitamin B_{12}, and folate deficiencies as well as possible effects of a drug, known infection, well-characterized autoimmune disease, hemolytic anemia, or splenomegaly. Most such patients do not require a BM biopsy. However, when cytopenia is chronic, refractory to treatment, or if clinical work-up is unrevealing, hematologists often perform a BM biopsy to rule out MDS or a BM infiltrative process.[3,4] A listing of the many non-MDS causes of various cytopenias is provided in **Table 2**.

Isolated anemia is most common and can be attributed to nutritional deficiency, systemic diseases (infections, chronic liver disease, kidney disease, collagen vascular diseases, or tumor

Table 2
Causes of clinical cytopenia not attributed to myelodysplastic syndromes

Isolated Anemia	Isolated Thrombocytopenia	Isolated Neutropenia	Bicytopenia and Pancytopenia
Iron deficiency (including blood loss)	Idiopathic thrombocytopenia purpura	Post infectious	Post infectious
Vitamin B$_{12}$ and folate deficiency	Post infectious	Drug-induced	Drug-induced
Anemia of systemic diseases	Drug/toxin	Primary immune disorders	Nutritional deficiency
Infections	Chemotherapy/ radiation	Antineutrophil antibodies	Aplastic anemia
Drug/toxin	Alcohol	Transfusion alloantibodies	Paroxysmal nocturnal hemoglobinuria
Hypersplenism	Hypersplenism	Antibodies to G-CSF	Macrophage activation syndrome
Hemolysis	Congenital/inherited BM disorders	Complement activation	Hemaphagocytosis
Aplastic anemia	LGL leukemia	Hypersplenism	Hypersplenism
Paroxysmal nocturnal hemoglobinuria		Congenital neutropenia	LGL leukemia
Low hormone:		Cyclic neutropenia	BM infiltrate:
Erythropoietin (chronic renal failure)		LGL leukemia	Hairy cell leukemia
Thyroid hormone			Other hematological/ non-hematological malignancy
Androgens (hypogonadism)			Granulomas
Undiagnosed hemoglobinopathy			
Pure red cell aplasia (often due to thymoma)			
Congenital/inherited BM disorders			
Large granular lymphocytic (LGL) leukemia			

paraneoplastic syndromes), peripheral destruction/consumption (hemolysis, splenomegaly, or microangiopathy), undiagnosed hemoglobinopathy, AA, or paroxysmal nocturnal hemoglobinuria (PNH). MDS should be a diagnosis of exclusion in these cases.

Isolated thrombocytopenia is mostly due to ITP. In children, most cases of ITP are acute, manifesting a few weeks after a viral illness. In adults, most cases of ITP are chronic, manifesting with an insidious onset, and typically occur in middle-aged women. In these patients, ITP is mediated by autoantibodies that are directed against platelet GPIIb/IIIa or GPIb/IX GP complexes (in 75% of cases).[53]

Isolated thrombocytopenia is less commonly a presenting manifestation of MDS, acute leukemia, or BM failure syndromes.[54] Isolated thrombocytopenia with minimal morphologic dysplasia may occur in indolent forms of MDS, particularly in patients with a del(20q)[7] cytogenetic abnormality.

Isolated neutropenia is an uncommon presentation of MDS. The most common causes of isolated neutropenia are chemical exposure, infections, autoimmune diseases, side effect of drugs, lymphoid neoplasms, and thyroid disease.[55] The drugs associated with isolated neutropenia include the antipsychotic medication clozapine; immunosuppressive drugs, such as sirolimus, mycophenolate mofetil, tacrolimus, and cyclosporine; interferons used to treat multiple sclerosis and hepatitis C; antidepressant drugs; antibiotics; antiepilepsy drugs; and arsenic. Autoimmune neutropenia can be either primary or secondary: primary autoimmune neutropenia is often seen in children, whereas secondary autoimmune leukopenia is usually seen in adults and is associated with systemic autoimmune diseases, infections, or malignancies. Antineutrophil autoantibodies may not be detectable, because the sensitivity for antibody detection varies depending on the tests, and in some patients, autoantibodies disappear even before the patient recovers. Cyclic neutropenia is an autosomal dominant disorder of unknown etiology in which 3 to 6 days of neutropenia occur every 21 to 30 days in a periodic pattern. Of the lymphoid neoplasms, large granular lymphocytic (LGL) leukemia often presents as an isolated neutropenia.

Chronic bicytopenia and pancytopenia are more clinically suggesting of MDS, but the most common causes are still of secondary (nonhematopoietic stem cell) origin, such as infection, chronic systemic diseases, toxins or drugs, nutritional deficiencies, or hemophagocytic syndromes. In patients who have received chemotherapy for primary malignancies, complete blood counts often recover within 3 to 4 weeks. Prolonged myelosuppression may occur in some patients, however. The severity and duration of anemia, thrombocytopenia, and neutropenia differ with each patient and with each chemotherapy regimen and its schedule, intensity, and duration.[56] In addition, cytopenia may be attributed directly or indirectly to the primary malignancy, as a result of blood loss, paraneoplastic syndromes, malnutrition/malabsorption, altered metabolism, autoimmune phenomena, microangiopathic hemolysis,[57] secondary infection, anemia of chronic inflammation, or other causes.

ROLE OF BONE MARROW EVALUATION IN DIFFERENTIAL DIAGNOSIS

Cytopenia due to a BM infiltrative process, such as metastatic carcinoma, lymphoma, multiple myeloma, or acute leukemia, is usually relatively straightforward for pathologists to diagnose when incorporating information from FCI and IHC. Hairy cell leukemia and LGL leukemia can be diagnostically challenging, because interstitial infiltration patterns may be subtle in the early stages of these diseases. On FCI, hairy cells in the BM samples may be underrepresented due to a poor or dry aspirate. On FCI, LGL leukemia exhibits increased numbers of LGLs, but they often have a normal immunophenotype. If there is suspicion of hairy cell leukemia or LGL leukemia,

IHC for CD20, DBA-44, and annexin A1 (hairy cell leukemia) and/or for CD4, CD8, granzyme, TIA-1, and CD57 (LGL leukemia) can be helpful. BM infiltration by lymphomas can elicit a sympathetic morphologic dysplasia in the hematopoietic elements and may lead to misdiagnosis of MDS.[58,59] Most reactive morphologic dysplasia is limited to the erythroid lineage, although mild dysplasia in granulocytes and megakaryocytes can also be observed.

Cytopenia due to peripheral destruction or consumption often shows a hyperplastic and/or regenerative BM. In a briskly regenerating BM, dysplastic features may be observed. In patients with hemolytic anemia, dyserythropoiesis (so-called stress erythropoiesis) is a common feature. Dysplastic features in myeloid and megakaryocytic cells may be present in regenerating BM after chemotherapy or other marrow insults, but the changes are usually mild. In patients with drug/toxin- or autoimmune-related neutropenia, however, the myeloid series is often left-shifted and may demonstrate hypogranulation or contain abnormally coarse granules (**Fig. 6**). FCI can be particularly helpful in these cases. In patients with ITP, many young megakaryocytes are often present that are monolobated but hypergranular; these megakaryocytes should not be confused with dysplastic megakaryocytes that are both monolobated and hypogranular. Unlike MDS, which usually exhibits architectural disorganization of hemopoiesis, reactive BM samples typically maintain a relatively normal BM topography, with intact clusters of erythroid elements and megakaryocytes located away from the bone trabeculae and not forming clusters. In BM of cytopenia due to peripheral destruction, cytopenia correlates with specific lineage hyperplasia. For example, anemia is associated with erythroid hyperplasia, and thrombocytopenia is usually associated with megakaryocytic hyperplasia. It is important to document the number or proportion of each lineage as supporting evidence of cytopenia secondary to peripheral destruction. Reactive BM often contains increased hematogones and shows no abnormalities in CD34+ cells (see the previous FCI description), whereas MDS shows decreased or absent hematogones with aberrant expression of certain markers on myeloblasts.[60] In most cases, regenerating BM can be differentiated from MDS on a careful BM examination and a thorough review of the laboratory data.

Cytopenia due to BM suppression is more diagnostically challenging. Similar to MDS, BM samples can show increased histiocytes, apoptotic cells, and an altered stroma. These

Fig. 6. Drug-induced neutropenia. There is myeloid maturation arrest with most of the cells in the promyelocyte, myelocyte, and metamyelocytes stages, seen in both the biopsy (*A*) and aspirate smear (*B*). Maturation arrest can share many clinical and morphologic features with MDS.

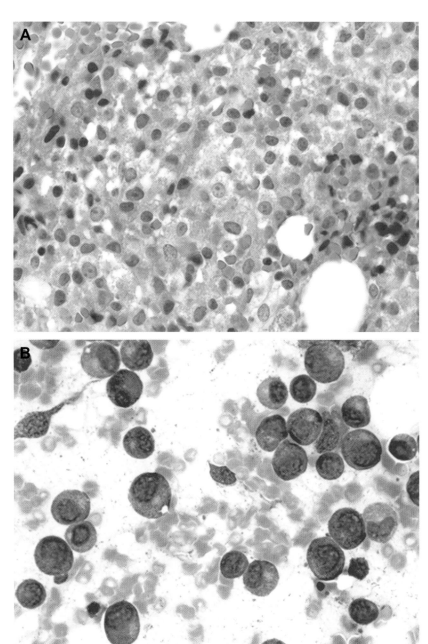

changes are particularly apparent in the BM of patients with HIV, hepatitis C virus, or systemic lupus erythematosus (**Fig. 7**) or in those who have undergone chemotherapy for malignancies. Dyserythropoiesis is commonly observed but is often mild. Dysgranulopoiesis and dysmegakaryopoiesis, if present, are also usually mild. Iron staining is helpful for identifying RS; however, storage iron is often increased in both MDS and anemia of chronic inflammation. Erythroid hypoplasia or aplasia may be indicative of a viral infection (parvovirus B19) or thymoma, but this does not exclude MDS, because erythroid hypoplasia or aplasia can be present in a subset of patients with MDS and is often associated with a clonal T-cell expansion (see **Fig. 2**C, D).[25] A cytogenetic abnormality characteristic of MDS confirms an MDS diagnosis, but cytogenetic abnormalities

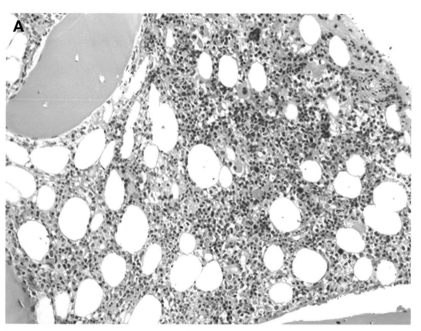

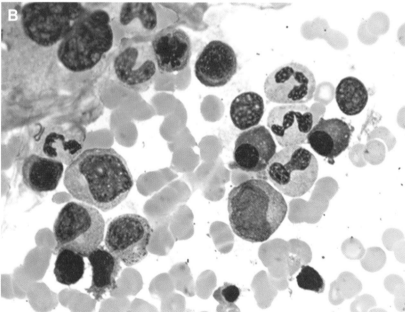

Fig. 7. Systemic lupus erythematosus. (*A*) The BM biopsy shows altered marrow stroma and some dysplastic-appearing small megakaryocytes, mimicking MDS. (*B*) Dyserythropoiesis with karyorrhexis of erythroid precursors is also present in the aspirate smear; plasma cells are increased, a clue to the diagnosis of an autoimmune disease.

are only seen in 5% to 20% of patients with low-grade MDS[5] and are especially infrequent in those with RCUD (2% to 5% of cases). Alternatively, after chemotherapy and autologous stem cell transplantation, transient chromosomal abnormalities can be observed and do not predict development of t-MDS.[61,62] Therefore, these findings must be interpreted with caution. On FCI, maturing myelomonocytic cells in reactive and suppressed BM may show alterations, such as a left-shifted maturation pattern; altered CD33, CD10, CD11b, CD16, CD15, or HLA-DR expression; and/or increased CD56 expression. The CD34+ precursors are immunophenotypically normal, however, and hematogones are preserved. Nevertheless, unless the diagnosis of MDS is clear-cut, it is prudent to raise the possibility of MDS without rendering a definitive diagnosis, especially in patients who have undergone chemotherapy or stem cell transplantation. Clinical follow-up often eventually confirms a diagnosis of true MDS by establishing the chronicity of the abnormality and by allowing time for excluding other possible reactive/reversible causes.

Cytopenias treated with growth factors can be problematic if the growth factors are administrated empirically before a BM biopsy is conducted. The effect of growth factors complicates a BM evaluation. Granulocyte colony-stimulating factor (G-CSF) and its derivatives are widely used to reduce the duration of neutropenia induced by chemotherapy. The changes associated with G-CSF include left-shifted myeloid maturation with increased myeloid precursors, including ALIPs in some cases as a result of rapid myeloid regeneration. Cytoplasmic hypergranulation and circulating myeloid precursors and blasts can also be observed. In MDS or AML BM samples, myeloblasts can increase significantly on G-CSF stimulation and drop back to baseline after G-CSF is stopped. Thus, it is important not to overdiagnose RAEB or AML in patients who recently started G-CSF treatment. G-CSF administration causes alteration of some of flow cytometric markers, such as increased CD64 and CD14 expression and decreased CD16 expression on neutrophils, decreased side scatter of maturing myeloid cells,[63] and increased CD7+ myeloid precursors. Erythropoietin is often administrated to anemia patients with a low erythropoietin level or patients with MDS who do not have significantly increased endogenous erythropoietin levels. In reactive BM, erythropoietin often increases the proportion of erythroid cells but does not cause significant morphologic dysplasia. In contrast, erythropoietin treatment in MDS patients often leads to a decreased, rather than an increased, proportion of erythroid cells as a result of reducing apoptosis and promoting effective hematopoiesis.[64]

AA may be difficult to distinguish from hypoplastic MDS. The low cellularity (**Fig.** 8A, B) and often poor-quality aspirates obtained from such specimens make the identification of dyspoiesis and the enumeration of blasts challenging; in some cases, it may be impossible to distinguish hypocellular MDS from AA.[65] In blood smears, macrocytic red blood cells are often found in both conditions, but the presence of neutrophils with pseudo-Pelger-Huët nuclei and/or hypogranular cytoplasm favor a diagnosis of MDS. Similarly, in BM samples, dysplastic

granulopoiesis and megakaryopoiesis favor an MDS diagnosis, whereas dyserythropoiesis is less specific and can occur in AA (see **Fig.** 8C). In hypoplastic MDS, BM biopsy samples have sparsely scattered dysgranulopoietic cells, patchy islands of immature erythropoiesis, and, in most cases, decreased megakaryopoiesis with some micromegakaryocytes.[66] The BM can be completely acellular in some areas, whereas discernible dysplastic cellular islands are present in other areas. A larger and deeper biopsy may help establish a more definitive diagnosis in equivocal cases. Normal or increased CD34+ cells in the BM are more likely seen in MDS, whereas CD34+ cells are markedly decreased in AA (see **Fig.** 8D). Although the identification of a clonal chromosomal abnormality at the time of presentation is generally considered indicative of MDS, clonal chromosomal abnormalities may occasionally be seen in AA,[67] particularly in cases associated with Fanconi anemia (discussed further in Pediatric Bone Marrow Interpretation by Dr Mihaela Onciu elsewhere in this issue).[68]

Biologically, an overlap between acquired AA and hypoplastic MDS has been suggested.[69] Moreover, MDS develops in 10% to 15% of patients with AA who are not treated with hematopoietic stem cell transplantation. Small populations of clones deficient in glycophosphatidylinositol (GPI)-anchored proteins on their cell surface may be detected in 40% to 50% of patients with AA by flow cytometric analysis in the absence of clinical signs of PNH.[70] These GPI-mutated cells likely reflect an independent clonal expansion that arises because of a selective growth advantage under immune-mediated destruction of BM hematopoietic cells. However, such small clones have been detected in approximately 20% of adults with low-grade MDS.[71,72] Therefore, the presence of such a PNH cell population does not exclude a diagnosis of MDS.

Dysplastic features in inherited BM failure syndromes may mimic MDS, particularly in pediatric patients. Congenital dyserythropoietic anemia, Noonan syndrome, Dobowitz syndrome, mitochondrial disorders (Pearson syndrome),[73] reticular dysgenesis, thrombocytopenia with absent radii syndrome, and congenital amegakaryocytic thrombocytopenia[14] can share some morphologic and clinical features with MDS but are not necessarily associated with an increased risk of acute leukemia. Many inherited BM failure disorders cannot be separated from MDS by morphologic criteria and, to make this distinction, careful physical examination, past medical

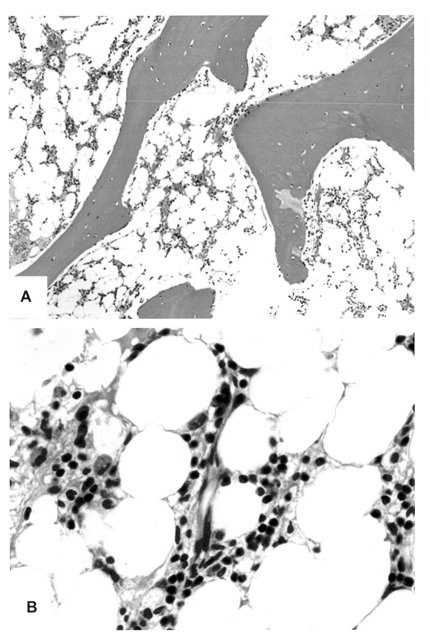

Fig. 8. Aplastic anemia. (*A*) BM biopsy shows marked hypocellularity. (*B*) The cellular elements are predominantly lympho-cytes, plasma cells, stromal cells and some maturing erythroid precursors.

history and family history analysis, and other appropriate laboratory tests are required. An associated constitutional abnormality is present in 29% to 45% of all pediatric MDS patients.[74] In patients with congenital BM failure disorders, hematopoiesis can show dysplastic features, in particular dyserythropoiesis. Therefore, evolution of MDS in such a setting can only be diagnosed if a persistent clonal chromosomal abnormality is present or if hypercellularity in the BM develops

Fig. 8. Aplastic anemia. (*C*) Some dysplastic features can be seen in the bone marrow aspirate (*arrows*). (*D*) CD34 precursors are decreased on a CD34 immunohistochemical stain, in contrast to hypocellular MDS, in which CD34+ cells would be relatively increased.

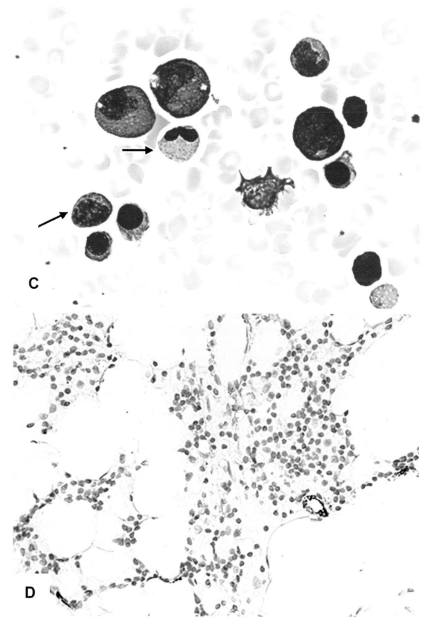

Differential Diagnosis
MYELODYSPLASTIC SYNDROMES

MDS Versus	Helpful Distinguishing Features
Hairy cell leukemia	• CD20 immunostain reveals neoplastic B-cells in BM biopsy in an interstitial pattern
Peripheral destruction (hemolytic anemia or immune thrombocytopenia)	• Retained normal BM topography • Hyperplasia of cytopenic lineage • Normal or increased hematogones
BM suppression (infection, autoimmune disease, status post chemotherapy)	• Absence of cytogenetic abnormalities • Normal immunophenotype of CD34+ blasts • Normal or increased hematogones • Clinical history
Growth factor therapy	• Clinical history • Hypergranulation of neutrophils • Minimal or no true morphologic dysplasia
Aplastic anemia	• No increase of CD34+ cells by IHC of BM biopsy dysplasia often mild and confined to erythroid
Congenital marrow failure syndromes	• Clinical history • Absence of clonal cytogenetic abnormality • Significant morphologic dysplasia usually absent

in the presence of persistent unexplained peripheral cytopenia. Diagnosis of MDS in pediatric patients is discussed in more detail in Pediatric Bone Marrow Interpretation by Dr Mihaela Onciu elsewhere, in this issue.

Pitfalls
IN MYELODYSPLASTIC SYNDROMES

! Establishing an initial diagnosis of low-grade MDS can be challenging, because cytogenetic alterations are infrequent and non-MDS cytopenias can mimic MDS morphologically

! Because lymphomas and plasma cell myeloma may share a similar cytopenic presentation with MDS, flow cytometry panels used to evaluate cytopenic patients should include markers capable of detecting clonal B cells, aberrant T cells, and clonal plasma cells.

! The presence of a cytogenetic abnormality is not necessarily indicative of MDS.

! Patients with idiopathic cytopenia of undetermined significance (ICUS) need close clinical follow-up.

! Aplastic anemia, especially after therapy, can share many features with hypoplastic MDS.

PROGNOSIS

The most significant causes of mortality in patients with MDS are BM failure and transformation to acute leukemia, which is almost always AML with rare cases of B lymphoblastic leukemia reported.[75,76] The overall incidence of transformation to AML in MDS is approximately 30% but varies significantly by subtype—5% to 35% for patients with RAEB compared with only 2% for refractory anemia.[77] The IPSS 4-tier score combining the percentage of marrow blasts, specific cytogenetic abnormalities, and number of cytopenias effectively predicts overall survival and evolution to AML. The median survival of patients in the IPSS-high group is only 0.4 years versus 5.7 years for patients in the IPSS-low group.[14] Several other clinical and pathologic factors have been shown to add significant prognostic information to that provided by the IPSS, such as patient age, performance status, transfusion dependence, WHO disease subtype, presence of marrow fibrosis, clustering of CD34+ myeloblasts, presence of ALIPs, and presence of molecular alterations involving FLT3, KIT, TP53, and RAS genes.[77–81] Although the presence of 20% blasts in PB or BM distinguishes AML from high-grade MDS (RAEB) according to the 2008 WHO Classification of MDS in adults, patients with lower blast counts may still be treated as AML, especially in the pediatric population. Therapeutic algorithms are currently based on a complex matrix of patient age, performance status, and risk and benefit assessment.

REFERENCES

1. Adams PF, Hendershot GE, Marano MA. Current estimates from the National Health Interview Survey, 1996. Vital Health Stat 10 1999;200:1−203.

2. DeMaeyer E, Adiels-Tegman M. The prevalence of anaemia in the world. World Health Stat Q 1985;38: 302−16.

3. Dubois RW, Goodnough LT, Ershler WB, et al. Identification, diagnosis, and management of anemia in adult ambulatory patients treated by primary care physicians: evidence-based and consensus recommendations. Curr Med Res Opin 2006;22:385−95.

4. Goldstein KH, Abramson N. Efficient diagnosis of thrombocytopenia. Am Fam Physician 1996;53: 915−20.

5. Swerdlow SH, Campo E, Harris NL, et al, editors. WHO classification of tumours of haematopoietic and lymphoid tissues. 4th edition. Lyon (France): IARC press; 2008. p. 87.

6. Vardiman JW, Harris NL, Brunning RD. The World Health Organization (WHO) classification of the myeloid neoplasms. Blood 2002;100:2292−302.

7. Gupta R, Soupir CP, Johari V, et al. Myelodysplastic syndrome with isolated deletion of chromosome 20q: an indolent disease with minimal morphological dysplasia and frequent thrombocytopenic presentation. Br J Haematol 2007;139:265−8.

8. Kuroda J, Kimura S, Kobayashi Y, et al. Unusual myelodysplastic syndrome with the initial presentation mimicking idiopathic thrombocytopenic purpura. Acta Haematol 2002;108:139−43.

9. Vardiman JW. Hematopathological concepts and controversies in the diagnosis and classification of myelodysplastic syndromes. Hematology Am Soc Hematol Educ Program 2006;199−204.

10. Schmitt-Graeff A, Mattern D, Kohler H, et al. [Myelodysplastic syndromes (MDS). Aspects of hematopathologic diagnosis]. Pathologe 2000;21:1−15 [in German].

11. Sole F, Espinet B, Sanz GF, et al. Incidence, characterization and prognostic significance of chromosomal abnormalities in 640 patients with primary myelodysplastic syndromes. Grupo Cooperativo Espanol de Citogenetica Hematologica. Br J Haematol 2000;108:346−56.

12. Young NS, Calado RT, Scheinberg P. Current concepts in the pathophysiology and treatment of aplastic anemia. Blood 2006;108:2509−19.

13. Konoplev S, Medeiros LJ, Lennon PA, et al. Therapy may unmask hypoplastic myelodysplastic syndrome that mimics aplastic anemia. Cancer 2007;110: 1520−6.

14. Greenberg P, Cox C, LeBeau MM, et al. International scoring system for evaluating prognosis in myelodysplastic syndromes. Blood 1997;89:2079−88.

15. Valent P, Horny HP, Bennett JM, et al. Definitions and standards in the diagnosis and treatment of the myelodysplastic syndromes: consensus statements and report from a working conference. Leuk Res 2007;31:727−36.

16. Verburgh E, Achten R, Louw VJ, et al. A new disease categorization of low-grade myelodysplastic syndromes based on the expression of cytopenia and dysplasia in one versus more than one lineage improves on the WHO classification. Leukemia 2007;21:668−77.

17. Verburgh E, Achten R, Maes B, et al. Additional prognostic value of bone marrow histology in patients subclassified according to the International Prognostic Scoring System for myelodysplastic syndromes. J Clin Oncol 2003;21:273−82.

18. Mangi MH, Mufti GJ. Primary myelodysplastic syndromes: diagnostic and prognostic significance of immunohistochemical assessment of bone marrow biopsies. Blood 1992;79:198−205.

19. Mangi MH, Salisbury JR, Mufti GJ. Abnormal localization of immature precursors (ALIP) in the bone marrow of myelodysplastic syndromes: current state of knowledge and future directions. Leuk Res 1991; 15:627−39.

20. Ogata K, Nakamura K, Yokose N, et al. Clinical significance of phenotypic features of blasts in patients with myelodysplastic syndrome. Blood 2002;100:3887−96.

21. Oriani A, Annaloro C, Soligo D, et al. Bone marrow histology and CD34 immunostaining in the prognostic evaluation of primary myelodysplastic syndromes. Br J Haematol 1996;92:360−4.

22. Mufti GJ, Bennett JM, Goasguen J, et al. Diagnosis and classification of myelodysplastic syndrome: International Working Group on Morphology of myelodysplastic syndrome (IWGM-MDS) consensus proposals for the definition and enumeration of myeloblasts and ring sideroblasts. Haematologica 2008;93:1712−7.

23. Hasserjian RP, Zuo Z, Garcia C, et al. Acute erythroid leukemia: a reassessment using criteria refined in the 2008 WHO classification. Blood 2010;115(10):1985−92.

24. Wang SA, Tang G, Fadare O, et al. Erythroid-predominant myelodysplastic syndromes: enumeration of blasts from nonerythroid rather than total marrow cells provides superior risk stratification. Mod Pathol 2008;21:1394−402.

25. Wang SA, Yue G, Hutchinson L, et al. Myelodysplastic syndrome with pure red cell aplasia shows characteristic clinicopathological features and clonal T-cell expansion. Br J Haematol 2007;138:271−5.

26. Shimamoto T, Iguchi T, Ando K, et al. Successful treatment with cyclosporin A for myelodysplastic syndrome with erythroid hypoplasia associated with T-cell receptor gene rearrangements. Br J Haematol 2001;114:358–61.

27. Kussick SJ, Fromm JR, Rossini A, et al. Four-color flow cytometry shows strong concordance with bone marrow morphology and cytogenetics in the evaluation for myelodysplasia. Am J Clin Pathol 2005;124:170–81.

28. Stachurski D, Smith BR, Pozdnyakova O, et al. Flow cytometric analysis of myelomonocytic cells by a pattern recognition approach is sensitive and specific in diagnosing myelodysplastic syndrome and related marrow diseases: emphasis on a global evaluation and recognition of diagnostic pitfalls. Leuk Res 2008;32:215–24.

29. Wells DA, Benesch M, Loken MR, et al. Myeloid and monocytic dyspoiesis as determined by flow cytometric scoring in myelodysplastic syndrome correlates with the IPSS and with outcome after hematopoietic stem cell transplantation. Blood 2003;102:394–403.

30. Truong F, Smith BR, Stachurski D, et al. The utility of flow cytometric immunophenotyping in cytopenic patients with a non-diagnostic bone marrow: a prospective study. Leuk Res 2009;33:1039–46.

31. Ogata K, Della Porta MG, Malcovati L, et al. Diagnostic utility of flow cytometry in low-grade myelodysplastic syndromes: a prospective validation study. Haematologica 2009;94:1066–74.

32. van de Loosdrecht AA, Alhan C, Bene MC, et al. Standardization of flow cytometry in myelodysplastic syndromes: report from the first European LeukemiaNet working conference on flow cytometry in myelodysplastic syndromes. Haematologica 2009; 94:1124–34.

33. Ogata K, Kishikawa Y, Satoh C, et al. Diagnostic application of flow cytometric characteristics of CD34+ cells in low-grade myelodysplastic syndromes. Blood 2006;108:1037–44.

34. Haase D, Germing U, Schanz J, et al. New insights into the prognostic impact of the karyotype in MDS and correlation with subtypes: evidence from a core dataset of 2124 patients. Blood 2007;110: 4385–95.

35. Pozdnyakova O, Miron PM, Tang G, et al. Cytogenetic abnormalities in a series of 1,029 patients with primary myelodysplastic syndromes: a report from the US with a focus on some undefined single chromosomal abnormalities. Cancer 2008;113: 3331–40.

36. Sole F, Luno E, Sanzo C, et al. Identification of novel cytogenetic markers with prognostic significance in a series of 968 patients with primary myelodysplastic syndromes. Haematologica 2005;90: 1168–78.

37. Haase D. Cytogenetic features in myelodysplastic syndromes. Ann Hematol 2008;87:515–26.

38. Beyer V, Castagne C, Muhlematter D, et al. Systematic screening at diagnosis of -5/del(5)(q31), -7, or chromosome 8 aneuploidy by interphase fluorescence in situ hybridization in 110 acute myelocytic leukemia and high-risk myelodysplastic syndrome patients: concordances and discrepancies with conventional cytogenetics. Cancer Genet Cytogenet 2004;152:29–41.

39. Yang W, Stotler B, Sevilla DW, et al. FISH analysis in addition to G-band karyotyping: Utility in evaluation of myelodysplastic syndromes? Leuk Res 2010; 34(4):420–5.

40. Cuneo A, Bigoni R, Roberti MG, et al. Detection and monitoring of trisomy 8 by fluorescence in situ hybridization in acute myeloid leukemia: a multicentric study. Haematologica 1998;83:21–6.

41. Paulsson K, Heidenblad M, Strombeck B, et al. High-resolution genome-wide array-based comparative genome hybridization reveals cryptic chromosome changes in AML and MDS cases with trisomy 8 as the sole cytogenetic aberration. Leukemia 2006;20: 840–6.

42. Evers C, Beier M, Poelitz A, et al. Molecular definition of chromosome arm 5q deletion end points and detection of hidden aberrations in patients with myelodysplastic syndromes and isolated del (5q) using oligonucleotide array CGH. Genes Chromosomes Cancer 2007;46:1119–28.

43. Maciejewski JP, Mufti GJ. Whole genome scanning as a cytogenetic tool in hematologic malignancies. Blood 2008;112:965–74.

44. Makishima H, Rataul M, Gondek LP, et al. FISH and SNP-A karyotyping in myelodysplastic syndromes: improving cytogenetic detection of del(5q), monosomy 7, del(7q), trisomy 8 and del(20q). Leuk Res 2010;34(4):447–53.

45. Deguchi K, Gilliland DG. Cooperativity between mutations in tyrosine kinases and in hematopoietic transcription factors in AML. Leukemia 2002;16:740–4.

46. Bernasconi P. Molecular pathways in myelodysplastic syndromes and acute myeloid leukemia: relationships and distinctions-a review. Br J Haematol 2008; 142:695–708.

47. Sankar M, Tanaka K, Kumaravel TS, et al. Identification of a commonly deleted region at 17p13.3 in leukemia and lymphoma associated with 17 p abnormality. Leukemia 1998;12:510–6.

48. Pellagatti A, Esoof N, Watkins F, et al. Gene expression profiling in the myelodysplastic syndromes using cDNA microarray technology. Br J Haematol 2004;125:576–83.

49. Hofmann WK, de Vos S, Komor M, et al. Characterization of gene expression of CD34+ cells from normal and myelodysplastic bone marrow. Blood 2002;100:3553–60.

50. Wimazal F, Fonatsch C, Thalhammer R, et al. Idiopathic cytopenia of undetermined significance (ICUS) versus low risk MDS: the diagnostic interface. Leuk Res 2007;31:1461–8.

51. Schroeder T, Ruf L, Bernhardt A, et al. Distinguishing myelodysplastic syndromes (MDS) from idiopathic cytopenia of undetermined significance (ICUS): HUMARA unravels clonality in a subgroup of patients. Ann Oncol 2010;21(11):2267–71.

52. Soupir CP, Vergilio JA, Kelly E, et al. Identification of del(20q) in a subset of patients diagnosed with idiopathic thrombocytopenic purpura. Br J Haematol 2009;144:800–2.

53. Tani P, Berchtold P, McMillan R. Autoantibodies in chronic ITP. Blut 1989;59:44–6.

54. Sashida G, Takaku TI, Shoji N, et al. Clinico-hematologic features of myelodysplastic syndrome presenting as isolated thrombocytopenia: an entity with a relatively favorable prognosis. Leuk Lymphoma 2003;44:653–8.

55. Lima CS, Paula EV, Takahashi T, et al. Causes of incidental neutropenia in adulthood. Ann Hematol 2006; 85:705–9.

56. Daniel D, Crawford J. Myelotoxicity from chemotherapy. Semin Oncol 2006;33:74–85.

57. Lin YC, Chang HK, Sun CF, et al. Microangiopathic hemolytic anemia as an initial presentation of metastatic cancer of unknown primary origin. Southampt Med J 1995;88:683–7.

58. Pittaluga S, Verhoef G, Maes A, et al. Bone marrow trephines. Findings in patients with hairy cell leukaemia before and after treatment. Histopathology 1994;25: 129–35.

59. Castello A, Coci A, Magrini U. Paraneoplastic marrow alterations in patients with cancer. Haematologica 1992;77:392–7.

60. Maftoun-Banankhah S, Maleki A, Karandikar NJ, et al. Multiparameter flow cytometric analysis reveals low percentage of bone marrow hematogones in myelodysplastic syndromes. Am J Clin Pathol 2008;129:300–8.

61. Martinez-Climent JA, Comes AM, Vizcarra E, et al. Chromosomal abnormalities in women with breast cancer after autologous stem cell transplantation are infrequent and may not predict development of therapy-related leukemia or myelodysplastic syndrome. Bone Marrow Transplant 2000;25: 1203–8.

62. Imrie KR, Dube I, Prince HM, et al. New clonal karyotypic abnormalities acquired following autologous bone marrow transplantation for acute myeloid leukemia do not appear to confer an adverse prognosis. Bone Marrow Transplant 1998;21:395–9.

63. Carulli G. Effects of recombinant human granulocyte colony-stimulating factor administration on neutrophil phenotype and functions. Haematologica 1997;82:606–16.

64. Hellstrom-Lindberg E, Kanter-Lewensohn L, Ost A. Morphological changes and apoptosis in bone marrow from patients with myelodysplastic syndromes treated with granulocyte-CSF and erythropoietin. Leuk Res 1997;21:415–25.

65. Hasle H, Baumann I, Bergstrasser E, et al. The International Prognostic Scoring System (IPSS) for childhood myelodysplastic syndrome (MDS) and juvenile myelomonocytic leukemia (JMML). Leukemia 2004; 18:2008–14.

66. Meadows AT, Baum E, Fossati-Bellani F, et al. Second malignant neoplasms in children: an update from the late effects Study Group. J Clin Oncol 1985;3:532–8.

67. Bhatia S, Ramsay NK, Steinbuch M, et al. Malignant neoplasms following bone marrow transplantation. Blood 1996;87:3633–9.

68. Neglia JP, Friedman DL, Yasui Y, et al. Second malignant neoplasms in five-year survivors of childhood cancer: childhood cancer survivor study. J Natl Cancer Inst 2001;93:618–29.

69. Barrett J, Saunthararajah Y, Molldrem J. Myelodysplastic syndrome and aplastic anemia: distinct entities or diseases linked by a common pathophysiology? Semin Hematol 2000;37:15–29.

70. Maciejewski JP, Rivera C, Kook H, et al. Relationship between bone marrow failure syndromes and the presence of glycophosphatidyl inositol-anchored protein-deficient clones. Br J Haematol 2001;115:1015–22.

71. Wang SA, Pozdnyakova O, Jorgensen JL, et al. Detection of paroxysmal nocturnal hemoglobinuria clones in patients with myelodysplastic syndromes and related bone marrow diseases, with emphasis on diagnostic pitfalls and caveats. Haematologica 2009;94:29–37.

72. Wang H, Chuhjo T, Yasue S, et al. Clinical significance of a minor population of paroxysmal nocturnal hemoglobinuria-type cells in bone marrow failure syndrome. Blood 2002;100:3897–902.

73. Passmore SJ, Hann IM, Stiller CA, et al. Pediatric myelodysplasia: a study of 68 children and a new prognostic scoring system. Blood 1995;85:1742–50.

74. Bacigalupo A, Broccia G, Corda G, et al. Antilymphocyte globulin, cyclosporin, and granulocyte colony-stimulating factor in patients with acquired severe aplastic anemia (SAA): a pilot study of the EBMT SAA Working Party. Blood 1995;85: 1348–53.

75. Disperati P, Ichim CV, Tkachuk D, et al. Progression of myelodysplasia to acute lymphoblastic leukaemia: implications for disease biology. Leuk Res 2006;30: 233–9.

76. Zainina S, Cheong SK. Myelodysplastic syndrome transformed into Acute Lymphoblastic Leukaemia (FAB: L3). Clin Lab Haematol 2006;28:282–3.

77. Malcovati L, Germing U, Kuendgen A, et al. Time-dependent prognostic scoring system for predicting survival and leukemic evolution in myelodysplastic syndromes. J Clin Oncol 2007;25:3503–10.

78. Kantarjian H, O'Brien S, Ravandi F, et al. Proposal for a new risk model in myelodysplastic syndrome that accounts for events not considered in the original International Prognostic Scoring System. Cancer 2008;113:1351—61.

79. Balducci L. Transfusion independence in patients with myelodysplastic syndromes: impact on outcomes and quality of life. Cancer 2006;106: 2087—94.

80. Shih LY, Lin TL, Wang PN, et al. Internal tandem duplication of fms-like tyrosine kinase 3 is associated with poor outcome in patients with myelodysplastic syndrome. Cancer 2004;101:989—98.

81. Kita-Sasai Y, Horiike S, Misawa S, et al. International prognostic scoring system and TP53 mutations are independent prognostic indicators for patients with myelodysplastic syndrome. Br J Haematol 2001; 115:309—12.

ACUTE MYELOID LEUKEMIA WITH MYELODYSPLASIA-RELATED CHANGES: A NEW DEFINITION

Olga K. Weinberg, MD, Daniel A. Arber, MD*

KEYWORDS

- Acute myeloid leukemia • Myelodysplasia-related changes • Multilineage dysplasia
- 2008 WHO classification

ABSTRACT

Acute myeloid leukemia (AML) with multilineage dysplasia was introduced in the 2001 World Health Organization (WHO) classification to encompass cases of AML characterized by myelodysplastic syndrome—like features. The 2008 WHO classification revised this group into a new category, AML with myelodysplasia-related changes (AML-MRC). The category now includes patients with at least 20% blasts in peripheral blood or bone marrow and any of the following: (1) AML arising from a previous MDS or mixed MDS/myeloproliferative neoplasm, (2) AML with a specific MDS-associated cytogenetic abnormality and/or (3) AML with multilineage dysplasia. Up to 48% of all patients with AML are encompassed within the AML-MRC subgroup. AML-MRC patients have worse prognosis compared with patients with AML, not otherwise specified.

Key Features
OF ACUTE MYELOID LEUKEMIA WITH MYELODYSPLASIA-RELATED CHANGES

1. Diagnostic criteria are the presence of 20% blood or marrow blasts and any of the following: (a) previous history of MDS or MDS/myeloproliferative neoplas (MDS/MPN), (b) MDS-associated cytogenetic abnormality, or (c) multilineage morphologic dysplasia.

2. Dysplasia must be present in at least 50% of the cells in at least two bone marrow lines to diagnose using morphologic multilineage dysplasia criteria.

3. Cases of AML after cytotoxic chemotherapy or radiotherapy or with any of the specific cytogenetic abnormalities qualifying for AML with recurrent genetic abnormalities are excluded.

4. AML-MRC is an aggressive leukemia with a poor prognosis.

OVERVIEW

Classification of acute myeloid leukemia (AML) was first standardized in 1976 by the French-American-British working group in what came to be known as the FAB classification, based primarily on morphology and cytochemistry.[1–5] Morphologic dysplastic changes had been observed both in patients with de novo AML as well as those with AML arising from myelodysplastic syndrome (MDS),[6] but the FAB classification did not assign significance to such findings. De novo AML cases with dysplasia were initially labeled as AML with

Department of Pathology, Stanford University Medical Center, 300 Pasteur Drive L235, Stanford, CA 94305, USA
* Corresponding author.
E-mail address: darber@stanford.edu

Surgical Pathology 3 (2010) 1153–1164
doi:10.1016/j.path.2010.09.012

surgpath.theclinics.com

trilineage myelodysplasia and were reported to account for 10% to 15% of all AML.[7] Early studies showed that AML with trilineage myelodysplasia could occur in young patients who presented with low peripheral blood and bone marrow blast counts.[6] These patients had a higher incidence of AML-M4 (myelomonocytic) and -M6 (erythro-leukemia) subtypes using FAB criteria.[6] The rate of achieving complete remission in patients with AML with trilineage myelodysplasia was reported to be poor in multiple studies.[6–11] Furthermore, relapses of leukemia occurred earlier and more frequently as compared with other AML types.[8,9] Specifically, Goasguen and colleagues[10] found that the presence of dysgranulopoiesis was associated with a lower likelihood of achieving complete remission, whereas Gahn and colleagues[11] found that dysplastic changes of granulocytes and megakaryocytes were associated with a worse event-free survival in a series of 102 patients. Other studies, however, did not find dysplasia to have an impact on outcome.[12,13] Some of these differences could be due to inclusion of different AML subtypes in these studies and absence of standardized criteria for morphologic dysplasia.

With improvements in treatment and newer biologic studies of AML, it became clear that the FAB classification had limited clinical relevance. Cytogenetic and molecular genetic features, as well as history of a prior MDS and prior therapy, were shown to have significant prognostic impact and did not correlate well with FAB categories.[14] A new classification was proposed by the World Health Organization (WHO) in 2001 that was based more on a biology-oriented understanding of AML.[14] This classification was based on three major determinants: cytogenetics, the presence or absence of dysplastic features in nonblast cells, and preceding history of cytotoxic chemotherapy or radiotherapy. Cases with none of these features were categorized as AML, not otherwise specified (AML-NOS), where criteria from the FAB classification were maintained. Cases with dysplastic features were placed in a new category of AML with multilineage dysplasia in that edition of the WHO classification. Although later studies have validated this system,[15–17] including the importance of multilineage dysplasia, others have suggested that multilineage dysplasia correlates with unfavorable cytogenetics and has no independent impact on prognosis.[18,19]

In 2008, a revision of the WHO classification incorporated recently acquired genetic information into an updated classification scheme of AML.[20] One of the revisions includes a new group, AML with myelodysplasia-related changes (AML-MRC), that replaced the previous category of AML with multilineage dysplasia. Patients are now assigned to this group for any one or combination of three reasons[20]:

1. AML arising from previous MDS or an MDS/myeloproliferative neoplasm (MDS/MPN), such as chronic myelomonocytic leukemia
2. AML with a specific MDS-related cytogenetic abnormality
3. AML with multilineage dysplasia.

Cases that have one of the entity-defining recurring cytogenetic abnormalities are excluded and are considered to represent AML with recurrent genetic abnormalities. This group includes AML with t(8;21)(q22;q22), inv(16) (p13.1q22), t(16;16)(p13.1;q22), t(15;17)(q22;q12), or t(9;11) (q22;q23) as well as new entities in the 2008 classification of AML with t(1;22)(p13;q13), inv(3) (q21q26.2), t(3;3)(q21;q26.2), or t(6;9)(p23;q34). The latter three abnormalities commonly show multilineage dysplasia and may resemble AML-MRC on morphology but are now considered specific entities within the subgroup of AML with recurrent genetic abnormalities and are excluded from AML-MRC.

CLINICAL FEATURES

In past literature, the definition of multilineage dysplasia has been variable, resulting in variable reported incidences. Early studies reported that trilineage dysplasia occurred in 10% to 15% of all de novo AML cases. Using 2001 WHO criteria for AML with multilineage dysplasia, Arber and colleagues[16] found that AML with multilineage dysplasia comprised 32% of all cases. Similarly, Yanada and colleagues[15] found that AML with multilineage dysplasia accounted for 29% of all AML cases. With the new definition outlined in the 2008 WHO classification, the number of patients included in the AML-MRC group is higher due to inclusion of AML patients with specific MDS-related cytogenetic abnormalities. The authors recently evaluated the clinical, pathologic, cytogenetic, and molecular features of 100 AML patients using the 2008 WHO criteria and found that AML-MRC comprised 48% of all AML cases.[21]

Early studies found no significant age difference between those with trilineage dysplasia and other AML cases.[6,22] More recently, Wandt and colleagues[19] found no difference in age between AML patients with multilineage dysplasia as defined by 2001 WHO and other types of AML. Applying the 2008 WHO criteria, the authors found that patients with AML-MRC were significantly older as compared with patients with AML-NOS.[21] Patients with AML-MRC also presented with lower hematocrit and their blasts more frequently expressed CD14 when compared with AML-NOS.[21] Earlier studies showed that patients with AML with tri-lineage dysplasia had higher platelet counts, fewer blasts in peripheral blood and bone marrow, fewer so-called Auer bodies and less myeloperoxidase positivity of the leukemic blasts.[22] Cases that evolve to AML-MRC after a preceding diagnosis of MDS or MDS/MPN often have low bone marrow blast counts of 20% to 30%.

DIAGNOSTIC CRITERIA

The diagnosis of AML-MRC requires the presence of 20% or more blasts in peripheral blood or bone marrow. In addition, one of the following must be present: morphologic evidence of multilineage dysplasia; prior history of MDS or MDS/MPN; or the presence of MDS-related cytogenetic abnormalities (Table 1). A case may be assigned to this group for one, two or all three of these reasons.[20] Important exclusions include prior cytotoxic therapy for an unrelated disease that designate a case as therapy-related AML and the presence of a specific cytogenetic abnormality that qualifies a case as AML with recurring genetic abnormalities. An algorithm to apply when classifying cases of newly diagnosed AML is shown in Fig. 1.

Table 1
Diagnostic criteria for acute myeloid leukemia with myelodysplasia-related changes

Qualifying Feature[a]	Diagnostic Criteria
Multilineage dysplasia	Morphologic dysplasia present in at least 50% of the cells in at least 2 cell lines
History of MDS or MDS/MPN	Documented history of a prior MDS or MDS/MPN
MDS-related cytogenetic abnormalities	Any of the following identifying by conventional cytogenetics: Complex karyotype[b] Unbalanced abnormalities −7/del(7q) −5/del(5q) i(17q)/t(17p) −13/del(13q) del(11q) del(12p)/t(12p) del(9q) idic(X)(q13) Balanced abnormalities t(11;16)(q23;p13.3) t(3;21)(q26.2;q22.1) t(1;3)(p36.3;q21.1) t(2;11)(p21;q23) t(5;12)(q33;p12) t(5;7)(q33;q11.2) t(5;17)(q33;p13) t(5;10)(q33;q21) t(3;5)(q25;q34)

[a] AML-MRC can be diagnosed if one, two, or all three of the qualifying features are present.
[b] Defined as three or more unrelated clonal abnormalities that do not include any of the specific abnormalities of AML with recurrent genetic abnormalities.

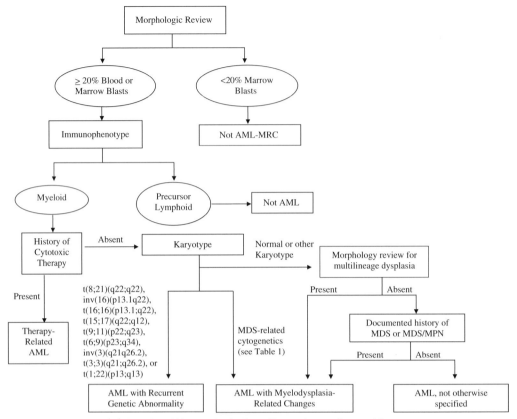

Fig. 1. Diagnostic algorithm that should be applied when diagnosing patients with AML.

DIAGNOSIS: MICROSCOPIC FEATURES

Morphologic dysplasia described by Bennett and colleagues[23] in MDS has been used in most studies that evaluated the significance of AML with dysplasia. In the bone marrow, dyserythropoiesis is defined as erythroids with multinuclearity, nuclear fragments of various sizes, abnormal nuclear shape, abnormal cytoplasmic features, such as nuclear-cytoplasmic dyssynchrony, and the presence of ring sideroblasts.[23] Changes in red blood cell morphology can be seen in peripheral blood, including hypochromasia and anisopoikilocytosis. Dysgranulopoiesis in peripheral blood is defined by agranular or hypogranular neutrophils. Abnormalities in nuclear segmentation may be seen in the form of hyposegmentation (Pelger-Huët–like anomaly) or hypersegmentation with bizarre shapes. In the bone marrow, abnormally staining primary (azurophilic) granules in promyelocytes and myelocytes, as well as absence of granules in some cells, are also common. In addition, secondary granules may be absent or reduced in the myelocytes and later forms, including mature granulocytes.[23] Similar nuclear abnormalities to those seen in the peripheral blood

are often present in the mature granulocytes. Abnormalities among megakaryocytes include the presence of micromegakaryocytes, large mononuclear megakaryocytes, and megakaryocytes with multiple small, separated nuclei. Occasionally megakaryocytes with giant and/or abnormal granules are seen.[23] Giant platelets and hypogranular platelets as well as micromegakaryocytes can be seen in peripheral blood.[23] The aforementioned descriptions of dysplastic changes are included in the definitions of AML-MRC in both the 2001 and 2008 editions of the WHO classification. An example of a typical AML-MRC case is shown in **Fig. 2**.

The earliest definitions of AML with multilineage dysplasia (so-called AML with trilineage dysplasia) required morphologic evidence of dysplasia in all three lineages.[6–11] In the 2001 WHO classification, the criteria of multilineage dysplasia were lowered to require the presence of dysplastic features in two cell lines, but such dysplasia must be seen in at least 50% of the cells in each of the two cell lines.[14] Applying this new definition, Arber and colleagues[16] found that these less rigid criteria retained clinical significance. The criteria for morphologic evidence of dysplasia have not changed in the 2008 WHO

Fig. 2. AML-MRC (multilineage dysplasia). (*A*) The marrow aspirate shows blasts, neutrophils with hypogranular cytoplasm, and small, hypolobated megakaryocytes as well as erythroid precursors with nuclear irregularities. (*B*) Higher power of the aspirate smear showing dysplastic megakaryocytes.

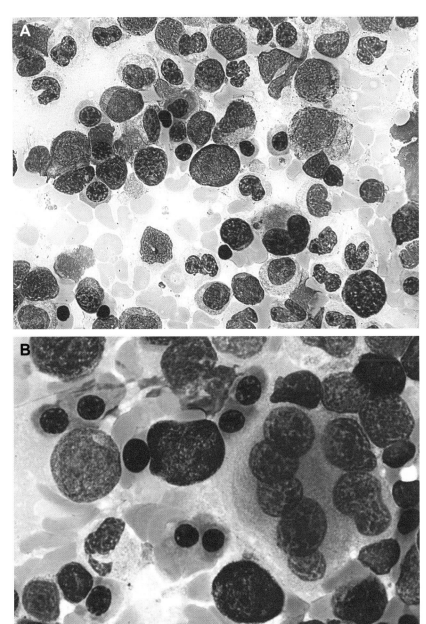

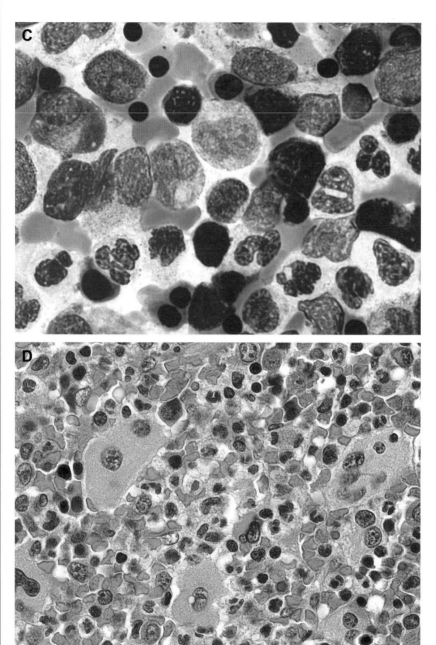

Fig. 2. AML-MRC (multilineage dysplasia). (*C*) Higher power of dysplastic neutrophils with clumped nuclear chromatin and hypogranular cytoplasm. (*D*) A bone marrow biopsy section shows dysplastic megakaryocytes with separated nuclei and admixed mononuclear cells consistent with blasts.

classification[20]: to classify a case as AML-MRC based on morphology, dysplasia must be present in at least 50% of cells in at least two bone marrow cell lines. This must be assessed on well-stained peripheral blood and bone marrow smears. The number of cells that must be present to be considered sufficient for evaluation is not specified[20]; in particular, megakaryocytes may be sparse and it is prudent to carefully evaluate both biopsy and aspirate material to fully assess the megakaryocytes present for dysplasia. The blast morphology of AML-MRC has not been well-studied, but in general these have similar morphologic features to myeloblasts found in other AML groups.

DIAGNOSIS: ANCILLARY STUDIES

Immunophenotyping results in these cases are also variable. Blasts often express panmyeloid markers, such as CD13 and CD33.[20] Those cases with antecedent MDS frequently have an aberrant expression of CD56 and CD7 and only partial expression of CD34, CD38 and HLA-DR.[24] Similarly, in cases with aberrations of chromosomes 5 and 7, a high incidence of CD34, terminal deoxynucleotidyl transferase, and CD7 expression is seen.[25] In comparison with AML-NOS, blasts in AML-MRC express CD14 more frequently.[21]

Cytogenetic studies of AML with dysplasia found that the frequency of morphologic dysplasia was higher in cases falling within adverse cytogenetic risk groups, although normal karyotype was still the most frequent finding in these patients.[18,21,26] Some of the common abnormalities include complex karyotype, −7/del(7q) and −5/del(5q).[20] Multilineage dysplasia is rare in the favorable cytogenetic risk groups AML with inv(16), t(15;17), and t(8;21). Abnormal features in the maturing myeloid elements, however, are frequent in AML with t(8;21). Such cases often show abnormally large Chédiak-Higashi–like granules, homogeneous pink cytoplasm, and abnormal nuclear lobation, including pseudo–Pelger-Huët cells. Unlike AML-MRC, however, these changes are limited to only one lineage (myeloid). In the authors' experience, CEBPA mutations, generally associated with a favorable prognosis in AML,[27] seem to be absent in AML-MRC, whereas the distribution of other mutations, including NPM1 and FLT3, are similar to AML-NOS.[21]

DIFFERENTIAL DIAGNOSIS

It is important to differentiate AML-MRC from refractory anemia with excess blasts, acute erythroid leukemia, acute megakaryoblastic leukemia, and other categories of AML-NOS.[20] According to the 2008 WHO classification scheme, acute erythroid leukemia cases with myeloblasts comprising 20% or more of all bone marrow cells and fulfilling AML-MRC criteria are classified as AML-MRC, whereas cases with blasts comprising less than 20% of total marrow cells but 20% or more of the nonerythroid cells are classified as acute erythroid leukemia, provided erythroid precursors are 50% or greater of all cells.[20] Thus, the distinction of acute erythroid leukemia from AML-MRC with erythroid hyperplasia is based solely on the number of blasts, calculated as the proportion of nonerythroid cells in acute erythroid leukemia but as the proportion of total bone marrow cells in AML-MRC (Fig. 3A). A recent study

suggests that acute erythroid leukemia, AML-MRC, and MDS with erythroid hyperplasia are likely biologically related diseases that seem to be arbitrarily separated into different entities in the current WHO classification scheme.[28] Acute megakaryoblastic leukemia often contains immature cells with cytoplasmic blebs (megakaryoblasts) and may show background dysplasia. It is unclear whether or not distinguishing acute megakaryoblastic leukemia in adults from AML-MRC has any clinical or prognostic significance; therefore, cases of AML displaying a megakaryocytic blast lineage that meet criteria for AML-MRC should be diagnosed as such using the 2008 WHO criteria. Finally, AML with t(8;21) may show abnormal myeloid granulation and pseudo–Pelger-Huët cells, but these dysplastic changes are limited to the myeloid lineage (see Fig. 3B). History of previous therapy for an unrelated disease classifies a case as therapy-related myeloid neoplasm (see Fig. 3C); it is thus critical to be aware of any antecedent history of cytotoxic chemotherapy or radiotherapy to correctly classify AML cases.

Chromosome abnormalities in AML-MRC are similar to MDS, with the common presence of complex karyotypes, monosomy 7, del(7q), monosomy 5, and del(5q).[20] Although trisomy 8 and del (20q) are common in MDS, they are not considered disease specific and by themselves are not sufficient for a diagnosis of AML-MRC. Cases with inv(3)(q21q26.2), t(3;3)(q21;q26.2), or t(6;9)(p23;q34) may contain multilineage dysplasia, but they are now classified as AML with recurrent genetic abnormalities (see Fig. 3D).[20] These recurrent cytogenetic categories of AML effectively trump a diagnosis of AML-MRC in the WHO classification, irrespective of the presence of qualifying levels of background morphologic dysplasia. The cytogenetic abnormalities, t(11;16)(q23;p13.3), t(3;21) (q26.2;q22.1), and t(2;11)(p21;q23), are more commonly associated with therapy-related AML than with de novo AML-MRC and these cytogenetic abnormalities should elicit a diligent search of the clinical history for any antecedent therapy. If there is no history of therapy, AML cases with any of these abnormalities are classified as AML-MRC.

Cases of AML with multilineage dysplasia may have NPM1 and FLT3 mutations. A recent study suggests that there is no survival difference between NPM1-mutated AML cases with multilineage dysplasia compared with NPM1-mutated AML cases without dysplasia[29]; however, this group has also not found the presence of multilineage dysplasia to have prognostic significance in any setting independent of cytogenetic findings (discussed later). Until further studies are preformed to evaluate the significance of NPM1

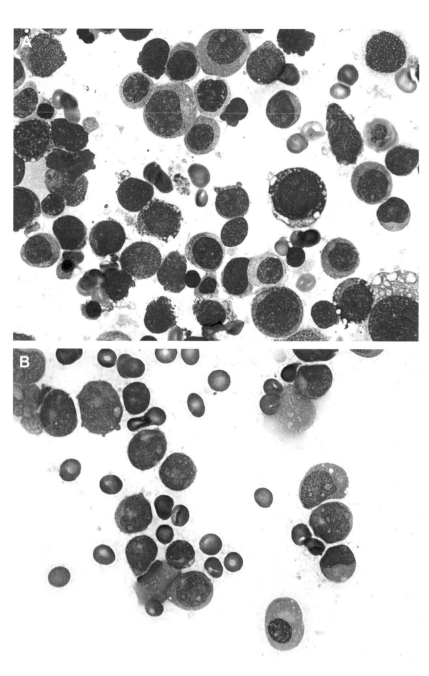

Fig. 3. Dyspoiesis in AML types other than AML-MRC. (*A*) This case of acute erythroid leukemia (a subtype of AML-NOS) demonstrates multilineage dysplasia, but myeloblasts represent less than 20% of nucleated marrow cells. Cases with similar features, but 20% or more myeloblasts, are classified as AML-MRC. (*B*) AML with t(8;21)(q22;q22); RUNX1-RUNX1T1 often shows so-called pelgeroid neutrophils with clumped nuclear chromatin without hyposegmentation (*lower right*). Multilineage dysplasia, however, is uncommon in this AML type and the detection of t(8;21) supercedes a diagnosis of AML-MRC.

Fig. 3. Dyspoiesis in AML types other than AML-MRC. (*C*) Therapy-related AML often has multilineage dysplasia, but a history of prior cytotoxic chemotherapy places this case into the group of therapy-related myeloid neoplasms. (*D*) AML with inv(3)(q21q26.2); *RPN1-EVI1* frequently shows multilineage dysplasia, with hypolobated mega-karyocytes predominating. This entity is now included in the category of AML with recurring genetic abnormalities and, in spite of the presence of multilineage dysplasia, this specific diagnosis should be made in the context of an inv(3) cytogenetic abnormality rather than AML-MRC.

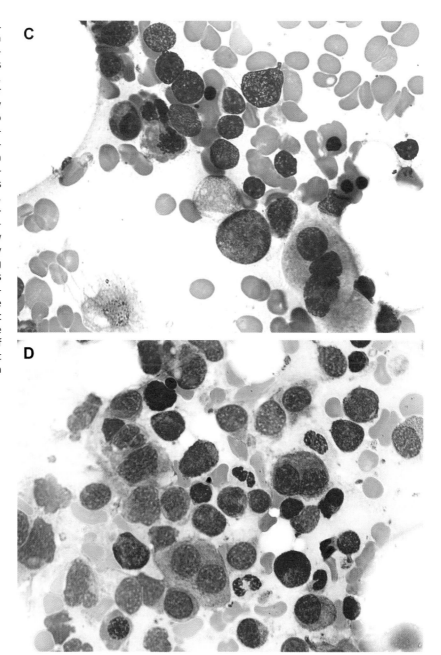

⚠️ DIFFERENTIAL DIAGNOSIS AML-MRC

AML-MRC Versus	Helpful Distinguishing Features
Refractory anemia with excess blasts	Myeloblasts comprise less than 20% of all nucleated cells; does not meet criteria for acute erythroid leukemia
Acute erythroid leukemia	Myeloblasts comprise less than 20% of all nucleated cells; however, erythroid elements comprise 50% or greater of all cells and myeloblasts comprise 20% or greater of the nonerythroid cells.
Acute megakaryoblastic leukemia	Blasts express megakaryocytic markers (CD41 and/or CD61) and defining features of AML-MRC are absent
AML with recurrent cytogenetic abnormalities, especially AML with t(6;9) and AML with inv(3) or t(3;3)	Cytogenetic, fluorescence in situ hybridization, or reverse transcriptase–polymerase chain reaction confirmation of one of the cytogenetic abnormalities defining a specific entity within the category of AML with recurrent cytogenetic abnormalities
Therapy-related AML and MDS	Clinical history of antecedent cytotoxic chemotherapy and/or radiotherapy

mutations in this disease group, the 2008 WHO recommends reporting the mutation status in the context of a diagnosis of AML-MRC for cases that fulfill WHO criteria for this entity.

The presence of chronic cytopenia without a definitive diagnosis of MDS preceding the development of AML is not sufficient for a diagnosis of AML-MRC. Similarly, AML cases with low blast counts (20% to 30%, which are categorized as a type of MDS—refractory anemia with excess blasts in transformation—in the FAB classification)

should not be classified as AML-MRC in the absence of a documented antecedent history of MDS, sufficient morphologic dysplasia, or qualifying cytogenetic abnormality.

PROGNOSIS

AML with myelodysplastic features generally has a poor prognosis with lower rate of achieving complete remission when compared with other AML types.[6,10,11,15,16,21,30,31] The definition of

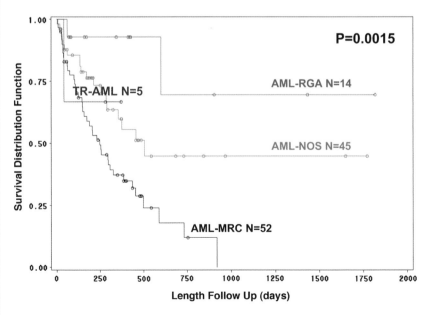

Fig. 4. Patients with AML-MRC have worse overall survival as compared with other types of AML, including AML-NOS, AML with recurrent genetic abnormalities (AML-RGAN), and therapy-related AML (TR-AML).

multilineage dysplasia applied in these studies has been variable, however. Although some studies using 2001 WHO criteria found that AML with multilineage dysplasia has a worse survival,[16] others have suggested that multilineage dysplasia correlates with unfavorable cytogenetics and has no independent impact on prognosis.[18,19] Applying 2008 WHO criteria to 100 AML patients, the authors found that patients with AML-MRC had a significantly worse overall survival, progression-free survival, and complete response when compared with AML-NOS using multivariate analysis (**Fig. 4**).[21] Even after excluding the 14 patients with unfavorable cytogenetics from the AML-MRC group, the remaining AML-MRC patients had significantly worse outcomes compared with all patients with AML-NOS, confirming the relevance of morphologic dysplasia as an important parameter in defining this group of AML.[21] In addition, among 65 patients with intermediate-risk cytogenetics, the outcome difference between the AML-MRC and AML-NOS remained significant,[21] also indicating prognostic significance of multilineage dysplasia. This finding confirms the previously observed clinical significance of multilineage dysplasia[15–17] when strictly defined by the WHO criteria. The clinical outcome of patients with a history of MDS was not significantly different from the remaining cases of AML-MRC, also consistent with prior studies.[16] Cases with dysplastic changes alone and lower blast counts may exhibit clinically less aggressive disease.[20] Although blast transformation of MPNs has a dismal prognosis, AML cases occurring after a diagnosis of MPN are not included in the AML-MRC group[31] and are considered separately in the WHO classification as blast transformation of the MPN.

Pitfalls
AML-MRC

! Careful and accurate blast count should be performed on all cases using well-stained peripheral blood and bone marrow aspirate smears.

! Maturing cells from each hematopoietic lineage (myeloid, erythroid, and megakaryocytic) should be carefully examined in the peripheral and bone marrow smear and bone marrow biopsy to determine if sufficient (>50%) dysplasia is present in at least two of the lineages.

! Cytogenetic evaluation should performed in all cases to exclude AML with recurrent genetic abnormalities.

! Clinical history must be examined to exclude therapy-related AML and to elicit any history of antecedent MDS or MDS/MPN.

REFERENCES

1. Bennett JM, Catovsky D, Daniel MT, et al. Proposals for the classification of the acute leukaemias. French-American-British (FAB) Co-operative Group. Br J Haematol 1976;33(4):451–8.
2. Bennett JM, Catovsky D, Daniel MT, et al. Proposed revised criteria for the classification of acute myeloid leukemia. A report of the French-American-British Cooperative Group. Ann Intern Med 1985;103(4):620–5.
3. Bennett JM, Catovsky D, Daniel MT, et al. Proposal for the recognition of minimally differentiated acute myeloid leukaemia (AML-MO). Br J Haematol 1991;78(3):325–9.
4. Bennett JM, Catovsky D, Daniel MT, et al. Criteria for the diagnosis of acute leukemia of megakaryocyte lineage (M7). A report of the French-American-British Cooperative Group. Ann Intern Med 1985;103(3):460–2.
5. Bennett JM, Catovsky D, Daniel MT, et al. A variant form of hypergranular promyelocytic leukaemia (M3). Br J Haematol 1980;44(1):169–70.
6. Brito-Babapulle F, Catovsky D, Galton DA. Clinical and laboratory features of de novo acute myeloid leukaemia with trilineage myelodysplasia. Br J Haematol 1987;66(4):445–50.
7. Kuriyama K, Tomonaga M, Matsuo T, et al. Poor response to intensive chemotherapy in de novo acute myeloid leukaemia with trilineage myelodysplasia. Japan Adult Leukaemia Study Group (JALSG). Br J Haematol 1994;86(4):767–73.
8. Jinnai I, Tomonaga M, Kuriyama K, et al. Dysmegakaryocytopoiesis in acute leukaemias: its predominance in myelomonocytic (M4) leukaemia and implication for poor response to chemotherapy. Br J Haematol 1987;66(4):467–72.
9. Estienne MH, Fenaux P, Preudhomme C, et al. Prognostic value of dysmyelopoietic features in de novo acute myeloid leukaemia: a report on 132 patients. Clin Lab Haematol 1990;12(1):57–65.
10. Goasguen JE, Matsuo T, Cox C, et al. Evaluation of the dysmyelopoiesis in 336 patients with de novo acute myeloid leukemia: major importance of dysgranulopoiesis for remission and survival. Leukemia 1992;6(6):520–5.
11. Gahn B, Haase D, Unterhalt M, et al. De novo AML with dysplastic hematopoiesis: cytogenetic and prognostic significance. Leukemia 1996;10(6):946–51.
12. Ballen KK, Gilliland DG, Kalish LA, et al. Bone marrow dysplasia in patients with newly diagnosed

acute myelogenous leukemia does not correlate with history of myelodysplasia or with remission rate and survival. Cancer 1994;73(2):314–21.

13. Fenaux P, Preudhomme C, Laï JL, et al. Cytogenetics and their prognostic value in de novo acute myeloid leukaemia: a report on 283 cases. Br J Haematol 1989;73(1):61–7.

14. Jaffe ES, Stein H, Vardiman DW, et al. Pathology and genetics of tumours of haematopoietic and lymphoid tissues: world health organization classification of tumours. Lyon (France): IARC Press; 2001. p. 351.

15. Yanada M, Suzuki M, Kawashima K, et al. Long-term outcomes for unselected patients with acute myeloid leukemia categorized according to the world health organization classification: a single center experience. Eur J Haematol 2005;74:418–23.

16. Arber DA, Stein AS, Carter NH, et al. Prognostic impact of acute myeloid leukemia classification: importance of detection of recurring cytogenetic abnormalities and multilineage dysplasia on survival. Am J Clin Pathol 2003;119:672–80.

17. Wakui M, Kuriyama K, Miyazaki Y. Diagnosis of acute myeloid leukemia according to the WHO classification in the Japan adult leukemia study group AML-97 protocol. Int J Hematol 2008;87:144–51.

18. Haferlach T, Schoch C, Loffler H, et al. Morphological dysplasia in de novo acute myeloid leukemia (AML) is related to unfavorable cytogenetics but has no independent prognostic relevance under the conditions of intensive induction therapy: results of a multiparameter analysis from the German AML Cooperative Group Studies. J Clin Oncol 2003;21: 256–65.

19. Wandt H, Schakel U, Kroschinsky F, et al. MLD according to the WHO classification in AML has no correlation with age and no independent prognostic relevance as analyzed in 1766 patients. Blood 2008; 111:1855–61.

20. Swerdlow SH, Campo E, Harris NL, et al, editors. WHO classification of tumours of haematopoietic and lymphoid tissues. Lyon (France): IARC Press; 2008. p. 109–38.

21. Weinberg OK, Seetharam M, Ren L, et al. Clinical characterization of acute myeloid leukemia with myelodysplasia-related changes as defined by the 2008 WHO classification system. Blood 2009; 113(9):1906–8.

22. Taguchi J, Miazaki Y, Yoshida S, et al. Allogeneic bone marrow transplantation improves outcome of de novo AML with trilineage dysplasia (AML-TLD). Leukemia 2000;14:1861–6.

23. Bennett JM, Catovsky D, Daniel MT, et al. Proposals for the classification of the myelodysplastic syndromes. Br J Haematol 1982;51(2):189–99.

24. Ogata K, Nakamura K, Yokose N, et al. Clinical significance of phenotypic features of blasts in patients with myelodysplastic syndrome. Blood 2002;100(12):3887–96.

25. Venditti A, Del Poeta G, Buccisano F, et al. Prognostic relevance of the expression of Tdt and CD7 in 335 cases of acute myeloid leukemia. Leukemia 1998;12(7):1056–63.

26. Miyazaki Y, Kuriyama K, Miyawaki S, et al. Japan adult leukaemia study group. cytogenetic heterogeneity of acute myeloid leukaemia (AML) with trilineage dysplasia: Japan Adult Leukaemia Study Group-AML 92 Study. Br J Haematol 2003;120(1):56–62.

27. Fröhling S, Schlenk RF, Stolze I, et al. CEBPA mutations in younger adults with acute myeloid leukemia and normal cytogenetics: prognostic relevance and analysis of cooperating mutations. J Clin Oncol 2004;22:624–33.

28. Hasserjian RP, Zuo Z, Garcia C, et al. Acute erythroid leukemia: a reassessment using criteria refined in the 2008 WHO classification. Blood 2010;115(10):1985–92.

29. Falini B, Macijewski K, Weiss T, et al. Multilineage dysplasia has no impact on biological, clinicopathological and prognostic features of AML with mutated nucleophosmin (NPM1). Blood 2010;115: 3776–86.

30. Leith CP, Kopecky KJ, Godwin J, et al. Acute myeloid leukemia in the elderly: assessment of multidrug resistance (MDR1) and cytogenetics distinguishes biologic subgroups with remarkably distinct responses to standard chemotherapy. A Southwest Oncology Group Study. Blood 1997;89(9):3323–9.

31. Tam CS, Nussenzveig RM, Popat U, et al. The natural history and treatment outcome of blast phase BCR-ABL-myeloproliferative neoplasms. Blood 2008;112(5):1628–37.

HISTIOCYTIC AND DENDRITIC CELL NEOPLASMS

Dan Jones, MD, PhD

KEYWORDS

• Dendritic cells • Lymph node sarcomas • Transdifferentiation • Plasticity • Lineage infidelity

ABSTRACT

This article reviews the features of dendritic cells (DCs) of myeloid-derived, plasmacytoid, and follicle-associated types and tumors of these cells, as well as myeloid sarcoma. The morphologic and immunophenotypic features in this group of neoplasms is featured, including mature neoplasms such as Langerhans cell histiocytosis, its malignant counterpart Langerhans cell sarcoma, and S100-negative histiocytic proliferations. More immature or precursor malignancies in this group include myeloid and monocytic leukemias presenting in extramedullary tissues as well as the newly codified blastic plasmacytoid dendritic cell neoplasm. Although likely not related histogenetically to myeloid-derived DCs, mesenchymal-type lymph node tumors including follicular dendritic cell and fibroblastic reticulum sarcomas are also discussed. All of these neoplasms can exhibit a range of immunophenotypic and morphologic features that underscore the plasticity of the non-neoplastic precursors from which they are derived.

OVERVIEW

Histiocytic and dendritic cell (DC) neoplasms represent some of the most difficult to classify lesions among hematolymphoid tumors. This is in part related to their rarity but also to the plasticity of their non-neoplastic counterparts and to their largely uncertain histogenesis. This complexity and uncertainty is reflected in the many names that exist in the literature for similar histiocytic and DC tumor types.

SUBSETS OF DENDRITIC CELLS

The preponderance of current data suggests that all histiocytic and dendritic lineages arise from multipotential progenitor cells that mostly reside in the bone marrow. These include classical (myeloid-type) DCs, Langerhans cells, and monocytic and histiocytic forms that arise from a common myeloid-monocytic progenitor, as well as the plasmacytoid dendritic cells (PDCs) that give rise to the DC2 interferon-producing cells.[1] The germinal center-resident stromal population of follicular dendritic cells likely has a different histogenesis closely related to lymph node fibroblastic reticular cells.

> ### Pathologic Key Features
> #### HISTIOCYTIC AND DENDRITIC CELL NEOPLASMS
>
> 1. Mature histiocytic and dendritic cell neoplasms exhibit variable clinical behavior and can show considerable immunophenotypic variability, likely related to the effects of admixed tumor-associated inflammatory cells and their cytokines.
>
> 2. Immature histiocytic and dendritic cell neoplasms have a nearly uniformly aggressive clinical behavior and exhibit a tendency to shift lineages, especially upon relapse.
>
> 3. An extended panel of immunostains is often required to accurately type these tumors.
>
> 4. The greatest difficulty in classification is in the group of localized and systemic histiocytic (non-Langerhans cell) neoplasms.

Quest Diagnostics Nichols Institute, 14207 Newbrook Drive, Chantilly, VA 20153, USA
E-mail address: dajones@mdanderson.org

Surgical Pathology 3 (2010) 1165–1183
doi:10.1016/j.path.2010.09.008

Although schema have been developed for stages of DC differentiation (**Fig. 1**), bone marrow transplantation studies (in humans and in rodent models) as well as ex vivo expansion studies demonstrate a considerable plasticity inherent to all of the bone marrow-derived histiocytic and dendritic cell lineages. The number and phenotype of mature DC subsets that are produced appear to be dependent on microenvironmental influences as well as systemic circulating cytokine levels reflecting the overall immune state.[2,3] The subsets of antigen-presenting and processing DCs include the circulating CD11c+ "veiled cell" and more mature forms such as the Langerhans cell (LC). LCs are found in skin and are characterized ultrastructurally by the presence of striated cytoplasmic "tennis racket"-like structures called Birbeck granules, as well as by immunohistochemical expression of S100, CD1a, langerin (CD207), and pan-DC markers like CD83. An apparently related DC type, the "indeterminate cell" shows expression of S100 and CD1a, but lacks Birbeck granules. LCs migrate along with activated lymphocytes from skin and mucosal sites to lymph nodes following immune activation where they undergo stepwise maturation as well as immunophenotypic changes in transit. Massive accumulations of these transiting LCs or indeterminate cells in the paracortical areas of lymph node characterize dermatopathic lymphadenitis.[4] This condition is most commonly seen in lymph nodes draining sites of skin inflammation or mucosal breakdown (**Fig. 2**) but can also accompany nodal involvement by cutaneous T-cell lymphomas.

A more recently elucidated lineage of antigen-presenting dendritic cells includes the PDCs, which express the interleukin (IL)-3 receptor CD123 and surface lectins, such as blood-derived dendritic cell antigen (BDCA)-2 and BDCA-4, but are negative for CD11c and CD1a. The production of interferon by PDCs is critical to their role in innate immunity, particularly in rapid response to viral infections.[5] Mature PDCs (also referred to as DC2) migrate into lymph nodes and other tissues across activated endothelium[6] where they accumulate around blood vessels as cohesive cell clusters with characteristic pale-staining cytoplasm (**Fig. 3**).

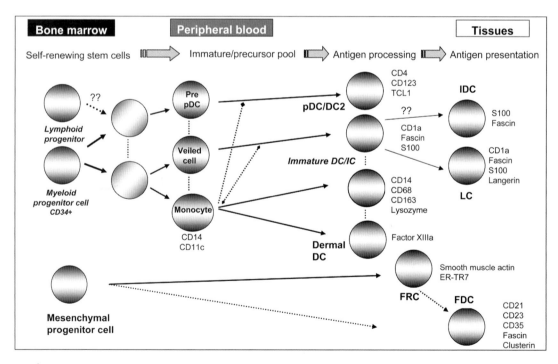

➡ Default differentiation pathway

...... Shifts, dependent on specific microenvironmental influences

Fig. 1. Proposed schema for dendritic cell and histiocytic maturation. The interrelationship and differentiation schema for histiocytes, myeloid-type dendritic cells, and mesenchymal-type dendritic cells is shown. These default and alternate pathways of differentiation are provisional and may be further refined as better experimental models to study tissue-based DC maturation are developed. DC, dendritic cell; FDC, follicular dendritic cell; FRC, fibroblastic reticular cell; IC, indeterminate cell; IDC, interdigitating dendritic cell; LC, Langerhans cell; pDC, plasmacytoid dendritic cell.

Fig. 2. Dermatopathic lymphadenitis. A proliferation of transitional dendritic/histiocytic cells and Langerhans cells migrating from skin to lymph node expands the paracortical areas. (*Inset*) Higher power view shows the oval nuclei and pale cytoplasm of the DC.

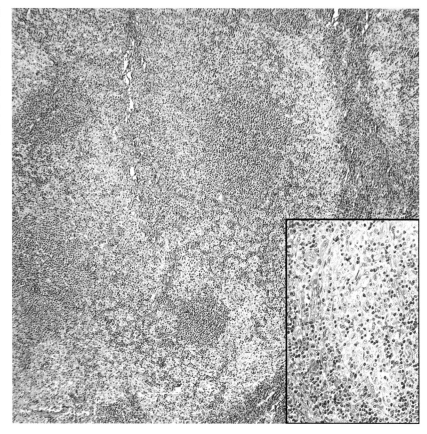

Fig. 3. Plasmacytoid dendritic cells in reactive lymph node. Aggregates of large cells with prominent central nuclei and pale-staining cytoplasm accumulate around high endothelial venules.

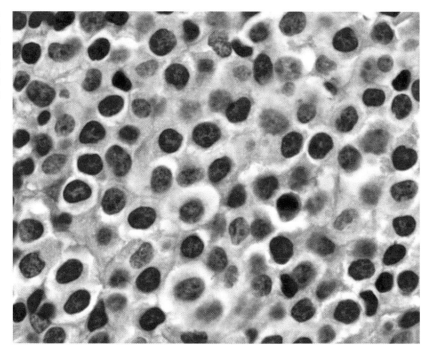

Another less well-defined DC subtype is the Factor XIIIa+, CD163+ interstitial DC/histiocyte, often found in high numbers in the dermis.[7] The relationship of this cell type to specialized lymph node and splenic interstitial DC/histiocytic populations and myeloid-type DCs is still unclear. Indeed, for all DC subtypes, ex vivo cell culture studies demonstrate an inherent ability of these cells to shift to from one type to another under the influence of different cytokine cocktails. These include the ability of FLT3 ligand to drive PDC maturation and granulocyte-macrophage colony stimulating factor (GM-CSF) and IL-4 to redirect both mature monocytes and immature precursor cells toward classical myeloid-type DCs.[8]

SUBSETS OF HISTIOCYTES

The term "histiocyte" is relatively imprecise, but generally refers to tissue-based antigen-presenting and -processing cells that also have a variety of biosynthetic, metabolic, inflammatory, and antimicrobial functions. The term can also encompass the various subsets of tissue and body fluid macrophages (eg, those found in the peritoneal cavity and within pulmonary alveoli), as well as cells with immune and phagocytic function scattered throughout the lymph nodes and spleen. Most histiocytes arise from circulating monocytes in response to cytokine signals in inflammatory states and then undergo apoptosis following cessation of the immune activation. However, they may persist for many years or undergo reprogramming or redifferentiation,[9] particularly within the walls of blood vessels.[10] Similar to subsets of committed T-helper cell subsets, macrophages resident at a particular site may become progressively more uniform and specialized in their function because of microenvironmental influences in a process of imprinting.[9] However, the stability of macrophage phenotypes or even their average life span within tissues is largely unknown.

Concordant with their antigen-processing functions, histiocytes are positive for lysosomal markers including CD68, CD163, and lysozyme and have variable expression of S100. However, given that lysosomes are also found in other cell types, these commonly used histiocytic markers lack specificity; thus, definitive immunophenotyping of histiocytes requires exclusion of other cell types, including DCs. Collections of histiocytes (occasionally with alarmingly atypical cytomorphology) accumulate in tissues in response to various different conditions, including persistent inflections (such as the granulomas in mycobacterial infections), inflammatory states (eg, sarcoidosis), genetic and acquired immune activation states, and certain immune-activating neoplasms (particularly Hodgkin lymphomas, T-cell lymphomas, and inflammatory carcinomas). Distinguishing these reactive histiocytic proliferations from neoplastic ones can be extremely difficult.

Many mature histiocytic and DC neoplasms retain the cytomorphology and migratory properties and express (at least partially) the typical immunophenotype of their presumed cell of origin (see Pathologic Key Features Box). These mature histiocytic and dendritic cell tumors include Langerhans cell histiocytosis, Langerhans cell sarcoma, inderdigitating dendritic cell sarcoma, non-Langerhans cell mature histiocytic tumors, and histiocytic sarcoma. Although the most mature of these DC and histiocytic neoplasms behave indolently, immature monocytic and DC tumors are in contrast aggressive neoplasms. The plasticity seen in non-neoplastic histiocytes and DC subtypes also appears to be retained in immature monocytic and DC neoplasms. These include extramedullary myeloid tumors and blastic plasmacytoid dendritic cell neoplasm.

LANGERHANS CELL HISTIOCYTOSIS AND RELATED ENTITIES

CLINICAL FEATURES

Langerhans cell histiocytosis (LCH) includes several variants that are distinguished mainly by their clinical presentation (age, localized vs multifocal, and unisystem vs multisystem disease). Localized LCH ("histiocytosis X") predominantly affects adults. Systemic forms primarily affect male infants (predominantly as multisystem Litterer-Siwe disease)[11] or young children (unisystem, multifocal Hand-Schüller-Christian syndrome), multifocal, multisystem LCH can also occur in adults (**Fig. 4**).[12] The bone is the most common site of involvement of all types of LCH; other common sites of involvement include the skin and lymph nodes, with the liver and spleen commonly affected in multisystem disease.

The nomenclature and distinguishing features of non-LC mature histiocytic neoplasms remains confusing and most relate to clinically defined syndromes.[13] The best-delineated entity is the nodular skin lesion termed juvenile xanthogranuloma,[14] which occurs predominantly in infants with a median age of 24 months; some cases are associated with neurofibromatosis type I or juvenile myelomonocytic leukemia, suggesting a genetic origin. Other non-LC mature histiocytoses can occur in both children and adults

Fig. 4. Langerhans cell histiocytosis in lymph node. (*A*) An interfollicular proliferation of Langerhans cells admixed with eosinophils. (*B*) Immunohistochemical stain for langerin is positive in the tumor cells.

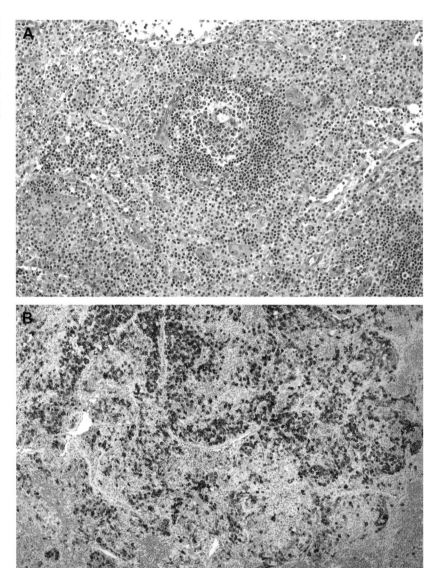

and may present variously as cutaneous lesions, cutaneous lesions with systemic disease, or primarily in extracutaneous locations. Some non-LC histiocytoses may resemble LCH clinically, with bone, lymph node, and skin involvement, but differ from LCH in terms of their immunophenotypic profile (see later in this article).[15]

DIAGNOSIS: MICROSCOPIC FEATURES AND ANCILLARY STUDIES

Langerhans cells are medium-sized cells with pale, eosinophilic cytoplasm and indented or grooved nuclei. All LCH types show a proliferation of Langerhans cells with minimal cytologic atypia in a polymorphous background containing admixed eosinophils as well as variable numbers of neutrophils, small histiocytes, lymphocytes, and multinucleated giant cells. When the lymph nodes are involved, LCH is present within the sinuses, while in the spleen the red pulp is mainly involved. The tumor cells in LCH are positive for S100, CD1a, and langerin[16]; however, similar to migrating LC, neoplastic proliferations can show variable positivity for these markers. LCH cells are also positive for CD68 and vimentin, but are negative for lysozyme. Unlike non-neoplastic LC, the tumor cells of LCH are positive for fascin.[17] Electron microscopy can demonstrate the characteristic Birbeck granules, but this is seldom needed to confirm the diagnosis. Whereas LCH is generally a clonal disease,[18] the localized, inflammatory cell-rich collection of LC in the lung most commonly affecting female smokers (also

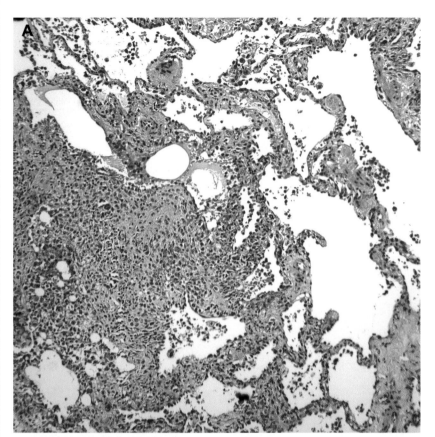

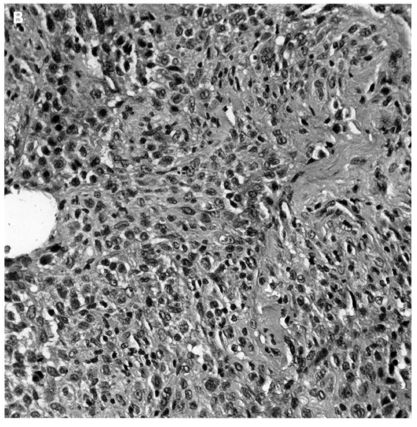

Fig. 5. Langerhans cell histiocytosis involving the lung. (*A*) There is a stellate-shaped lesion in the pulmonary parenchyma. (*B*) The lesion contains Langerhans cells as well as other inflammatory cells.

called eosinophilic granuloma) is usually poly-clonal and may regress with cessation of smoking (**Fig. 5**).[19,20]

The non-LC histiocytic proliferations are negative for CD1a and are negative or only dimly or variably positive for S100; they have varied histologic appearances. Juvenile xanthogranuloma is composed of dermal-based cohesive histiocytoid or spindled cells with foamy or xanthomatous cytoplasm admixed with giant cells showing characteristic "wreathlike" nuclei and inflammatory cells (**Fig. 6**A).[21] The histiocytes are positive for CD68, CD163, fascin, vimentin, and Factor XIIIa, but are negative for CD1a, S100, and langerin. The clonality of juvenile xanthogranuloma is uncertain. Other non-LC histiocytic proliferations may exhibit variably spindled or foamy histiocytes and are generally classified based on their clinical picture of presentation. The histogenetic relationship of these lesions to the more common atypical fibroxanthoma that occurs in adults (often at sites

of prior sun damage or in association with overlying squamous cell lesions) remains unclear (see **Fig. 6**B). Other proliferations include the multifocal Erdheim-Chester disease that involves bone and soft tissues and solitary and multifocal reticulohistiocytomas of skin and soft tissues (see **Fig. 6**C) that may have a genetic basis in some cases.[22]

DIFFERENTIAL DIAGNOSIS

In LCH, the eosinophils and/or neutrophils may be so numerous as to simulate an infectious process or abscess; careful attention is needed in such cases to recognize the admixed LCs. Dermatopathic lymphadenitis is a reactive proliferation of lymph node dendritic cells and LCs, often associated with a cutaneous inflammatory process. Helpful clues to separate this from nodal LCH are location within the paracortex (rather than intrasinusoidal involvement that characterizes LCH), preserved lymph node architecture, lack of

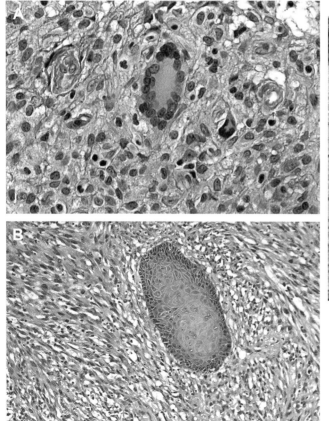
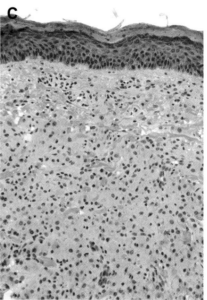

Fig. 6. Xanthogranulomas of presumed dermal dendritic cell origin. (*A*) Juvenile xanthogranuloma is a dermal-based tumor composed of histiocytoid cells with abundant granular cytoplasm admixed with giant cells. The tumor cells were uniformly positive for vimentin and Factor XIIIa (not shown). (*B*) Adult atypical fibroxanthoma is composed of a superficial dermal-based proliferation of spindle cells that are variably positive for Factor XIIIa; this lesion arose in a 70-year-old man associated with sun-damaged skin. (*C*) Adult reticulohistiocytoma shows a dense dermal infiltration of eosinophilic tumor cells with histiocytoid appearance. Tumor cells were uniformly positive for CD68 and CD163, and negative for S100 and Factor XIIIa (not shown).

prominent eosinophilia, and the presence of admixed melanin-laden and/or hemosiderin-laden macrophages in dermatopathic lymphadenitis. Paraneoplastic LCH proliferations may also occur as reactions to Hodgkin or non-Hodgkin lymphomas and may be so prominent as to obscure the underlying lymphoid neoplasm.

The prominent intrasinusoidal infiltration of LCH may mimic other intrasinusoidal proliferations, including sinus histiocytosis with massive lymphadenopathy (SHML, also known as Rosai-Dorfman disease), anaplastic large cell lymphoma, and metastatic carcinoma or melanoma. The combination of the immunohistochemical profile (in particular, positivity for langerin and CD1a, as melanomas share S100 positivity with LCH) and cytologic features help distinguish these entities from LCH. Finally, in the lung, localized LCH must be distinguished from sarcoidosis, lymphomas with abundant histiocytes, such as lymphomatoid granulomatosis, and mycobacterial or fungal infections that may present with granulomas and/or histiocytic infiltration.

LCH and related entities must be distinguished from macrophage activation syndromes, such as hemophagocytic syndromes. In contrast to LCH,

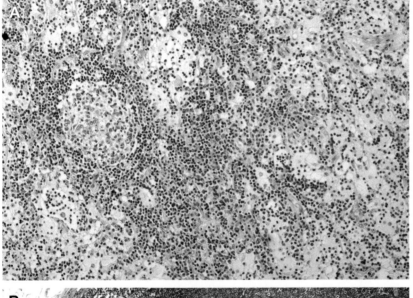

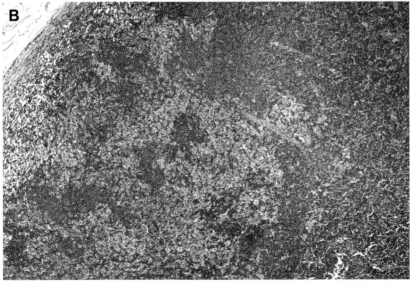

Fig. 7. Sinus histiocytosis with massive lymphadenopathy (Rosai-Dorfman disease). (*A*) Interfollicular and intrasinusoidal large histiocytes with abundant pale and often foamy cytoplasm containing intact lymphocytes. (*B*) Rosai-Dorfman-type histiocytes associated with lymphoma: pale-staining sheets of histiocytes with engulfed lymphocytes on the left part of the image are adjacent to lymph node involvement by small lymphocytic lymphoma. The histiocytes were uniformly positive for S100 (not shown).

these usually have an acute presentation and are often associated with viral infections (in particular Epstein-Barr virus [EBV]) or lymphomas. One distinct macrophage activation syndrome producing tumor masses composed of histiocytes of uniform appearance and phenotype is sinus histiocytosis with massive lymphadenopathy (SHML). This condition, also known as Rosai-Dorfman disease, is composed of sheets of S100+, CD163+, CD68+, and CD1a− macrophages with abundant pale cytoplasm containing engulfed lymphocytes.[13] SHML can be seen focally in association with neoplasms that activate adjacent lymphocytes, such as lymphocyte-predominant Hodgkin lymphoma,[23] suggesting a cytokine-driven etiology (**Fig. 7**). In support of this reactive origin, Rosai-Dorfman lesions have not been

shown to be clonal[24] and often regress over time without cytoreductive therapy. However, one recent study has shown that SHML may occur together with LCH, suggesting some relationship between these two entities.[25] The differential diagnosis of LCH with other histiocytic/dendritic proliferation is shown in the table "Differential Diagnosis of Dendritic/Histiocytic Neoplasms."

PROGNOSIS

Focal LCH has an excellent prognosis, with long-term survival above 95%. Multifocal or multisystem LCH behaves more aggressively. In particular, involvement of multiple organ systems at presentation, more than 3 bone lesions, hepatosplenomegaly, and failure to respond to

△△ DIFFERENTIAL DIAGNOSIS OF DENDRITIC/HISTIOCYTIC NEOPLASMS

Tumor	Sites Commonly Involved	Immunohistochemistry								
		S100	CD1a	Langerin	CD21	CD35	CD123	CD163	FXIIIa	Lysozyme
LCH	Skin, bone, lung, lymph nodes	++	++	++	−	−	−	−	−	−
JXG	Skin	−	−	−	−	−	−	−/+	++	−
Non-LCH histiocytosis	Variable	−/+	−	−	−	−	−	++	−/+	+
Histiocytic sarcoma	Variable	−/+	−	−	−	−	−	++	−	++
IDC sarcoma	Lymph nodes, various extranodal sites	++	−	−	−	−	−	−/+	−/+	−
BPDCN	Skin, lymph nodes, bone marrow	−	−	−	−	−	++	−	−	−
Myeloid sarcoma	Oral mucosa, skin, spleen	−/+	−	−	−	−	−/+	−/+	−	+
FDC sarcoma	Peripheral and mesenteric lymph nodes, tonsil, gut	−/+	−	−	++	++	−	−	−/+	−

Abbreviations: BPDCN, blastic plasmacytoid dendritic cell neoplasm; FDC, follicular dendritic cell; IDC, interdigitating dendritic cell; JXG, juvenile xanthogranuloma; LCH, Langerhans cell histiocytosis.

chemotherapy are adverse prognostic features. Localized therapy such as surgery, radiation, or topical steroids for cutaneous lesions can be effective for focal LCH, whereas multisystem multifocal disease is usually treated with chemotherapy.[12] The clinical behavior of the non-LC histiocytoses is uncertain; although many cases appear to have an indolent or relapsing course, cases with multifocal disease, particularly when involving the cerebrospinal fluid (CSF), may have an aggressive course.

LANGERHANS CELL, INTERDIGITATING DENDRITIC CELL, AND HISTIOCYTIC SARCOMAS

CLINICAL FEATURES

Sarcomas of dendritic and histiocytic cells are exceedingly rare. Fewer than 20 cases of LC sarcoma have been reported. This tumor typically involves skin and lymph nodes, as well as liver, spleen, and lung. Interdigitating dendritic cell sarcomas (IDCs) mainly involve lymph nodes and affect older adult males with a median age of 70. Likewise, histiocytic sarcomas are extremely rare: most cases previously reported as such appear to represent extramedullary manifestations

of monocytic leukemias or poorly differentiated B-cell malignancies.

DIAGNOSIS: MICROSCOPIC FEATURES AND ANCILLARY STUDIES

Langerhans cell sarcoma resembles LCH immunophenotypically, with S100+, CD1a+, and langerin+ tumor cells but, unlike LCH, these have bizarre cytomorphology or anaplastic appearance and a high mitotic rate.[26] Interdigitating dendritic cell sarcomas involve the lymph node paracortex and are composed of a proliferation of atypical spindled cells in whorls or fascicles. The tumor cells are strongly positive for S100 but lack CD1a expression[27]; they are also negative for CD163 and markers of follicular dendritic cells (CD21, CD23, and CD35) (**Fig. 8**). The proposed histogenesis of IDC sarcoma is from a population of transitional S100+ interdigitating DCs found in activated lymph nodes.[28] However, given its spindled appearance and ultrastructural findings in some cases suggesting partial myoid differentiation, some have suggested that this tumor may be a phenotypic variant of follicular dendritic cell (FDC) sarcoma or nodal reticular cell tumor, as discussed later.[29] Histiocytic sarcomas appear as cytologically malignant proliferations resembling

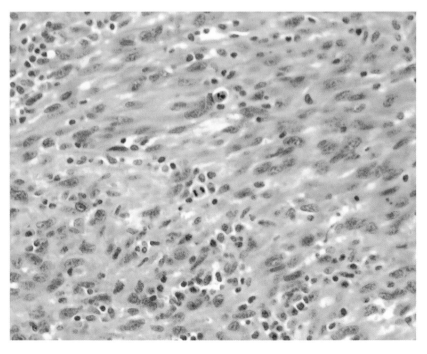

Fig. 8. Interdigitating dendritic cell sarcoma. The tumor is composed of spindled cells with only occasional admixed lymphocytes. Tumor cells were strongly uniformly positive for S100 and negative for CD1a and CD21 (not shown).

mature histiocytes in terms of their morphology and immunophenotype (CD68+, CD163+).[30,31]

DIFFERENTIAL DIAGNOSIS

The main difficulty is in differentiating IDC sarcomas from other malignant neoplasms. FDC sarcomas (discussed later in this article) may show a similarly spindled appearance but, unlike IDC sarcomas, should express of CD21, CD23, and/or CD35 and also should show desmosomes on electron microscopy. Metastatic melanoma shares S100 positivity with IDC sarcomas and may exhibit a spindled appearance; expression of melanoma-specific markers and a clinical history of melanoma are helpful in this distinction. In cases of presumed histiocytic sarcoma, the clinical history should be carefully searched for evidence of prior B-cell lymphoma, as some cases appear to represent "transdifferentiated" B-cell malignancies. These cases may show an immunoglobulin heavy chain (*IGH*) gene rearrangement shared with the B-cell lymphoma, indicating a clonal relationship.[31,32] Histiocytic sarcoma must also be distinguished from myeloid/monocytic sarcoma; this differential diagnosis is discussed later in this article. The differential diagnosis of dendritic/histiocytic sarcomas is listed in the "Differential Diagnosis of Dendritic/Histiocytic Neoplasms" table.

PROGNOSIS

Langerhans cell sarcoma has a poor prognosis with high mortality. Survival of IDC sarcoma is variable, with about one-third of patients dying within 2 years of the initial diagnosis; bulky disease and extranodal disease at presentation are poor prognostic factors. Data on the clinical behavior of the rare "true" histiocytic sarcomas are very limited, but these also appear to be aggressive neoplasms.[33]

MYELOID SARCOMA

CLINICAL FEATURES

Myeloid sarcoma or extramedullary myeloid cell tumor (MS) is the most commonly encountered immature histiocytic/dendritic neoplasm. MS is a localized extramedullary presentation of systemic acute myeloid, monocytic, or myelomonocytic leukemia (AML) (**Fig. 9**). Myeloid sarcoma can affect patients of any age and most frequently presents in skin or mucosal sites, with systemic involvement present at diagnosis or soon thereafter in most cases.[34] Monocytic leukemias have a particular propensity to involve the skin as

nodules or palpable purpura and can involve the oral cavity as gum hypertrophy.[35]

DIAGNOSIS: MICROSCOPIC FEATURES AND ANCILLARY STUDIES

Myeloid or monocytic sarcoma presents as sheets of blasts infiltrating the tissue and forming a mass lesion. In the skin, the blasts often infiltrate as single cells with a prominent perivascular growth and sparing of the epidermis. Despite the often striking nodular or purpuric clinical appearances of skin or gum lesions, tissue involvement in monocytic leukemia can be histologically subtle with only small nests of perivascular blasts and immature monocytes and occasionally associated vasculitis.[35] The blasts are positive for CD43 and are positive for one or more of the following markers: CD34, CD117, myeloperoxidase (MPO), lysozyme, or CD68. The bone marrow may or may not be involved at presentation; in those cases lacking increased blasts in bone marrow, myelodysplastic features can often be found.[36]

DIFFERENTIAL DIAGNOSIS

Distinguishing tissue involvement by chronic myelomonocytic leukemia (CMML) from MS is difficult; however, this separation may be of limited clinical value, because CMML involvement of tissues is often followed by acute leukemic transformation within a few weeks to months. A more difficult distinction is the separation of MS from histiocytic sarcoma. A cohesive growth pattern and uniformly mature histiocytic appearance without underlying bone marrow myelodysplastic changes would favor histiocytic sarcoma. Histiocytic sarcomas can remain localized to a single site or exhibit lymphoma-like multifocal lymph node involvement, but do not disseminate to blood and bone marrow, unlike most cases of MS.[37] Distinction between MS and BPDCN is discussed later in this article. The differential diagnosis of myeloid sarcoma with dendritic/histiocytic proliferations is listed in the "Differential Diagnosis of Dendritic/Histiocytic Neoplasms" table.

PROGNOSIS

Myeloid sarcoma is treated systemically as acute myeloid leukemia, irrespective of whether the marrow is involved at presentation. Localized therapy is ineffective, as patients eventually relapse with systemic leukemia. Presentation as MS appears to be an adverse prognostic feature in acute myeloid leukemia.

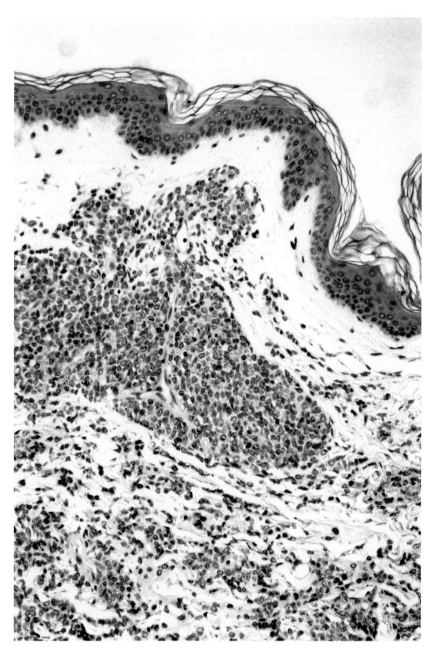

Fig. 9. Myeloid sarcoma of skin. There is dermal infiltration by sheets and perivascular collections of blasts and immature monocytes. This patient developed systemic acute monocytic leukemia with circulating blasts within 2 weeks of this biopsy.

BLASTIC PLASMACYTOID DENDRITIC CELL NEOPLASM

CLINICAL FEATURES

Blastic plasmacytoid dendritic cell neoplasm (BPDCN) is an uncommon tumor that arises from an immature dendritic cell. BPDCN can occur at any age (including children) with a median age of 67 years and a male predominance. It involves skin and lymph node (**Fig. 10**A, B), with subsequent, usually rapid, dissemination to spleen and bone marrow.[38] The cutaneous involvement is usually as patches, plaques, or purpuric lesions that may be ulcerated. BPDCN can occur de novo, or may precede or coincide with other myeloid neoplasms, in particular CMML, AML, and myelodysplastic syndromes.[39]

DIAGNOSIS: MICROSCOPIC FEATURES AND ANCILLARY STUDIES

BPDCN has an immature, blastic cytomorphology, high mitotic rate, and sheetlike growth. In the skin, it

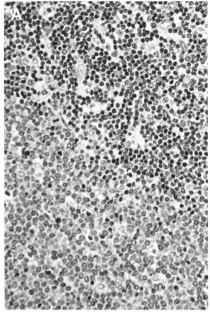

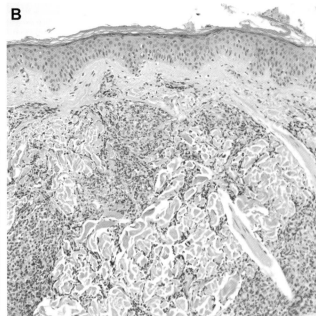

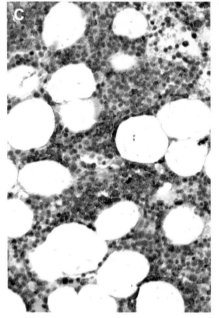

Fig. 10. Blastic plasmacytoid dendritic cell neoplasm. (*A*) The lymph node is infiltrated by large blastoid tumor cells (top part of image shows normal lymphocytes for comparison). (*B*) Skin involvement shows sheetlike dermal infiltration with sparing of the epidermis. (*C*) CD123 immunohistochemical stain highlights groups of neoplastic cells infiltrating the bone marrow biopsy.

involves the dermis, often with prominent perivascular and periadnexal infiltration, and spares the epidermis. The chromatin is finely dispersed and blastlike and nucleoli vary from indistinct to prominent. In the bone marrow aspirate smear, the tumor cells often show vacuolated cytoplasm and/or cytoplasmic blebs. By immunohistochemistry, expression of the PDC markers CD123 (see **Fig. 10**C), TCL1, and BDCA2 is characteristic.[40] These neoplasms also express CD4 and CD56,

giving rise to their alternate designation as "CD4+ CD56+ hematodermic tumor."[41,42] Expression of CD45RA in the absence of other B-cell markers is an additional diagnostically helpful feature of BPDCN. BPDCN is most positive for CD43 and CD68, whereas CD33, CD7, and TdT may be variably expressed; however, the tumor cells are negative for CD34, B-cell markers, the specific T-cell marker CD3, and the myelomonocytic antigens CD117, CD14, MPO, and lysozyme.[43]

DIFFERENTIAL DIAGNOSIS

The typical cutaneous presentation of BPDCNs, their cytomorphology, and their expression of CD4 and CD56 raises the differential diagnosis of a T/natural killer (NK) cell lymphoma. However, these lymphomas usually show angioinvasion and necrosis (unusual in BPDCN), should be positive for the specific T-cell marker CD3, and are negative for CD123 and TCL1; additionally, NK cell lymphomas/leukemias are usually EBV positive. Because of its blastic appearance and not infrequent expression of TdT, BPDCN may be mistaken for a T-lymphoblastic lymphoma; unlike BPDCN, T-lymphoblastic lymphoma should be negative for CD123 and may be positive for CD34 and/or CD1. Perhaps the most difficult differential is with myelomonocytic leukemias or myeloid sarcoma, which may express CD123 and/or CD56, but are TCL1 negative. Performing a full immunohistochemical panel should help resolve this distinction, as myeloid sarcomas usually express lysozyme and often express MPO, markers that should be negative in BPDCN. Neoplasms with definitive expression of markers of myelomonocytic differentiation, such as lysozyme, CD14, and MPO, are best diagnosed as myeloid sarcoma. The differential diagnosis of BPDCN with other histiocytic/dendritic neoplasms is listed in the "Differential Diagnosis of Dendritic/Histiocytic Neoplasms" table.

PROGNOSIS

Nearly all cases of BPDCN pursue an extremely aggressive course, recurring soon after chemotherapy,[42] but a few localized, indolent variants have recently been reported. Some cases may relapse as acute myeloid leukemia, underscoring the relationship of PDCs to the myeloid lineage and their lineage plasticity.

FOLLICULAR DENDRITIC CELL SARCOMA AND ITS VARIANTS

CLINICAL FEATURES

Although grouped with other DC tumor types based on its dendritic morphology, FDC sarcoma has a clinical behavior, morphology, and immunophenotype completely distinct from other DC tumors.[44] FDC sarcoma has a median age of 44 years at presentation and affects males and females equally. This neoplasm can involve any secondary lymphoid tissue, including tonsil/Waldeyer ring and gut,[45] but is most common in peripheral or abdominal lymph nodes, particularly cervical, axillary, and mesenteric nodes.[29]

DIAGNOSIS: MICROSCOPIC FEATURES AND ANCILLARY STUDIES

Follicular dendritic cell sarcomas can show a variety of spindled, epithelioid, or myxoid appearances, with more poorly differentiated cells and overtly malignant cytomorphology more common at relapse (Fig. 11). The spindled and epithelioid whorls of tumor cells are usually admixed with numerous small lymphocytes and tumor cells often colonize preexisting germinal centers; lymphocytes may be sparse in extranodal tumor implants, however. Some cases may show anaplastic or giant-cell morphology. The characteristic immunophenotype of FDC sarcoma cells is CD21+, CD23+, CD35+: at least 2 of these markers are positive in more than 90% of cases.[13] The tumor cells are also positive for CXCL13, EMA, podoplanin (D240), and fascin. The definitive diagnostic feature of FDC sarcoma is the ultrastructural demonstration of desmosomes, which supports its derivation from germinal center-derived FDC that acquire desmoplakin+ cell connections during follicle development (Fig. 11C). The ultimate histogenesis of non-neoplastic FDCs remains unresolved, but experimental data have tended to suggest that these cells develop dynamically in B-cell follicles from locally derived fibroblastic reticular cells. The tight association of FDC sarcoma with sites of mature B-cell expansions suggests that development of FDC tumors is also dependent on supportive interactions with B-cell growth factors. Further evidence of this microenvironmental requirement is that FDC tumors sometimes develop in patients with a preexisting history of hyaline vascular Castleman disease (HVCD), a localized benign lymph node expansion characterized by numerous hyperstimulated and regressed follicles with dysplastic-appearing FDCs.[46–48] Some cases of FDC sarcoma show incomplete FDC differentiation, with partial loss of CD21 and/or CD35 and upregulation of myofibroblastic markers.[49] This finding is reminiscent of the apparent stromal overgrowth of reticular cells and angiomyoid proliferations occasionally seen in HVCD (Fig. 12). Because of their presumed shared histogenesis, fibroblastic tumors arising in lymph nodes ("fibroblastic reticular cell tumors")[50,51] have been grouped with FDC sarcoma in the current 2008 WHO classification.[52] These tumors lack FDC markers and exhibit immunophenotypic features of myofibroblasts, with expression of smooth muscle actin and vimentin and variable expression of desmin and cytokeratins 8 and 18 (detected by keratin antibody Cam5.2). Fibroblastic reticular cell tumors are rare and poorly characterized, with variable clinical behavior.

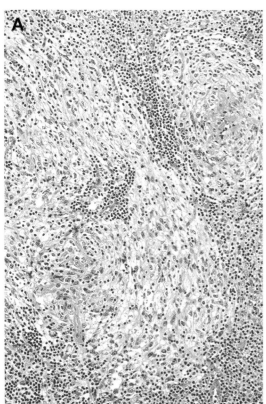

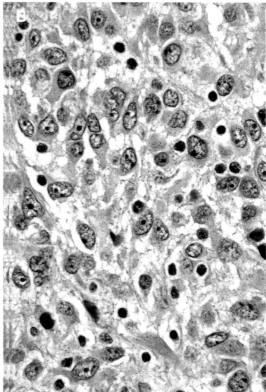

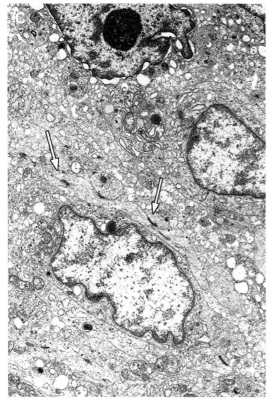

Fig. 11. Follicular dendritic cell sarcoma. (*A*) FDC sarcoma with prominent spindle cell morphology, showing colonization of an adjacent lymphoid follicle (*top right of image*) and frequent admixed small lymphocytes. (*B*) High-grade cytologic appearance and more epithelioid morphology with myxoid stroma is seen in a case of recurrent FDC sarcoma. (*C*) Electron micrograph of a case with intercellular junctions (desmosomes) highlighted by the arrows.

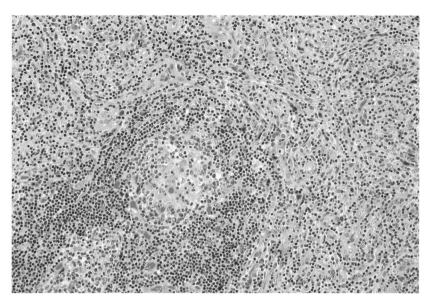

Fig. 12. Stromal-rich variant of hyaline vascular Castleman disease. The interfollicular area of the lymph node is expanded by a proliferation of blood vessels and myofibroblasts. A regressed follicle (*bottom left portion of image*) shows mantle zone expansion with multiple germinal centers ("twinning"), a characteristic feature of Castleman disease.

DIFFERENTIAL DIAGNOSIS

Cases of FDC sarcoma presenting in intra-abdominal locations in females often show a prominent reactive lymphoplasmacytic infiltrate with relatively sparse spindled tumor cells resembling inflammatory myofibroblastic tumors (so-called "inflammatory pseudotumor-like variant"). Immunostains are usually necessary to disclose the characteristic FDC phenotype: inflammatory myofibroblastic tumors express ALK protein and are negative for FDC markers. The spindled tumor cell pattern can also mimic spindle-cell melanoma, sarcomas, and sarcomatoid carcinomas. Again, immunohistochemistry to demonstrate positivity for FDC markers may be necessary to resolve this differential diagnosis. Whereas FDC sarcomas can show variable staining for S100, they are negative for other melanoma markers such as Melan-A and HMB-45. Distinction from IDC sarcoma can be more difficult, but demonstrating expression of CD21, CD23, and/or CD35 is critical. The presence of admixed lymphocytes, which are usually numerous in FDC sarcomas but infrequent in IDC sarcomas, can also be helpful. In ambiguous cases, electron microscopy can be used to show the presence of desmosomes, characteristic of FDC sarcoma and absent in IDC sarcoma. Some cases of HVCD may show florid proliferations of FDCs that are reminiscent of FDC sarcoma. However, these are usually only small microscopic foci as opposed to the gross tumor masses that characterize FDC sarcoma; the remaining areas of lymph node in such cases should show otherwise typical features of HVCD, including hypervascularity and regressed follicles.[53] The differential diagnosis of FDC sarcomas with histiocytic/dendritic neoplasms is listed in the "Differential Diagnosis of Dendritic/Histiocytic Neoplasms" table.

PROGNOSIS

The clinical course of FDC sarcoma is typically slowly progressive, with initial response to CHOP-type chemotherapy (cyclophosphamide, doxorubicin, vincristine, and prednisone) and/or radiotherapy, but with frequent relapses in a pattern resembling lymphoma.[54] Mortality is often related to invasion into abdominal viscera. An intra-abdominal location, large tumor size (>6 cm), tumor cell pleomorphism, high mitotic rate, and necrosis appear to be correlated with an adverse prognosis.[54] A variety of paraneoplastic phenomena have been reported in association with FDC sarcoma, including amyloidosis and pemphigus,[47] which contribute to morbidity. These findings suggest that FDC sarcoma retains many functional properties of its non-neoplastic counterpart, including B-cell costimulation.

FUTURE DIRECTIONS IN THE CLASSIFICATION AND PATHOPHYSIOLOGY OF DENDRITIC AND HISTIOCYTIC NEOPLASMS

Much remains to be understood about the complex interrelationships and functional properties of different histiocytic and DC subsets. As these data are gathered, they will likely affect the

Table 1
Reported synchronous or metachronous neoplasms with histiocytic and dendritic cell neoplasms: evidence for "transdifferentiation" or phenotypic plasticity

Tumor Type	Other Neoplasm(s)/Condition(s)
BPDCN	Myelodysplasia, AML
Histiocytic and DC neoplasms	Follicular lymphoma
Histiocytic sarcoma	T-lymphoblastic leukemia/lymphoma (especially those with *CALM-AF10* translocations)
LCH	T-lymphoblastic leukemia/lymphoma (especially those with *NOTCH1* mutation)
LCH	SHML (Rosai-Dorfman disease)

Abbreviations: AML, acute myeloid leukemia; BPDCN, blastic plasmacytoid dendritic cell neoplasms; DC, dendritic cell; LCH, Langerhans cell histiocytosis; SHML, sinus histiocytosis with massive lymphadenopathy (Rosai-Dorfman disease).

classification of neoplasms derived from these cells. There are limited data currently on the genomic and proteomic properties of these tumors that seem to support the implied histogenic derivations summarized in this article. However, one of the curious features of a number of histiocytic and DC neoplasms is their association with precedent or subsequent hematolymphoid neoplasms of other types (**Table 1**).[32,39,55–57] This suggests once again that the plasticity of non-neoplastic progenitors is often maintained during the process of neoplastic transformation[58] and that certain oncogenic processes may be common to DC/histiocytic neoplasms and the more commonly encountered leukemias and lymphomas.

Pitfalls
HISTIOCYTIC AND DENDRITIC CELL NEOPLASMS

! Immature monocytic infiltrates in the skin that represent cutaneous presentations of acute monocytic leukemia may be mistaken for reactive monocytic infiltrates.

! Localized histiocytic proliferations in skin, lung, and other tissues may be overcalled as neoplasms.

! Histiocyte-rich T-cell lymphoma or anaplastic large cell lymphoma may be misdiagnosed as histiocytic sarcoma, which is an exceedingly rare entity.

! Follicular dendritic cell sarcoma should be considered in any poorly differentiated epithelioid neoplasm that contains admixed lymphocytes.

REFERENCES

1. Ito T, Liu YJ, Kadowaki N. Functional diversity and plasticity of human dendritic cell subsets. Int J Hematol 2005;81(3):188–96.

2. Tian F, Grimaldo S, Fugita M, et al. The endothelial cell-produced antiangiogenic cytokine vascular endothelial growth inhibitor induces dendritic cell maturation. J Immunol 2007;179(6):3742–51.

3. Angelot F, Seillès E, Biichlé S, et al. Endothelial cell-derived microparticles induce plasmacytoid dendritic cell maturation: potential implications in inflammatory diseases. Haematologica 2009;94(11):1502–12.

4. Asano S, Muramatsu T, Kanno H, et al. Dermatopathic lymphadenopathy. Electron microscopic, enzyme-histochemical and immunohistochemical study. Acta Pathol Jpn 1987;37(6):887–900.

5. Facchetti F, Vermi W, Mason D, et al. The plasmacytoid monocyte/interferon producing cells. Virchows Arch 2003;443(6):703–17.

6. Cella M, Jarrossay D, Facchetti F, et al. Plasmacytoid monocytes migrate to inflamed lymph nodes and produce large amounts of type I interferon. Nat Med 1999;5(8):919–23.

7. Zaba LC, Fuentes-Duculan J, Steinman RM, et al. Normal human dermis contains distinct populations of CD11c+BDCA-1+ dendritic cells and CD163+FXIIIA+ macrophages. J Clin Invest 2007;117(9):2517–25.

8. Comeau MR, Van der Vuurst de Vries AR, Maliszewski CR, et al. CD123bright plasmacytoid predendritic cells: progenitors undergoing cell fate conversion? J Immunol 2002;169(1):75–83.

9. Stout RD, Suttles J. Functional plasticity of macrophages: reversible adaptation to changing microenvironments. J Leukoc Biol 2004;76(3):509–13.

10. Han JW, Shimada K, Ma-Krupa W, et al. Vessel wall-embedded dendritic cells induce T-cell

autoreactivity and initiate vascular inflammation. Circ Res 2008;102(5):546—53.

11. Stein SL, Paller AS, Haut PR, et al. Langerhans cell histiocytosis presenting in the neonatal period: a retrospective case series. Arch Pediatr Adolesc Med 2001;155(7):778—83.

12. Arico M, Girschikofsky M, Genereau T, et al. Langerhans cell histiocytosis in adults. Report from the International Registry of the Histiocyte Society. Eur J Cancer 2003;39(16):2341—8.

13. Pileri SA, Grogan TM, Harris NL, et al. Tumours of histiocytes and accessory dendritic cells: an immunohistochemical approach to classification from the International Lymphoma Study Group based on 61 cases. Histopathology 2002;41(1):1—29.

14. Zelger B, Cerio R, Orchard G, et al. Juvenile and adult xanthogranuloma. A histological and immunohistochemical comparison. Am J Surg Pathol 1994; 18(2):126—35.

15. Zelger BW, Sidoroff A, Orchard G, et al. Non-Langerhans cell histiocytoses. A new unifying concept. Am J Dermatopathol 1996;18(5):490—504.

16. Dziegiel P, Dolilnska-Krajewska B, Dumanska M, et al. Coexpression of CD1a, langerin and Birbeck's granules in Langerhans cell histiocytoses (LCH) in children: ultrastructural and immunocytochemical studies. Folia Histochem Cytobiol 2007;45(1):21—5.

17. Pinkus GS, Lones MA, Matsumura F, et al. Langerhans cell histiocytosis immunohistochemical expression of fascin, a dendritic cell marker. Am J Clin Pathol 2002;118(3):335—43.

18. Willman CL, Busque L, Griffith BB, et al. Langerhans'-cell histiocytosis (histiocytosis X)—a clonal proliferative disease. N Engl J Med 1994;331(3): 154—60.

19. Howarth DM, Gilchrist GS, Mullan BP, et al. Langerhans cell histiocytosis: diagnosis, natural history, management, and outcome. Cancer 1999;85(10): 2278—90.

20. Yousem SA, Colby TV, Chen YY, et al. Pulmonary Langerhans' cell histiocytosis: molecular analysis of clonality. Am J Surg Pathol 2001;25(5):630—6.

21. Weitzman S, Jaffe R. Uncommon histiocytic disorders: the non-Langerhans cell histiocytoses. Pediatr Blood Cancer 2005;45(3):256—64.

22. Zelger B, Cerio R, Soyer HP, et al. Reticulohistiocytoma and multicentric reticulohistiocytosis. Histopathologic and immunophenotypic distinct entities. Am J Dermatopathol 1994;16(6):577—84.

23. Lu D, Estalilla OC, Manning JT, et al. Sinus histiocytosis with massive lymphadenopathy and malignant lymphoma involving the same lymph node: a report of four cases and review of the literature. Mod Pathol 2000;13(4):414—9.

24. McClain KL, Natkunam Y, Swerdlow SH. Atypical cellular disorders. Hematology Am Soc Hematol Educ Program Book 2004;283—96.

25. Duong A, O'Malley DP, Barry TS, et al. Coexistence of Langerhans Cell histiocytosis and Rosai-Dorfman disease: related-disorders? Mod Pathol 2010;23 (Suppl 1):294A.

26. Bohn OL, Ruiz-Arguelles G, Navarro L, et al. Cutaneous Langerhans cell sarcoma: a case report and review of the literature. Int J Hematol 2007;85(2): 116—20.

27. Gaertner EM, Tsokos M, Derringer GA, et al. Interdigitating dendritic cell sarcoma. A report of four cases and review of the literature. Am J Clin Pathol 2001;115(4):589—97.

28. Angel CE, Chen CJ, Horlacher OC, et al. Distinctive localization of antigen-presenting cells in human lymph nodes. Blood 2009;113(6):1257—67.

29. Fonseca R, Yamakawa M, Nakamura S, et al. Follicular dendritic cell sarcoma and interdigitating reticulum cell sarcoma: a review. Am J Hematol 1998; 59(2):161—7.

30. Vos JA, Abbondanzo SL, Barekman CL, et al. Histiocytic sarcoma: a study of five cases including the histiocyte marker CD163. Mod Pathol 2005;18(5): 693—704.

31. van Heerde P, Feltkamp CA, Hart AA, et al. Malignant histiocytosis and related tumors. A clinicopathologic study of 42 cases using cytological, histochemical and ultrastructural parameters. Hematol Oncol 1984;2(1):13—32.

32. Feldman AL, Arber DA, Pittaluga S, et al. Clonally related follicular lymphomas and histiocytic/dendritic cell sarcomas: evidence for transdifferentiation of the follicular lymphoma clone. Blood 2008;111(12):5433—9.

33. Sun W, Nordberg ML, Fowler MR. Histiocytic sarcoma involving the central nervous system: clinical, immunohistochemical, and molecular genetic studies of a case with review of the literature. Am J Surg Pathol 2003;27(2):258—65.

34. Pileri SA, Ascani S, Cox MC, et al. Myeloid sarcoma: clinico-pathologic, phenotypic and cytogenetic analysis of 92 adult patients. Leukemia 2007;21(2): 340—50.

35. Jones D, Dorfman DM, Barnhill RL, et al. Leukemic vasculitis: a feature of leukemia cutis in some patients. Am J Clin Pathol 1997;107(5):637—42.

36. Audouin J, Comperat E, Le Tourneau A, et al. Myeloid sarcoma: clinical and morphologic criteria useful for diagnosis. Int J Surg Pathol 2003;11(4):271—82.

37. Paydas S, Zorludemir S, Ergin M. Granulocytic sarcoma: 32 cases and review of the literature. Leuk Lymphoma 2006;47(12):2527—41.

38. Chaperot L, Perrot I, Jacob MC, et al. Leukemic plasmacytoid dendritic cells share phenotypic and functional features with their normal counterparts. Eur J Immunol 2004;34(2):418—26.

39. Khoury JD, Jedeiros LJ, Manning JT, et al. CD56(+) TdT(+) blastic natural killer cell tumor of the

skin: a primitive systemic malignancy related to myelomonocytic leukemia. Cancer 2002;94(9): 2401–8.

40. Jaye DL, Geigerman CM, Herling M, et al. Expression of the plasmacytoid dendritic cell marker BDCA-2 supports a spectrum of maturation among CD4+ CD56+ hematodermic neoplasms. Mod Pathol 2006;19(12):1555–62.

41. Petrella T, Bagot M, Willemze R, et al. Blastic NK-cell lymphomas (agranular CD4+CD56+ hematodermic neoplasms): a review. Am J Clin Pathol 2005;123(5): 662–75.

42. Herling M, Jones D. CD4+/CD56+ hematodermic tumor: the features of an evolving entity and its relationship to dendritic cells. Am J Clin Pathol 2007; 127(5):687–700.

43. Reichard KK, Burks EJ, Foucar MK, et al. CD4(+) CD56(+) lineage-negative malignancies are rare tumors of plasmacytoid dendritic cells. Am J Surg Pathol 2005;29(10):1274–83.

44. Vermi W, Lonardi S, Bosisio D, et al. Identification of CXCL13 as a new marker for follicular dendritic cell sarcoma. J Pathol 2008;216(3):356–64.

45. Shia J, Chen W, Tang LH, et al. Extranodal follicular dendritic cell sarcoma: clinical, pathologic, and histogenetic characteristics of an underrecognized disease entity. Virchows Arch 2006;449(2): 148–58.

46. Pauwels P, Dal Cin P, Vlasveld LT, et al. A chromosomal abnormality in hyaline vascular Castleman's disease: evidence for clonal proliferation of dysplastic stromal cells. Am J Surg Pathol 2000; 24(6):882–8.

47. Lee IJ, Kim SC, Kim HS, et al. Paraneoplastic pemphigus associated with follicular dendritic cell sarcoma arising from Castleman's tumor. J Am Acad Dermatol 1999;40(2 Pt 2):294–7.

48. Chan AC, Chan KW, Chan JK, et al. Development of follicular dendritic cell sarcoma in hyaline-vascular Castleman's disease of the nasopharynx: tracing its evolution by sequential biopsies. Histopathology 2001;38(6):510–8.

49. Jones D, Amin M, Ordonez NG, et al. Reticulum cell sarcoma of lymph node with mixed dendritic and fibroblastic features. Mod Pathol 2001;14(10): 1059–67.

50. Schuerfeld K, Lazzi S, De Santi MM, et al. Cytokeratin-positive interstitial cell neoplasm: a case report and classification issues. Histopathology 2003; 43(5):491–4.

51. Andriko JW, Kaldjian EP, Tsokos M, et al. Reticulum cell neoplasms of lymph nodes: a clinicopathologic study of 11 cases with recognition of a new subtype derived from fibroblastic reticular cells. Am J Surg Pathol 1998;22(9):1048–58.

52. Jaffe R, Pileri SA, Facchetti F, et al. Histiocytic and dendritic cell neoplasms, introduction. In: Swerdlow SH, Campo E, Harris NL, et al, editors. WHO classification of tumours of hematopoietic and lymphoid tissues. Lyon (France): IARC; 2008. p. 354–5.

53. Lin O, Frizzera G. Angiomyoid and follicular dendritic cell proliferative lesions in Castleman's disease of hyaline-vascular type: a study of 10 cases. Am J Surg Pathol 1997;21(11):1295–306.

54. Chan JK, Fletcher CD, Nayler SJ, et al. Follicular dendritic cell sarcoma. Clinicopathologic analysis of 17 cases suggesting a malignant potential higher than currently recognized. Cancer 1997;79(2): 294–313.

55. Rodig SJ, Payne EG, Degar BA, et al. Aggressive Langerhans cell histiocytosis following T-ALL: clonally related neoplasms with persistent expression of constitutively active NOTCH1. Am J Hematol 2008;83(2):116–21.

56. Greif PA, Tizazu B, Krause A, et al. The leukemogenic CALM/AF10 fusion protein alters the subcellular localization of the lymphoid regulator Ikaros. Oncogene 2008;27(20):2886–96.

57. Nayer H, Murphy KM, Hawkins AL, et al. Clonal cytogenetic abnormalities and BCL2 rearrangement in interdigitating dendritic cell sarcoma. Leuk Lymphoma 2006;47(12):2651–4.

58. Mohty M, Jarrossay D, Lafage-Pochitaloff M, et al. Circulating blood dendritic cells from myeloid leukemia patients display quantitative and cytogenetic abnormalities as well as functional impairment. Blood 2001;98(13):3750–6.

SYSTEMIC MASTOCYTOSIS

Tracy I. George, MD[a],*, Hans-Peter Horny, MD[b]

KEYWORDS

- Systemic mastocytosis • Mast cell • KIT D816V • Mast cell leukemia

ABSTRACT

An unusual disease, mastocytosis challenges the pathologist with a variety of morphologic appearances and heterogeneous clinical presentations ranging from skin manifestations (pruritus, urticaria, dermatographism) to systemic signs and symptoms indicative of mast cell mediator release, including flushing, hypotension, headache, and anaphylaxis among others. In this article, we focus on recognizing the cytology, histopathology, clinical features, and prognostic implications of systemic mastocytosis, a clonal and neoplastic mast cell proliferation infiltrating extracutaneous organ(s) with or without skin involvement. Diagnostic pitfalls are reviewed with ancillary studies to help unmask the mast cell and exclude morphologic mimics.

OVERVIEW

Mast cell disease, or mastocytosis, includes a variety of disorders that are characterized by clonal, neoplastic proliferations of mast cells in one or multiple organs, ranging from indolent and isolated proliferations to aggressive and systemic disorders.[1] Mastocytosis is now included in the myeloproliferative neoplasms category in the 2008 World Health Organization (WHO) classification in recognition of the common theme of abnormal protein tyrosine kinase function that characterizes the myeloproliferative neoplasms. The hallmark of most mastocytosis cases is the Asp816Val (D816 V) somatic mutation in the catalytic domain of the *KIT* gene, resulting in enhanced mast cell survival and proliferation owing to constitutive activation of the *KIT* tyrosine kinase activity.[2]

The WHO classification of mastocytosis is as follows:

- Cutaneous mastocytosis
- Indolent systemic mastocytosis
- Systemic mastocytosis with associated clonal hematological non−mast cell lineage disease (SM-AHNMD)
- Aggressive systemic mastocytosis
- Mast cell leukemia
- Mast cell sarcoma
- Extracutaneous mastocytoma.

Clinical manifestations are caused by the release of chemical mediators and by infiltration of tissues by neoplastic mast cells. Morphologic detection and immunophenotypic confirmation of mast cells in tissue sections is essential for the diagnosis of mastocytosis. Mast cells can vary from collections of round cells with many fine basophilic granules to spindled forms with associated fibrosis to blastlike cells with large metachromatic granules, with the latter atypical forms correlating with the more aggressive clinical syndromes. The subtle nature of some mast cell infiltrates can be easily overlooked or masked by accompanying eosinophils, small lymphocytes, and plasma cells.

Classification of mastocytosis into systemic mastocytosis (SM) subtypes requires correlation with clinical and laboratory findings. The WHO classification of mastocytosis separates cutaneous from systemic forms and provides criteria to further subclassify the systemic forms of mastocytosis, based on the presence of specific clinical, laboratory, and pathologic findings (that are divided into "B" and "C" groups) (**Tables 1 and 2**).[2]

Disclosures: Drs George and Horny are on the Steering Committee for Study CPKC412D2201 for Novartis and are paid consultants.

[a] Department of Pathology, Stanford University School of Medicine, Stanford University Medical Center, 300 Pasteur Drive, Room H1501B, Stanford, CA 94305-5627, USA

[b] Institut für Pathologie, Klinikum Ansbach, Escherichstrasse 6 DE-91522, Ansbach, Germany

* Corresponding author.

E-mail address: tigeorge@stanford.edu

Surgical Pathology 3 (2010) 1185–1202
doi:10.1016/j.path.2010.09.003

Table 1
Criteria for systemic mastocytosis[a]
Diagnosis requires 1 major and 1 minor criterion or 3 minor criteria

Major	Multifocal dense infiltrates of mast cells in tissue sections[b]
Minor	>25% spindled, immature or atypical mast cells in tissue sections or bone marrow aspirate smears
	Detection of *KIT* D816 V mutation
	Expression of CD2 and/or CD25 in mast cells
	Serum total tryptase persistently exceeds 20 ng/mL[c]

[a] 2008 World Health Organization Diagnostic Criteria for Systemic Mastocytosis.
[b] Infiltrate is ≥15 mast cells in aggregates in bone marrow and/or extracutaneous organs.
[c] Not valid if there is an associated clonal myeloid disorder.

CLINICAL FEATURES

Mastocytosis is clinically heterogeneous, ranging from skin lesions that spontaneously regress to aggressive malignancies with short survival. It can occur at any age with a slight male predominance.[3] In cutaneous mastocytosis, mast cell infiltration is limited to the skin and typically presents in childhood with urticarial symptoms. It has a benign clinical course and may regress spontaneously, often around the time of puberty. In adults, cutaneous disease is more frequently associated with indolent rather than aggressive forms of SM (see the WHO classification listed previously). Thus, in adults presenting with cutaneous disease, careful staging for SM is recommended, including a physical examination, complete blood cell count, total serum tryptase, bone marrow examination, and molecular analysis for the D816 V *KIT* mutation; additional laboratory and radiographic studies may be indicated based on the patient's symptoms and signs of disease. Whereas the bone marrow is almost always involved in SM,[4] the spleen, lymph nodes, liver and gastrointestinal tract, and virtually any organ, can also be affected. Clinical manifestations of SM reflect either mediator release from mast cells or infiltration of mast cells into tissues; they include constitutional signs, skin lesions, mediator-related findings (flushing, syncope, diarrhea, hypotension, headache, and/or abdominal pain), and musculoskeletal disease.

Four major types of SM are known[5]:

1. Indolent systemic mastocytosis
2. Systemic mastocytosis accompanied by an associated hematological non–mast cell disorder (SM-AHNMD)
3. Aggressive systemic mastocytosis and variant lymphadenopathic mastocytosis with eosinophilia
4. Mast cell leukemia.

Table 2
"B Findings" and "C Findings" used to subcategorize systemic mastocytosis

B Findings	
1. Increased mast cell burden	>30% mast cell aggregates on bone marrow biopsy and/or total serum tryptase level >200 ng/mL
2. Dysplasia or myeloproliferation	Hypercellular marrow, signs of myelodysplasia or abnormal myeloid proliferation, and normal or slightly abnormal blood counts, without sufficient criteria to diagnose an AHNMD
3. Organomegaly	Palpable hepatomegaly without ascites or signs of liver dysfunction, palpable or radiologic lymphadenopathy (>2 cm), or palpable splenomegaly, without hypersplenism
C Findings	
1. Cytopenias	ANC <1.0 × 10⁹/L; Hb <10 g/dL; or platelets <100 × 10⁹/L
2. Liver	Palpable hepatomegaly with impaired liver function, ascites, and/or portal hypertension
3. Bone	Large osteolytic lesions and/or pathologic fractures
4. Spleen	Palpable splenomegaly with hypersplenism
5. Gastrointestinal	Malabsorption with weight loss and/or hypoalbuminemia

Abbreviations: AHNMD, associated clonal hematologic non–mast cell lineage disease; ANC, absolute neutrophil count; Hb, hemoglobin.

Indolent systemic mastocytosis involves skin and bone marrow and is the most common form of SM. Variants of indolent SM include *bone marrow mastocytosis,* in which no skin disease is present, *smoldering systemic mastocytosis* in which 2 or more "B findings" are present (see **Table 2**), and *well-differentiated (round cell) mastocytosis*, discussed later. Smoldering SM mainly affects older patients and is associated with more constitutional symptoms than the other types of indolent disease.

In *systemic mastocytosis accompanied by an associated hematological non–mast cell disorder* (SM-AHNMD), the associated non–mast cell disorder is usually a myeloid malignancy, but may also include lymphomas or plasma cell neoplasms. Symptoms and prognosis typically reflect the associated non–mast cell disease.

Aggressive systemic mastocytosis is a disorder typically lacking skin lesions and presenting with one or more "C findings" that indicate organ dysfunction owing to mast cell infiltration (see **Table 2**). A variant of aggressive SM is *lymphadenopathic mastocytosis with eosinophilia,* which presents with lymphadenopathy and eosinophilia. This subtype should be differentiated from myeloid/lymphoid neoplasms with *PDGFRA* rearrangements.

The last major type is the rare *mast cell leukemia* (comprising only 1% of SM cases), which also presents without skin lesions and shares the extremely poor prognosis of aggressive SM. Two localized extracutaneous mast cell neoplasms, mast cell sarcoma and extracutaneous mastocytoma, are exceedingly rare and are not discussed in this article.[5]

MICROSCOPIC FEATURES

Mast Cell Cytology

The spectrum of reactive and neoplastic mast cell appearances is presented in **Table 3**. Reactive tissue mast cells are small with round, centrally located nuclei, indistinct to absent nucleoli, and abundant cytoplasm containing faint cytoplasmic granules on hematoxylin and eosin (H&E)-stained tissue sections. In Romanowsky-stained smears, normal mast cells contain tightly packed uniform metachromatic granules with round to oval-shaped nuclei (**Fig. 1**). Neoplastic mast cell morphology has been classified into 3 subtypes (see **Fig. 1**) that are best recognized on bone marrow aspirate smears. The first subtype is the *atypical mast cell type I,* a spindled mast cell with elongated cytoplasmic projections, oval eccentric nuclei, and hypogranulated cytoplasm. The

second subtype is the *atypical mast cell type II* or *promastocyte*, with bilobed or polylobed nuclei and typically less cytoplasmic granulation than reactive mast cells. The third subtype is the *metachromatic blast,* which has a high nuclear to cytoplasmic ratio, fine nuclear chromatin, prominent nucleoli, and several metachromatic granules. Atypical type I mast cells are more commonly seen in indolent types of SM, whereas atypical type II mast cells and metachromatic blasts are more common in patients with mast cell leukemia and myelomastocytic leukemia; these latter disorders are associated with a poor prognosis and short survival.[6,7]

Histology

In most cases, histologic evaluation of a bone marrow biopsy, coupled with immunohistochemistry and/or special stains to identify mast cells, provides the best material to diagnose SM. The diagnostic criteria for SM include examination of tissue sections for multifocal aggregates of mast cells (see **Table 1**). Five patterns of bone marrow infiltration by mast cells are described.[8]

Pattern 1 is an *interstitial* pattern typically seen in mast cell hyperplasia (**Fig. 2**).

Patterns 2 through 4 involve *focal, dense infiltrates* of mast cells either alone (pattern 2) or coupled with additional interstitial mast cell components, located either preferentially around the focal infiltrates (pattern 3) or evenly distributed throughout the biopsy (pattern 4). Patterns 2, 3, and 4 characterize most SM cases (**Figs. 3** and **4**).

Pattern 5 represents *diffuse, dense* mast cell infiltrates that obliterate the marrow architecture, and is found in mast cell leukemia and smoldering SM (**Fig. 5**).

One type of focal, dense infiltrate is the *tryptase-positive compact round cell infiltrate of the bone marrow* (TROCI-BM) (**Fig. 6**). This particular pattern, while rare, brings the differential diagnosis of a specific set of myeloid neoplasms, including SM, mast cell leukemia, myelomastocytic leukemia, tryptase-positive acute myeloid leukemia, acute basophilic leukemia, and SM-AHNMD (**Table 4**).[9]

The dense infiltrates of mast cells in SM are typically perivascular and paratrabecular, formed by round or spindle-shaped mast cells and often accompanied by reticulin and collagen fibrosis (**Figs. 7** and **8**). Associated reactive lymphoid aggregates are quite common, as are accompanying eosinophils and plasma cells (**Figs. 9** and **10**). Immunophenotyping (flow cytometry, immunohistochemistry, and/or in situ hybridization) can separate reactive lymphocytes and

Table 3
Pathology key features of mast cell proliferations: mast cell morphology

Mast Cell Type	Size/Shape	Nucleus	Nuclear Chromatin	Cytoplasm	Nuclear to Cytoplasmic Ratio	Associated Disorders
Reactive	Small-medium, round or oval	Central, round or oval	Condensed	Well granulated, may be hypo- or degranulated	Low	Reactive mastocytosis
Atypical type I	Elongated cytoplasmic extensions (spindle shaped)	Central or eccentric, oval	Condensed	Hypogranulated, focal granule accumulation without degranulation	Variable	SM, SM-AHNMD
Atypical type II	Variable	Bi- or polylobed	Fine or condensed	Hypogranulated without degranulation	Variable	MCL, MML
Metachromatic[a] blast	Medium-large, round or oval	Prominent nucleoli	Fine	Few metachromatic granules	High	MCL, MML

Abbreviations: ASM, aggressive systemic mastocytosis; BM, bone marrow; MC, mast cell(s); MCL, mast cell leukemia; MML, myelomastocytic leukemia; SM-AHNMD, systemic mastocytosis with an associated clonal hematological non—mast cell lineage disease.

[a] Metachromatic refers to a cell that characteristically takes on a color different from that of the dye with which it is stained; a metachromatic blast has the nuclear features of a blast with many large basophilic cytoplasmic granules.

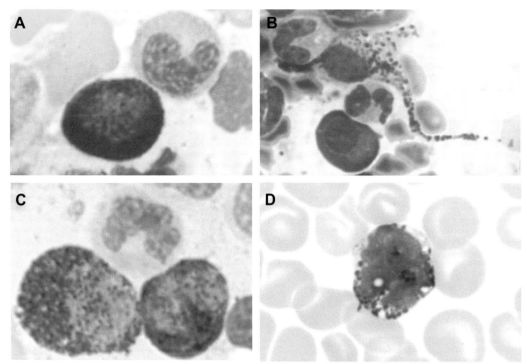

Fig. 1. Cytology of mast cells. (*A*) Typical mature tissue mast cell with well-granulated cytoplasm and a round to oval-shaped central nucleus adjacent to a band neutrophil. Basophils (not shown), in contrast, contain multilobated nuclei similar to a neutrophil. (*B*) Atypical mast cell type 1 with elongated cytoplasmic projections giving the cell a characteristic spindle shape containing reduced numbers of metachromatic granules. The nucleus is oval and eccentrically placed. (*C*) Two atypical mast cells type II with bilobed nuclei. Note the size of these atypical mast cells is larger than the adjacent neutrophil. (*D*) Metachromatic blast with high nuclear-to-cytoplasmic ratio, smooth chromatin, and scattered metachromatic granules from a patient with myelomastocytic leukemia. Bone marrow aspirate smears, Wright Giemsa stain, ×1000.

polytypic plasma cells from their neoplastic counterparts. Osteosclerosis and an increase in small capillaries (neoangiogenesis) also can accompany mastocytosis (**Fig. 11**). Finally, in cases of SM-AHNMD, recognizing the mast cell infiltrate can be of particular challenge when the infiltrate is quite focal or masked by the non-mast neoplasm (**Fig. 12**). Approximately 20% to 30% of patients with SM will develop a second hematologic disease, which is usually a clonal myeloid disorder (**Fig. 13**).[9,10]

ANCILLARY STUDIES

Normal mast cells stain with chloracetate esterase, Giemsa, and toluidine blue, but the latter stain is pH dependent and these stains are less specific than immunophenotypic studies. Mast cells express CD33, CD43, CD68, CD117, and tryptase.[5] Tryptase is the most lineage specific of these markers, but may show high background staining, particularly in patients with high serum tryptase levels. Neoplastic mast cells also aberrantly express CD2 and/or CD25, with CD25 more

easily detected with immunohistochemistry[11]; these markers are not present in normal or reactive mast cells. For practical purposes, an immunohistochemistry panel of CD117, tryptase, and CD25 is recommended to aid in confirming mast cell lineage and to identify an aberrant immunophenotype. For flow cytometry, a panel containing CD117, CD45, CD2, and CD25 is helpful, although mast cells may be underrepresented in flow cytometry samples and difficult to identify.[12]

Point mutations of the tyrosine kinase receptor gene *KIT* are the most common genetic abnormality in mastocytosis and the most common mutation results in a substitution of valine for aspartate at codon 816 of exon 17, termed Asp816Val or D816 V. More than 95% of patients with SM have this mutation.[13] Other mutations have been described in exons 11 and 17.[14] *KIT* mutations are less common in pediatric and cutaneous mast cell tumors, and more than one-half of these mutations occur outside of exon 17.[15] *KIT* mutations are not specific for mastocytosis and do occur in other diseases.[16,17] Even the D816 V

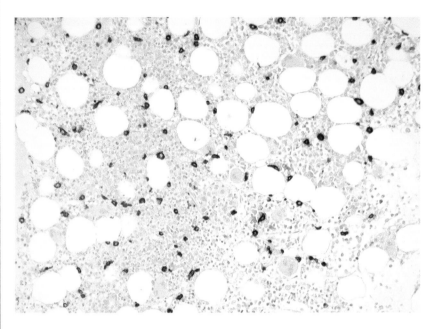

Fig. 2. Mast cell hyperplasia showing a diffuse interstitial increase in mast cells without any compact infiltrates (bone marrow biopsy, tryptase, ×200).

mutation is not disease specific, and for this reason, detection of the mutation represents only a minor diagnostic criterion (see **Table 1**). Molecular detection of *KIT* mutations can be performed on fresh bone marrow aspirate, clot sections or bone marrow biopsy sections; the latter should be fixed in formalin and decalcified in EDTA. Clot sections should be fixed in formalin. *KIT* mutation testing can be performed on peripheral blood if there are circulating mast cells or if the blood is involved by an AHNMD with the *KIT* mutation.

Given the overlap in morphology between SM and myeloid and lymphoid neoplasms with eosinophilia and *PDGFRA* and *PDGFRB* abnormalities (**Fig. 14**), it may be necessary to perform additional analysis to exclude neoplasms with these molecular abnormalities, especially in cases of SM with a marked eosinophilia and loose networks of CD25+ mast cells. The *FIP1L1-PDGFRA* fusion is cryptic and thus conventional cytogenetic analysis is usually normal; fluorescence in situ hybridization (FISH) analysis or reverse

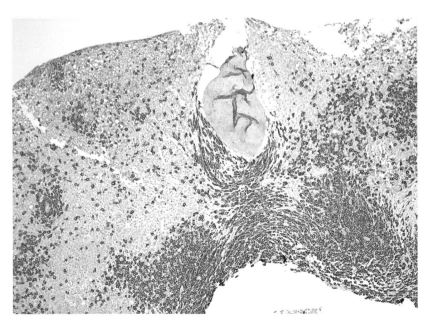

Fig. 3. Focal dense infiltrates of tryptase-positive mast cells around bone and vessels in a patient with SM and chronic myelomonocytic leukemia (bone marrow biopsy, tryptase, ×100).

Fig. 4. Rare focal dense infiltrates of CD25-positive mast cells in indolent SM occupying less than 10% of marrow cellularity (bone marrow biopsy, CD25, ×100).

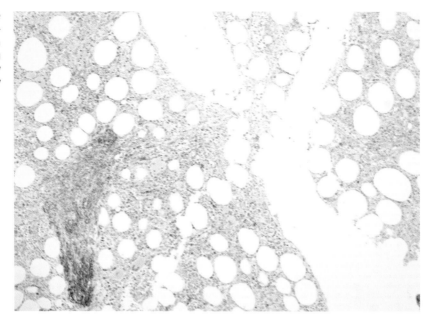

transcriptase–polymerase chain reaction (RT-PCR) can be performed to detect this fusion gene.[18] In myeloid neoplasms with *PDGFRB* rearrangements, typically a t(5;12)(q31-q33;p12) is present on cytogenetic testing; nevertheless, molecular confirmation of the *ETV6-PDGFRB* fusion gene is helpful.[19] This distinction between SM and neoplasms with *PDGFRA* and *PDGFRB* abnormalities is vitally important, given the latter neoplasms' excellent response to imatinib,[18] in contrast to SM.

DIFFERENTIAL DIAGNOSIS

When increased mast cells are noted on smears or histologic sections, recognizing the cytology of the mast cells (normal, atypical type I, atypical type II, metachromatic blast) and the pattern of mast cell infiltration (interstitial, diffuse dense, focal dense, TROCI-BM) can direct the pathologist to a differential diagnosis (see **Figs. 1—6**).

Interstitial pattern (mast cell hyperplasia, mast cell leukemia, acute basophilic leukemia,

Fig. 5. Diffuse dense infiltrates of immature mast cells efface normal marrow architecture in mast cell leukemia (bone marrow biopsy, H&E, ×400).

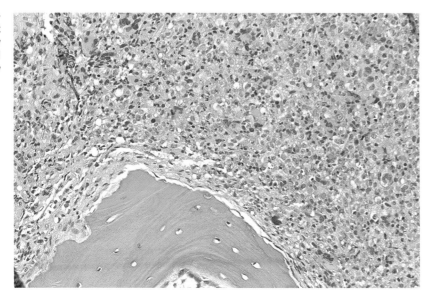

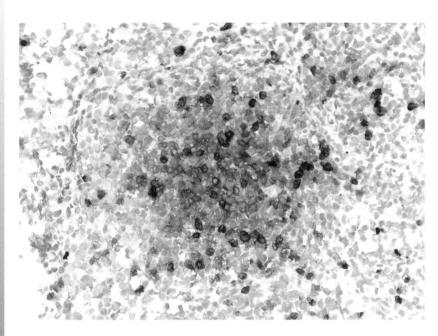

Fig. 6. Tryptase-positive compact round cell infiltrate of the bone marrow (TROCI-BM) in accelerated phase of chronic myeloid leukemia. These cells did not express CD117 (not shown) (bone marrow biopsy, tryptase, ×200).

tryptase-positive acute myeloid leukemia, myelomastocytic leukemia, myeloproliferative neoplasms with eosinophilia): Mast cell hyperplasia differs from the other neoplastic disorders by its normal mast cell cytology with small cell size, low nuclear-to-cytoplasm ratio, and round to oval nuclei. Histologically, reactive mast cells are increased in a loose scattered fashion without clusters or compact

Table 4
Differential diagnosis of systemic mastocytosis

Disease	Cell Pattern	Phenotype	KIT D816 V
Systemic mastocytosis	Compact, dense infiltrates meeting criteria for SM	Tryptase+, CD117+, CD25/CD2+[a]	+[b]
Acute basophilic leukemia	Interstitial	Tryptase weak+, CD117−/+, CD13/CD33+, 2D7+, BB1+, CD123+	−
Mast cell hyperplasia	Interstitial	Tryptase+, CD117+, CD25/CD2−	−
Myeloid neoplasms with eosinophilia and PDGFRA/PDGRFB abnormalities	Interstitial or clustered[c]	Tryptase+, CD117+, CD25+	−[d]
Myelomastocytic leukemia	Interstitial mast cells and blasts	Mast cells: tryptase+, CD117+, CD25/CD2− Blasts: CD34+, CD25−, CD117+	−
Tryptase-positive AML	Insterstitial	Tryptase+, CD117+, CD25−, CD34+, CD13/33+	−

Abbreviation: MC, mast cell.
[a] Some cases of systemic mastocytosis may lack CD25/CD2 expression.
[b] A small minority of cases lack the D816 V KIT mutation.
[c] Mast cells may be scattered, in loose clusters, or cohesive clusters.
[d] *FIP1L1-PDGFRA+* or *PDGFRB*-fusion variants.

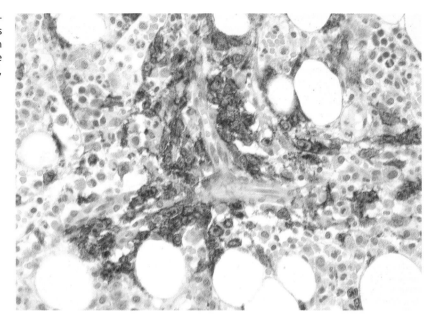

Fig. 7. Clusters of predominantly round mast cells surround this vessel in indolent SM (bone marrow biopsy, CD117, ×600).

infiltrates (see **Fig. 2**). In contrast, mast cell leukemia will show sheets of mast cells, typically with diffuse and focal dense areas, in addition to heavy interstitial infiltrates (see **Fig. 5**). On marrow smears, more than 20% of mast cells are detected and these are atypical, showing immature features including metachromatic blasts and/or atypical type II mast cells and criteria for SM are met. In the rare basophilic leukemia, the neoplastic cells are morphologically indistinguishable from the metachromatic

blasts of mast cell leukemia, but these cells do not mark as true mast cells (low tryptase expression, CD117 negative) and express myeloid markers (CD13 and CD33) and CD123; thus, immunophenotyping "saves the day" in distinguishing acute basophilic leukemia from SM.[1] Tryptase-positive acute myeloid leukemia, another rare disorder, can also show a diffuse interstitial pattern in areas and shows strong tryptase expression, but lacks other features of mastocytosis; moreover, the cells cytologically

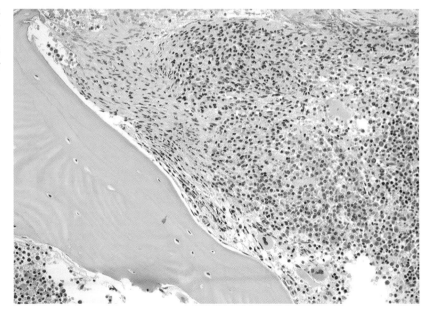

Fig. 8. Spindled mast cells comprise this paratrabecular aggregate in SM with adjacent clusters of reactive plasma cells (bone marrow biopsy, H&E, ×400).

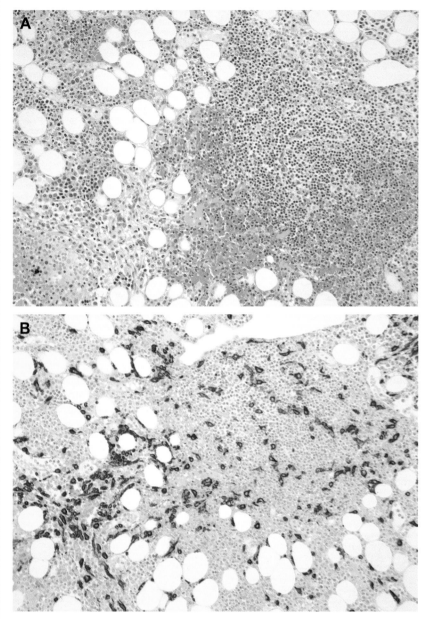

Fig. 9. A reactive lymphoid aggregate at right is adjacent to a loose collection of mast cells admixed with eosinophils in a case of indolent SM. Immunohistochemical staining for tryptase highlights a surprising number of clustered and single mast cells with cytoplasmic staining, including spindle forms. (*A*) H&E. (*B*) Tryptase. Bone marrow biopsy, ×500.

resemble myeloblasts, usually of the M0 or M1 FAB subtype.[20] Myelomastocytic leukemia is a rare disease described in patients with advanced myeloid neoplasms (most commonly refractory anemia with excess blasts or acute myeloid leukemia [AML]) with elevated numbers of atypical mast cells who do not meet full criteria for SM. Typically there are greater than 5% myeloblasts and greater than 10% metachromatic blasts in the blood and/or marrow without focal dense mast cell infiltrates, without mast cell coexpression of CD2 or CD25, and without evidence of the D816 V KIT mutation (**Fig. 15**).[21] Myelomastocytic leukemia is a controversial entity not widely recognized by pathologists and is not included in the 2008 WHO classification. In the myeloproliferative neoplasms associated with eosinophilia and *PDGFRA* abnormalities, loose aggregates of CD25+ spindled

Fig. 10. The spindle-shaped mast cells in this aggregate are admixed with numerous eosinophils. On H&E sections, mast cell granules are not visible and the cytoplasm typically has a light eosinophilic color (bone marrow biopsy, ×600).

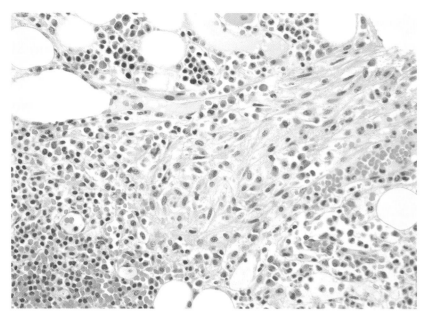

mast cells may be present in more than one-half of cases; CD25+ spindled mast cell infiltrates have also been described in myeloid neoplasms with *PDGFRB* abnormalities. However, criteria for SM are not fulfilled because the KIT D816 V mutation is absent and compact, dense mast cell infiltrates are lacking.[22]

Diffuse dense pattern (mast cell leukemia, smoldering SM): Although both mast cell leukemia and smoldering SM can show diffuse dense mast cell infiltrates in tissue sections with alteration of bone marrow architecture, as well as markedly elevated serum tryptase levels, mast cell leukemia exhibits "C findings," whereas smoldering SM does not.[1] Furthermore, mast cell leukemia shows marked atypia on cytologic smears, a feature that is lacking in smoldering SM.

Focal dense pattern (indolent SM, smoldering SM, well-differentiated SM, isolated bone marrow mastocytosis, mast cell hyperplasia, SM-AHNMD,

Fig. 11. Osteosclerosis with broad bands of bony trabeculae and paratrabecular collections of mast cells are present in this case of SM with associated chronic myelomonocytic leukemia (H&E, ×100).

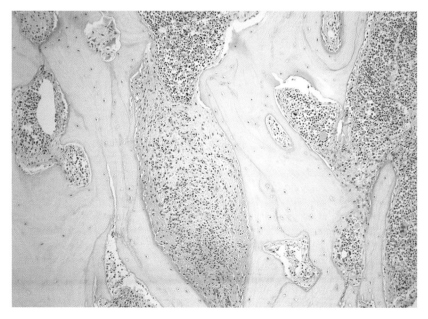

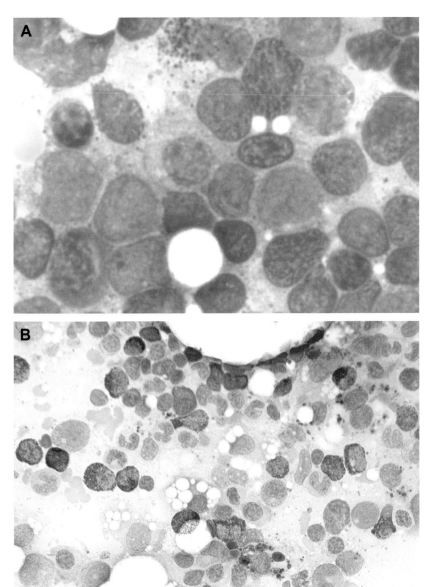

Fig. 12. (*A*) Acute myeloid leukemia with t(8;21)(q22; q22) was diagnosed in this bone marrow aspirate with sheets of blasts (Wright Giemsa, ×1000). (*B*) After induction chemotherapy, numerous atypical type II mast cells were unmasked (Wright Giemsa, ×600).

aggressive SM): Although many types of SM can show focal dense mast cell infiltrates, one can separate them into the more indolent disorders, aggressive SM, and SM-AHNMD. Rarely, mast cell hyperplasia may show focal dense mast cell infiltrates, but the mast cells lack atypia on smears and the cases do not fulfill criteria for SM. Indolent SM, the most common subtype of SM, shows focal dense mast cell infiltrates that minimally involve the bone marrow (<10% of marrow cellularity) with little effect on surrounding hematopoiesis; reactive lymphoid aggregates, plasmacytosis, and eosinophilia may be seen (see **Figs. 9** and **10**). The mast cells may be round or spindle shaped and skin lesions of urticaria pigmentosa are usually present (**Fig. 16**). Isolated bone marrow mastocytosis, smoldering SM, and well-differentiated mastocytosis all represent variants of indolent SM. In isolated bone marrow mastocytosis, there is no skin involvement and serum tryptase level is normal. Most of these cases were previously called *eosinophilic fibrohistiocytic bone marrow lesion.*[23] Smoldering SM has "B findings" and a greater degree of marrow infiltration

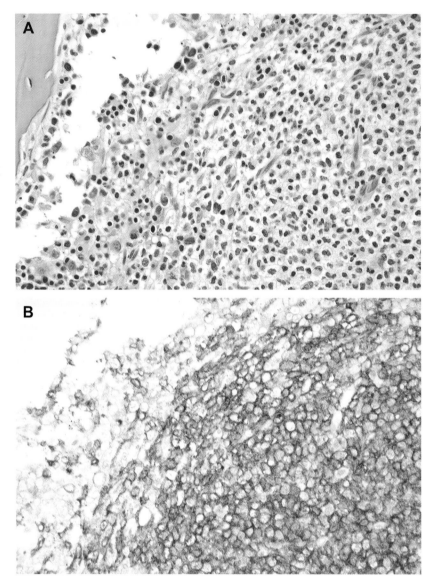

Fig. 13. Systemic mastocytosis with a mixed myelodysplastic/myeloproliferative neoplasm, unclassifiable. (*A*) Large aggregate of mast cells with clear cytoplasm and irregular nuclei admixed with eosinophils (H&E, ×400). (*B*) Crisp strong membrane staining with CD117 rings the mast cells (bone marrow biopsy, CD117, ×400).

than that seen in indolent SM (>30% of marrow cellularity) with a markedly elevated serum tryptase level. Well-differentiated SM is characterized by round mast cells with multifocal dense marrow infiltrates lacking CD25 and *KIT* D816 V mutation. A different, imatinib-sensitive *KIT* mutation has been described with this variant.[24] Aggressive SM has "C findings," atypical mast cells on smears and usually a markedly hypercellular marrow with focal dense and diffuse infiltration by atypical mast cells. Aggressive SM should be regarded as a diagnosis of exclusion because most cases are in fact SM-AHNMD when bone marrow and blood smears are carefully investigated. A variant

of aggressive SM, lymphadenopathic mastocytosis with eosinophilia, has generalized lymphadenopathy and marked eosinophilia.[25]

TROCI-BM pattern (SM, mast cell leukemia, myelomastocytic leukemia, tryptase-positive AML, basophilic leukemia, SM-AHNMD): Tryptase-positive compact round cell infiltrates of the bone marrow raise a specific differential diagnosis requiring the application of lineage-specific markers to determine whether the neoplastic cells are mast cells or basophilic granulocytes (see **Fig. 6**).[9] In cases of SM and mast cell leukemia, expression of CD117 is found. In myelomastocytic leukemia and tryptase-positive AML, expression

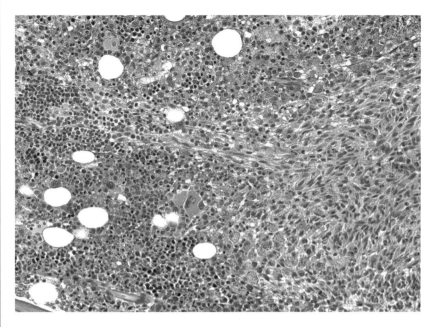

Fig. 14. Myeloid neoplasm with *PDGFRB* rearrangement and t(5;12). A compact clustered of spindled mast cells is present at right admixed with numerous eosinophils and fewer numbers of pigment-laden macrophages. At left an aggregate of lymphocytes is seen (H&E, ×200).

of CD34 and CD117 is found, whereas neither CD34 nor CD117 is detected in accelerated phases of chronic myeloid leukemia with numerous basophils ("basophilic leukemia"); basophil-related antigens such as 2D7 and CD123 are positive in the latter.

DIAGNOSIS AND CLASSIFICATION

In the 2008 WHO classification, SM is diagnosed when 1 major criterion and 1 minor criterion, or at least 3 minor criteria are present (see **Table 1**). The major diagnostic criterion for SM is fulfilled by the presence of multifocal dense mast cell infiltrates (≥15 mast cells per aggregate) detected histologically in the bone marrow or in another extracutaneous organ(s). Minor criteria include the following[2,3]:

1. Twenty-five percent or more of the mast cells in the infiltrate are spindle shaped or show atypical morphology, or 25% or more are immature or atypical on bone marrow aspirate smears.
2. Serum tryptase level is persistently greater than 20 ng/mL (note that this parameter is not valid if there is an associated clonal myeloid disorder).
3. The D816 V *KIT* mutation is detected in bone marrow, blood, or another extracutaneous organ.
4. There is expression of CD2, CD25, or both in the neoplastic mast cells.

Indolent forms of systemic mast cell disease may be characterized by one or more "B findings" (see **Table 2**). If 2 or more "B findings" are present, the disease is classified as smoldering SM. Treatment of mediator-related symptoms, when present, is commonly used in all SM variants, whereas cytoreductive agents are not prescribed. In contrast, aggressive SM and mast cell leukemia are characterized by 1 or more "C findings" (see **Table 2**); aggressive SM often requires cytoreductive therapy. In SM-AHNMD, WHO diagnostic criteria for both SM and a distinct non–mast cell hematologic neoplasm (such as a myelodysplastic syndrome, myeloproliferative neoplasm, acute leukemia, lymphoma, or plasma cell myeloma) are met.[7]

Mast cell leukemia is a rare subtype of SM characterized by leukemic spread of mast cells and an aggressive, rapidly progressing clinical course. By definition, mast cell leukemia meets criteria for SM with additional features, including (1) leukemic infiltration of the bone marrow and/or other extracutaneous organs by neoplastic mast cells, (2) at least 20% neoplastic mast cells in bone marrow and/or blood smears, and (3) high-grade cytologic findings.[2] "C findings" are commonly associated with mast cell leukemia.[26] Mast cell leukemia is the only advanced mastocytic disorder for which a cytologic diagnosis on an aspirate smear preparation is required to make the diagnosis.[27] To satisfy the major WHO criterion for SM, multifocal dense infiltrates in the bone marrow biopsy must be present, whereas mast cell leukemia is defined by diffuse and interstitial mast cell infiltrates.[2] Thus, the mast cell infiltrate in mast cell leukemia

Fig. 15. (*A*) Myelomastocytic leukemia with bone marrow biopsy effaced by immature mononuclear cells (H&E, ×500). Discrete subsets of the immature cells stain strongly with myeloperoxidase (*B*) and tryptase (*C*), the latter in an interstitial pattern. Flow cytometry confirmed 2 populations of cells: myeloblasts and mast cells. The D816 V KIT mutation was absent and criteria for SM were not met. Circulating blasts and metachromatic blasts were also seen (not shown). (Images *courtesy of* Luke Shier, MD, University of Alberta Hospital, Edmonton, Canada. Case originally published in Arredondo A, Gotlib J, Shier L, et al. Myelomastocytic leukemia versus mast cell leukemia versus systemic mastocytosis associated with acute myeloid leukemia: a diagnostic challenge. Am J Hematol 2010;85:600−6.)

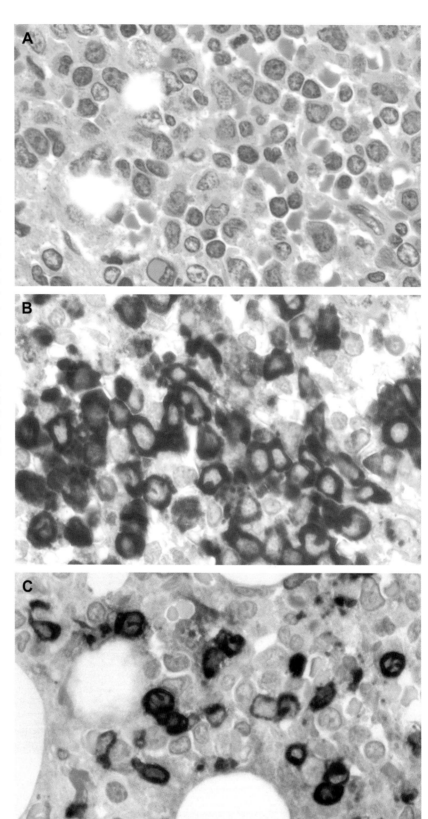

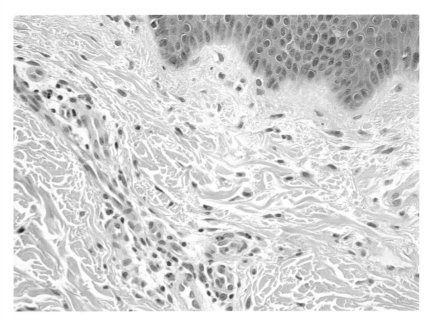

Fig. 16. A 27-year-old woman with urticaria pigmentosa and indolent SM. Histologic sections show a subtle superficial perivascular and interstitial infiltrate composed of mononuclear cells with pale eosinophilic cytoplasm (mast cells) and scattered eosinophils (skin, H&E, ×200).

is dense and multifocal, but also has an additional diffuse component, representing a mixed pattern. Mast cells typically show marked atypia and often express CD25 and there are persistently elevated serum tryptase levels. In more than 50% of mast cell leukemia cases, the *KIT* mutation D816 V is detectable.

PROGNOSIS

Prognosis in indolent SM is usually excellent and the course of the disease is typically benign. Advanced mast cell neoplasms such as aggressive SM and mast cell leukemia are notoriously difficult to manage and no curative treatments are currently available; the median survival time in mast cell leukemia is typically only 6 months. Patients should avoid triggers of mast cell activation, including exposure to extreme variations in temperature, excess exercise, and, in some patients, exposure to certain inciting drugs or alcohol. Treatment for advanced SM may include standard therapy to treat mediator symptoms,[7] along with cytoreductive therapy, such as interferon-α with or without corticosteroids, or cladribine in those who have slowly progressing aggressive SM.[5] However, major or partial responses are observed in only a subset of patients.[5,7] Rare patients have long-term survival after chemotherapy and bone marrow transplantation.[27,28] Importantly, the D816 V *KIT* mutation results in resistance to imatinib, thus this tyrosine

kinase inhibitor is ineffective at treating SM.[29] Alternative tyrosine kinase inhibitors have shown some promise and clinical trials are ongoing.[30–32] SM-AHNMD is treated in a dichotomous fashion, with the AHNMD being treated independently of the SM, and vice versa[7] The prognosis of SM-AHNMD is typically driven by the AHNMD rather than the SM.

Pitfalls
SYSTEMIC MASTOCYTOSIS

! Mast cell nuclei are typically round to oval, whereas basophils have lobulated nuclei similar to neutrophils

! Paratrabecular and perivascular spindle-shaped cells may mimic fibrosis: check for mastocytosis using immunostains for CD117 and tryptase

! CD117 is not specific for mast cells, and may be seen in myeloblasts and proerythroblasts in the bone marrow

! Marrows with marked eosinophilia and loose collections of CD25+ mast cells could represent *PDGFRA/PDGFRB*-associated myeloid neoplasms; these patients will respond to imatinib, but patients with SM will not

ACKNOWLEDGMENTS

The authors would like to thank Daniel A. Arber, MD, for his help and advice.

REFERENCES

1. Horny HP. Mastocytosis: an unusual clonal disorder of bone marrow-derived hematopoietic progenitor cells. Am J Clin Pathol 2009;132(3):438–47.

2. Horny HP, Akin C, Metcalfe DD, et al. Mastocytosis. In: Swerdlow S, Campo E, Harris NL, et al, editors. WHO classification of tumours of haematopoietic and lymphoid tissues. Lyon (France). IARC Press; 2008. p. 53–63.

3. Valent P, Sperr WR, Schwartz LB, et al. Diagnosis and classification of mast cell proliferative disorders: delineation from immunologic diseases and non-mast cell hematopoietic neoplasms. J Allergy Clin Immunol 2004;114(1):3–11.

4. Horny HP, Parwaresch MR, Lennert K. Bone marrow findings in systemic mastocytosis. Hum Pathol 1985; 16(8):808–14.

5. Horny HP, Sotlar K, Valent P. Mastocytosis: state of the art. Pathobiology 2007;74(2):121–32.

6. Valent P, Samorapoompichi P, Sperr WR, et al. Myelomastocytic leukemia: myeloid neoplasm characterized by partial differentiation of mast cell-lineage cells. Hematol J 2002;3(2):90–4.

7. Valent P, Horny HP, Escribano L, et al. Diagnostic criteria and classification of mastocytosis: a consensus proposal. Leuk Res 2001;25(7):603–25.

8. Krokowski M, Sotlar K, Krauth MT, et al. Delineation of patterns of bone marrow mast cell infiltration in systemic mastocytosis: value of CD25, correlation with sub-variations of the disease and separation from mast cell hyperplasia. Am J Clin Pathol 2005;124(4):560–8.

9. Horny HP, Sotlar K, Stellmacher F, et al. The tryptase positive compact round cell infiltrate of the bone marrow (TROCI-BM): a novel histopathological finding requiring the application of lineage specific markers. J Clin Pathol 2006;59(3):298–302.

10. Sperr WR, Horny HP, Lechner K, et al. Clinical and biological diversity of leukemias occurring in patients with mastocytosis. Leuk Lymphoma 2000; 37(5–6):473–86.

11. Sotlar K, Horny HP, Simonitsch I, et al. CD25 indicates the neoplastic phenotype of mast cells: a novel immunohistochemical marker for the diagnosis of systemic mastocytosis in routinely processed bone marrow biopsy specimens. Am J Surg Pathol 2004; 28(10):1319–25.

12. Escribano L, Diaz-Agustin B, López A, et al. Immunophenotypic analysis of mast cells in mastocytosis: when and how to do it. Proposals of the Spanish network on mastocytosis (REMA). Cytometry B Clin Cytom 2004;58(1):1–8.

13. Garcia-Montero AC, Jara-Acevedo M, Teodosio C, et al. KIT mutation in mast cells and other bone marrow hematopoietic cell lineages in systemic mast cell disorders: a prospective study of the Spanish network on mastocytosis (REMA) in a series of 113 patients. Blood 2006;108(7):2366–72.

14. Feger F, Ribadeau DA, Lerich L, et al. Kit and c-kit mutations in mastocytosis: a short overview with special reference to novel molecular and diagnostic concepts. Int Arch Allergy Immunol 2002;127(2): 110–4.

15. Bodemer C, Hermine O, Palmerini F, et al. Pediatric mastocytosis is a clonal disease associated with D816V and other activating c-KIT mutations. J Invest Dermatol 2010;130(3):804–15.

16. Lasota J, Miettinen M. Clinical significance of oncogenic KIT and PDGFRA mutations in gastrointestinal stromal tumours. Histopathology 2008;53(3): 245–66.

17. Beghini A, Ripamonti CB, Cairoli R, et al. KIT activating mutations: incidence in adult and pediatric acute myeloid leukemia, and identification of an internal tandem duplication. Haematologica 2004; 89(8):920–5.

18. Cools J, DeAngelo DJ, Gotlib J, et al. A tyrosine kinase created by fusion of the PDGFRA and FIP1L1 genes as a therapeutic target of imatinib in idiopathic hypereosinophilic syndrome. N Engl J Med 2003;348(13):1201–14.

19. Bain BJ, Fletcher SH. Chronic eosinophilic leukemias and the myeloproliferative variant of the hypereosinophilic syndrome. Immunol Allergy Clin North Am 2007;27(3):377–88.

20. Sperr WR, Jordan JH, Baghestanian M, et al. Expression of mast cell tryptase by myeloblasts in a group of patients with acute myeloid leukemia. Blood 2001;98(7):2200–9.

21. Arredondo A, Gotlib J, Shier L, et al. Myelomastocytic leukemia versus mast cell leukemia versus systemic mastocytosis associated with acute myeloid leukemia: a diagnostic challenge. Am J Hematol 2010;85(8):600–6.

22. Pardanani A, Ketterling RP, Brockman SR, et al. CHIC2 deletion, a surrogate for FIP1L1-PDGFRA fusion, occurs in systemic mastocytosis associated with eosinophilia and predicts response to imatinib mesylate therapy. Blood 2003;102(9):3093–6.

23. Rywlin AM, Hoffman EP, Ortega RS. Eosinophilic fibrohistiocytic lesion of bone marrow: a distinctive new morphologic finding, probably related to drug hypersensitivity. Blood 1972;40(4):464–72.

24. Akin C, Fumo G, Akif S, et al. A novel form of mastocytosis associated with a transmembrane c-kit mutation and response to imatinib. Blood 2004;103(8): 3222–5.

25. Frieri M, Linn N, Schweitzer M, et al. Lymphadenopathic mastocytosis with eosinophilia and biclonal

gammopathy. J Allergy Clin Immunol 1990;86(1): 126–32.

26. Noack F, Sotlar K, Notter M, et al. A leukemic mast cell leukemia with abnormal immunophenotype and c-kit mutation D816V. Leuk Lymphoma 2004; 45(11):2295–302.

27. Valentini CG, Rondoni M, Pogliani EM, et al. Mast cell leukemia: a report of ten cases. Ann Hematol 2008;87(16):505–8.

28. Sperr WR, Drach J, Hauswirth AW, et al. Myelomastocytic leukemia: evidence for the origin of mast cells from the leukemic clone and eradication by allogeneic stem cell transplantation. Clin Cancer Res 2005;11(19 Pt 1):6787–92.

29. Ma Y, Zeng S, Metcalfe DD, et al. The c-KIT mutation causing human mastocytosis is resistant to STI571 and other KIT kinase inhibitors; kinases with enzymatic site mutations show different inhibitor sensitivity profiles than wild-type kinases and those with regulatory-type mutations. Blood 2002;99(5):1741–4.

30. Gotlib J, Berube C, Growney JD, et al. Activity of tyrosine kinase inhibitor PKC412 in a patient with mast cell leukemia with the D816V KIT mutation. Blood 2005;106(8):2865–70.

31. Verstovsek S, Tefferi A, Cortes J, et al. Phase II study of dasatinib in Philadelphia chromosome-negative acute and chronic myeloid diseases, including systemic mastocytosis. Clin Cancer Res 2008; 14(12):3906–15.

32. Ustun C, Corless CL, Savage N, et al. Chemotherapy and dasatinib induce long-term hematologic and molecular remission in systemic mastocytosis with acute myeloid leukemia with KIT D816V. Leuk Res 2009;33(5):735–41.

Index

Note: Page numbers of article titles are in **boldface** type.

Surgical Pathology 3 (2010) 1203–1211
doi:10.1016/S1875-9181(10)00205-9
1875-9181/10/$ – see front matter © 2010 Elsevier Inc. All rights reserved.

United States Postal Service

Statement of Ownership, Management, and Circulation
(All Periodicals Publications Except Requestor Publications)

1. Publication Title	2. Publication Number	3. Filing Date
Surgical Pathology Clinics	0 2 5 - 4 7 8	9/15/10

4. Issue Frequency	5. Number of Issues Published Annually	6. Annual Subscription Price
Mar, Jun, Sep, Dec	4	$159.00

7. Complete Mailing Address of Known Office of Publication (Not printer) (Street, city, county, state, and ZIP+4®)

Elsevier Inc.
360 Park Avenue South
New York, NY 10010-1710

Contact Person: Stephen Bushing
Telephone (Include area code): 215-239-3688

8. Complete Mailing Address of Headquarters or General Business Office of Publisher (Not printer)

Elsevier Inc., 360 Park Avenue South, New York, NY 10010-1710

9. Full Names and Complete Mailing Addresses of Publisher, Editor, and Managing Editor (Do not leave blank)

Publisher (Name and complete mailing address)

Kim Murphy, Elsevier, Inc., 1600 John F. Kennedy Blvd. Suite 1800, Philadelphia, PA 19103-2899

Editor (Name and complete mailing address)

Joanne Husovski, Elsevier, Inc., 1600 John F. Kennedy Blvd. Suite 1800, Philadelphia, PA 19103-2899

Managing Editor (Name and complete mailing address)

Catherine Bewick, Elsevier, Inc., 1600 John F. Kennedy Blvd. Suite 1800, Philadelphia, PA 19103-2899

10. Owner (Do not leave blank. If the publication is owned by a corporation, give the name and address of the corporation immediately followed by the names and addresses of all stockholders owning or holding 1 percent or more of the total amount of stock. If not owned by a corporation, give the names and addresses of the individual owners. If owned by a partnership or other unincorporated firm, give its name and address as well as those of each individual owner. If the publication is published by a nonprofit organization, give its name and address.)

Full Name	Complete Mailing Address
Wholly owned subsidiary of	4520 East-West Highway
Reed/Elsevier, US holdings	Bethesda, MD 20814

11. Known Bondholders, Mortgagees, and Other Security Holders Owning or Holding 1 Percent or More of Total Amount of Bonds, Mortgages, or Other Securities. If none, check box ☐ None

Full Name	Complete Mailing Address
N/A	

12. Tax Status (For completion by nonprofit organizations authorized to mail at nonprofit rates) (Check one)
The purpose, function, and nonprofit status of this organization and the exempt status for federal income tax purposes:
☐ Has Not Changed During Preceding 12 Months
☐ Has Changed During Preceding 12 Months (Publisher must submit explanation of change with this statement)

PS Form 3526, September 2007 (Page 1 of 3 (Instructions Page 3)) PSN 7530-01-000-9931 PRIVACY NOTICE: See our Privacy policy in www.usps.com

---

13. Publication Title	14. Issue Date for Circulation Data Below
Surgical Pathology Clinics	June 2010

15. Extent and Nature of Circulation		Average No. Copies Each Issue During Preceding 12 Months	No. Copies of Single Issue Published Nearest to Filing Date
a. Total Number of Copies (Net press run)		1084	1349
b. Paid Circulation (By Mail and Outside the Mail)	(1) Mailed Outside-County Paid Subscriptions Stated on PS Form 3541. (Include paid distribution above nominal rate, advertiser's proof copies, and exchange copies)	522	521
	(2) Mailed In-County Paid Subscriptions Stated on PS Form 3541 (Include paid distribution above nominal rate, advertiser's proof copies, and exchange copies)		
	(3) Paid Distribution Outside the Mails Including Sales Through Dealers and Carriers, Street Vendors, Counter Sales, and Other Paid Distribution Outside USPS®	49	52
	(4) Paid Distribution by Other Classes Mailed Through the USPS (e.g. First-Class Mail®)		
c. Total Paid Distribution (Sum of 15b (1), (2), (3), and (4))	►	571	573
d. Free or Nominal Rate Distribution (By Mail and Outside the Mail)	(1) Free or Nominal Rate Outside-County Copies Included on PS Form 3541	42	36
	(2) Free or Nominal Rate In-County Copies Included on PS Form 3541		
	(3) Free or Nominal Rate Copies Mailed at Other Classes Through the USPS (e.g. First-Class Mail)		
	(4) Free or Nominal Rate Distribution Outside the Mail (Carriers or other means)		
e. Total Free or Nominal Rate Distribution (Sum of 15d (1), (2), (3) and (4))	►	42	36
f. Total Distribution (Sum of 15c and 15e)	►	613	609
g. Copies not Distributed (See instructions to publishers #4 (page #3))	►	471	740
h. Total (Sum of 15f and g)	►	1084	1349
i. Percent Paid (15c divided by 15f times 100)		93.15%	94.09%

16. Publication of Statement of Ownership

If the publication is a general publication, publication of this statement is required. Will be printed in the December 2010 issue of this publication. ☐ Publication not required.

17. Signature and Title of Editor, Publisher, Business Manager, or Owner

Stephen R. Bushing
Stephen R. Bushing – Fulfillment/Inventory Specialist

Date: September 15, 2010

I certify that all information furnished on this form is true and complete. I understand that anyone who furnishes false or misleading information on this form or who omits material or information requested on the form may be subject to criminal sanctions (including fines and imprisonment) and/or civil sanctions (including civil penalties).

PS Form 3526, September 2007 (Page 2 of 3)

Moving?

Make sure your subscription moves with you!

To notify us of your new address, find your **Clinics Account Number** (located on your mailing label above your name), and contact customer service at:

Email: journalscustomerservice-usa@elsevier.com

800-654-2452 (subscribers in the U.S. & Canada)
314-447-8871 (subscribers outside of the U.S. & Canada)

Fax number: 314-447-8029

Elsevier Health Sciences Division
Subscription Customer Service
3251 Riverport Lane
Maryland Heights, MO 63043

ELSEVIER